Hepatobiliary Manifestations of Diseases Involving Other Organ Systems

Guest Editor

KE-QIN HU, MD

CLINICS IN LIVER DISEASE

www.liver.theclinics.com

Consulting Editor
NORMAN GITLIN, MD

February 2011 • Volume 15 • Number 1

SAUNDERS an imprint of ELSEVIER, Inc.

W.B. SAUNDERS COMPANY

A Division of Elsevier Inc.

1600 John F. Kennedy Boulevard, Suite 1800 • Philadelphia, PA 19103-2899

http://www.theclinics.com

CLINICS IN LIVER DISEASE Volume 15, Number 1
February 2011 ISSN 1089-3261, ISBN-13: 978-1-4557-0526-9

Editor: Kerry Holland
Developmental Editor: Jessica Demetriou

Clinics in Liver Disease (ISSN 1089-3261) is published quarterly by Elsevier Inc., 360 Park Avenue South, New York, NY 10010-1710. Months of issue are February, May, August, and November. Business and Editorial Offices: 1600 John F. Kennedy Blvd., Ste. 1800, Philadelphia, PA 19103-2899. Customer Service Office: 3251 Riverport Lane, Maryland Heights, MO 63043. Periodicals postage paid at New York, NY and additional mailing offices. Subscription prices are $251.00 per year (U.S. individuals), $124.00 per year (U.S. student/resident), $343.00 per year (U.S. institutions), $333.00 per year (foreign individuals), $171.00 per year (foreign student/resident), $413.00 per year (foreign instituitions), $290.00 per year (Canadian individuals), $171.00 per year (Canadian student/resident), and $413.00 per year (Canadian institutions). Foreign air speed delivery is included in all *Clinics* subscription prices. All prices are subject to change without notice. **POSTMASTER:** Send address changes to *Clinics in Liver Disease*, Elsevier Health Sciences Division, Subscription Customer Service, 3251 Riverport Lane, Maryland Heights, MO 63043. **Customer Service: Telephone: 1-800-654-2452 (U.S. and Canada); 314-447-8871 (outside U.S. and Canada). Fax: 314-447-8029. E-mail: journalscustomer service-usa@elsevier.com (for print support); journalsonlinesupport-usa@elsevier.com (for online support).**

Reprints. For copies of 100 or more of articles in this publication, please contact the Commercial Reprints Department, Elsevier Inc., 360 Park Avenue South, New York, NY 10010-1710. Tel.: 212-633-3812; Fax: 212-462-1935; E-mail: reprints@elsevier.com.

Clinics in Liver Disease is covered in *MEDLINE/PubMed (Index Medicus)*, Science Citation Index Expanded, Journal Citation Reports/Science Edition, and Current Contents/Clinical Medicine.

Printed and bound by CPI Group (UK) Ltd, Croydon, CR0 4YY
Transferred to Digital Print 2011

Contributors

CONSULTING EDITOR

NORMAN GITLIN, MD, FRCP(London), FRCPE(Edinburgh), FACG, FACP,
Formerly, Professor of Medicine, Chief of Hepatology, Emory University; Currently,
Consultant, Atlanta Gastroenterology Associates, Atlanta, Georgia

GUEST EDITOR

KE-QIN HU, MD
Director, Hepatology Services; Associate Professor of Clinical Medicine, Division
of Gastroenterology and Hepatology, University of California, Irvine School of Medicine,
Orange, California

AUTHORS

ANDREW ARONSOHN, MD
Assistant Professor of Medicine, Center for Liver Disease, Section of Gastroenterology,
Hepatology and Nutrition, University of Chicago Medical Center, Chicago, Illinois

DAVID BERNSTEIN, MD, AGAF, FACP, FACG
Chief, Digestive Disease Institute, Department of Medicine, North Shore University
Hospital and Long Island Jewish Medical Center, Manhasset; Professor of Clinical
Medicine, Department of Medicine, Albert Einstein College of Medicine, Bronx, New York

MICHAEL B. FALLON, MD
Division Director and Professor of Medicine, Division of Gastroenterology, Hepatology and
Nutrition, The University of Texas Health Science Center at Houston, Houston, Texas

BRUCE L. GILLIAM, MD
Associate Professor of Medicine, Division of Infectious Diseases, Department of Medicine,
Institute of Human Virology, University of Maryland School of Medicine, Baltimore,
Maryland

TIMOTHY HALTERMAN, MD
Fellow in Gastroenterology, Department of Medicine, University of Washington, Seattle,
Washington

CHARLES HOWELL, MD
Professor of Medicine, Division of Gastroenterology and Hepatology, Department
of Medicine, University of Maryland School of Medicine; Director of Hepatology Research,
University of Maryland School of Medicine, Baltimore, Maryland

KE-QIN HU, MD
Director, Hepatology Services; Associate Professor of Clinical Medicine, Division
of Gastroenterology and Hepatology, University of California, Irvine School of Medicine,
Orange, California

IRA M. JACOBSON, MD
Professor of Medicine, Division of Gastroenterology and Hepatology, Weill Cornell Medical Center, New York Presbyterian Hospital, New York, New York

DONALD JENSEN, MD
Professor of Medicine, Center for Liver Disease, Section of Gastroenterology, Hepatology and Nutrition, University of Chicago Medical Center, Chicago, Illinois

RAJAN KOCHAR, MD, MPH
Assistant Professor of Medicine, Division of Gastroenterology, Hepatology and Nutrition, The University of Texas Health Science Center at Houston, Houston, Texas

KRIS V. KOWDLEY, MD
Director, Center for Liver Disease, Digestive Disease Institute, Virginia Mason Medical Center; Clinical Professor of Medicine, University of Washington, Seattle, Washington

ANURAG MAHESHWARI, MD
Institute for Digestive Health and Liver Diseases, Mercy Medical Center, Baltimore, Maryland

SHEHZAD N. MERWAT, MD
Fellow, Hepatology and Liver Transplantation Program, Baylor College of Medicine, and St Luke's Episcopal Hospital; Departments of Medicine and Surgery, Baylor College of Medicine, Houston, Texas

CALVIN PAN, MD
Associate Professor of Medicine, Division of Liver Diseases, Department of Medicine, Mount Sinai Medical Center, Mount Sinai School of Medicine, New York, New York

PONNI V. PERUMALSWAMI, MD
Assistant Professor of Medicine, Division of Liver Diseases, Department of Medicine, Mount Sinai Medical Center, Mount Sinai School of Medicine, New York, New York

PAUL J. POCKROS, MD
Head, Division of Gastroenterology/Hepatology, Scripps Clinic; Adjunct Associate Professor, The Scripps Research Institute, La Jolla, California

JASON B. SAMARASENA, MD
GI Fellow, Division of Gastroenterology, University of California Irvine Medical Center, Orange, California

SANJAYA K. SATAPATHY, MD, DM
Fellow, Gastroenterology, Long Island Jewish Medical Center at Albert Einstein College of Medicine, North Shore-Long Island Jewish Health System, New Hyde Park, New York

CHRISTINE SCHLENKER, MD
Fellow in Gastroenterology, Department of Medicine, University of Washington, Seattle, Washington

MARVIN M. SINGH, MD
Division of Gastroenterology and Hepatology, Scripps Clinic, La Jolla, California

ROHIT TALWANI, MD
Assistant Professor of Medicine, Division of Infectious Diseases, Department of Medicine, Institute of Human Virology, University of Maryland School of Medicine, Baltimore, Maryland

PAUL J. THULUVATH, MD, FRCP
Institute for Digestive Health and Liver Diseases, Mercy Medical Center, Baltimore, Maryland; Professor of Surgery and Medicine, Georgetown University School of Medicine, Washington, DC

JOHN M. VIERLING, MD
Professor of Medicine and Surgery; Chief of Hepatology; Director of Advanced Liver Therapies; Hepatology and Liver Transplantation Program, Baylor College of Medicine, and St Luke's Episcopal Hospital; Departments of Medicine and Surgery, Baylor College of Medicine, Houston, Texas

ILAN S. WEISBERG, MD, MSc
Clinical Fellow, Division of Gastroenterology and Hepatology, Weill Cornell Medical Center, New York Presbyterian Hospital, New York, New York

FLORENCE WONG, MD, FRACP, FRCPC
Department of Medicine, Toronto General Hospital, University of Toronto, Toronto, Ontario, Canada

Contents

The dual blood supply of the liver, originating from the portal vein and the hepatic artery, makes it relatively resistant to minor circulatory disturbances. However, hepatic manifestations of common cardiovascular disorders are frequently encountered in both the inpatient and outpatient setting. Beginning with the macro- and microcirculation of the liver, this article reviews the pathophysiology of hepatic blood flow and gives a detailed appraisal of ischemic hepatitis, congestive hepatopathy, and other less common hepatic conditions that arise when cardiovascular function is impaired.

Chronic liver disease is associated with many pulmonary complications. Several, including hepatopulmonary syndrome, portopulmonary hypertension, and hepatic hydrothorax have been extensively reviewed. However, hepatobiliary manifestations of primary pulmonary diseases have received less attention. This review focuses on hepatobiliary complications of respiratory failure, cystic fibrosis, α-1 antitrypsin deficiency, sarcoidosis, and tuberculosis.

Many liver diseases coexist with chronic renal disease, because many systemic conditions affect both the liver and the kidneys. Certain liver diseases are also common in patients with chronic renal disease, especially viral hepatitis, either because the renal disease occurs as a complication of viral hepatitis, or the viral hepatitis is acquired as a result of dialysis. Renal tubular dysfunction is also frequently observed with cholestasis. However, liver complications of renal diseases are extremely uncommon, notable examples include nephrogenic ascites and nephrogenic hepatic dysfunction. Nephrogenic ascites can mimic liver cirrhosis with ascites, and it improves with renal transplantation. Nephrogenic hepatic dysfunction is a manifestation of renal cell carcinoma, which settles with the removal of the renal cell carcinoma, but returns with the recurrence of the tumor. In general, the presence of liver disease in patients with chronic renal disease makes management of both conditions more challenging. Viral hepatitis should be treated, if possible, before renal transplant. If cirrhosis is present, renal transplant alone is contraindicated; combined liver and kidney transplantation is indicated in patients with end-stage renal disease and advanced cirrhosis.

> Liver disease and endocrine disorders, both common in the general population, have a bidirectional and complex relationship. Certain liver diseases are more commonly associated with endocrine disorders, including nonalcoholic fatty liver disease, autoimmune hepatitis, and primary biliary cirrhosis. There may be an association between hepatitis C and type 2 diabetes mellitus as well as thyroid disorders, and sex hormonal preparations may cause specific hepatic lesions. The presence of relative adrenal insufficiency in patients with end-stage liver disease may have therapeutic implications in patients admitted with acute-on-chronic liver failure. The objective of this review is to focus on the effect of endocrine disorders on liver.

> Malignant and nonmalignant disorders may affect the liver, causing signs and symptoms ranging from mild increases of liver tests to fulminant hepatic failure. This article discusses the most common hematologic and oncologic disorders and their effect on the liver. The section on nonmalignant hematologic disorders includes the anemias, paroxysmal nocturnal hemoglobinuria, disseminated intravascular coagulation, malaria, Banti syndrome, the porphyrias, thrombotic thrombocytopenic purpura, and hemolytic uremic syndrome. Malignant hematologic conditions include leukemias, lymphomas, and myeloproliferative disorders. Other conditions causing portal hypertension and hepatic metastases are also discussed. The most commonly encountered hepatic manifestations of hematologic and oncologic disorders are reviewed.

> Hepatobiliary manifestations of gastrointestinal and nutritional disorders can occur as part of the clinical spectrum of the underlying disease or as a consequence of the treatment of the disease. This article reviews aspects of pathogenesis, diagnosis, and management of hepatobiliary manifestations associated with a selection of gastrointestinal and nutritional disorders including inflammatory bowel disease, celiac disease, Whipple's disease, and parenteral nutrition associated disorders.

> The liver plays an important role in host defense against invasive microorganisms. The effect of microbial pathogens on the liver can vary greatly, presenting with a wide variety of manifestations from asymptomatic increases in aminotransaminases, acute liver failure, hepatic fibrosis, and cirrhosis. In evaluating the liver manifestations of a potential infectious pathogen, diagnosis of some of the less common infectious pathogens is dependent on a high level of suspicion and recognition of some of the key diagnostic clues. Successful diagnosis can only be accomplished through a careful history, including travel and exposures, physical examination,

and appropriate microbiologic studies. This article reviews the involvement of the liver during systemic infections with organisms that are not considered to be primarily hepatotropic.

Hepatitis C virus-Human immunodeficiency virus (HCV-HIV) coinfections are identified in up to 30% of patients infected with HIV and in 8% of patients infected with HCV. Now that progression of HIV and deaths due to AIDS can be prevented by highly active antiretroviral therapy (HAART), it is clear that HCV coinfection is associated with accelerated progression to cirrhosis and increased liver-related morbidity and mortality. Antiviral therapy with pegylated interferon and ribavirin for HCV in HCV-HIV coinfected patients is less successful than in patients with HCV monoinfection, and HAART can cause drug-induced liver injury. Multiple barriers limit the number of HCV-HIV coinfected patients who receive antiviral therapy for HCV, and the role of orthotopic liver transplantation (OLT) in HIV monoinfected and HCV-HIV coinfected patients remains controversial. Clinical trials of HCV-specific protease or polymerase inhibitors combined with pegylated interferon and ribavirin are needed urgently in coinfected patients, both before and after OLT.

Rheumatologic diseases such as rheumatoid arthritis, systemic lupus erythematosus, Sjögren syndrome, and scleroderma are immunologically mediated disorders that typically have multisystem involvement. Although clinically significant liver involvement is rare, liver enzyme abnormalities may be observed in up to 43% of patients. The biochemical abnormalities are typically mild and transient and the histologic abnormalities are usually nonprogressive. Such biochemical and histologic findings are typically ascribed to the primary rheumatologic condition and require no specific management. In a subset of patients with rheumatologic conditions and liver test abnormalities, further evaluation identifies a coexisting, primary liver disease or medication-related liver toxicity as the cause of the biochemical abnormality. Liver test abnormalities in patients with a coexisting primary liver disease are more likely to be persistent. In such cases, further workup using serologic tests, appropriate imaging studies and liver biopsy may be needed to accurately identify the cause of liver test abnormalities. This article reviews the spectrum of liver-related abnormalities associated with several rheumatologic diseases. Hepatotoxicity related to medications commonly prescribed in such conditions is also discussed.

Chronic liver disease is associated with several cutaneous manifestations. Although many of these changes are nonspecific, some are associated with distinct liver diseases and correlate with the severity of hepatic pathology. Often the first clue to a liver disease is manifested through skin. Although cirrhosis is associated with spider nevi and palmar erythema, disorders can result in noncirrhotic cutaneous manifestations. It is important for physicians to be familiar with the spectrum of these manifestations, to recognize, help detect, and treat the underlying hepatic disease. This article reviews the medical literature and discusses the spectrum of dermatologic manifestations of liver disorders and their pathogenesis, significance, and treatment.

Andrew Aronsohn and Donald Jensen

Liver dysfunction is common in both the critically ill and postoperative patient. Metabolic derangements secondary to sepsis, poor hepatic perfusion, total parenteral nutrition, in addition to hemodynamic and anesthetic-induced changes that occur during surgery, can cause liver damage ranging from small self-limited abnormalities in liver chemistries to acute liver failure. Early recognition, supportive care, and effective treatment of the underlying disease process are crucial steps in managing liver disease in a critically ill patient.

Calvin Pan and Ponni V. Perumalswami

Liver diseases related to pregnancy may be associated with preeclampsia (liver dysfunction related to preeclampsia; hemolysis, elevated liver enzymes, and low platelets with or without preeclampsia [HELLP syndrome]; and acute fatty liver of pregnancy) or may not involve preeclampsia (hyperemesis gravidarum and intrahepatic cholestasis of pregnancy). Liver diseases associated with pregnancy have unique presentations, but it can be difficult differentiating these from liver diseases that occur coincidentally with pregnancy. Recently, advances have been made in the disease mechanism and intervention of pregnancy-related liver diseases. Early diagnosis and delivery remains the key element in managing the liver diseases associated with preeclampsia, but emerging data suggest that incorporating advance supportive management into current strategies can improve both maternal and fetal outcomes.

THE CLINICS ARE NOW AVAILABLE ONLINE!

Access your subscription at:
www.theclinics.com

Preface

Hepatobiliary Manifestations of Systemic Diseases

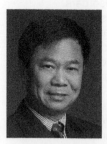

Ke-Qin Hu, MD
Guest Editor

Hepatobiliary manifestations can be the clinical presentation of other systemic disorders that are commonly seen in our daily practice and usually require gastroenterology or hepatology consultation. Understanding these clinical issues would enrich our knowledge and improve outcomes of the patient care. Some of these conditions have been well reviewed in a 2002 issue of *Clinics in Liver Disease* edited by Dr Herbert L. Bonkovsky. This issue of *Clinics in Liver Disease* denotes to an updated and systematic review on hepatobiliary manifestations of other systemic disorders. It has been my privilege and pleasure to assemble a group of expert clinicians to present their views and share their vast experiences in these complicated clinical issues.

The first review by Drs Weisberg and Jacobson provides an excellent summary on common hepatobiliary manifestations of cardiovascular diseases. The article begins by introducing a physiologic base of macro- and microcirculation of the liver, followed by most common clinical issues, such as ischemic hepatitis and congestive hepatopathy.

Both hepatopulmonary syndrome and portopulmonary hypertension are well-known pulmonary complications of liver diseases. The article by Drs Kochar and Fallon reviews hepatobiliary manifestations of some common pulmonary disorders, including respiratory failure and hepatic dysfunction, genetic and granulomatous disorders, and the liver.

Many liver diseases coexist with chronic renal disease. Dr Wong's article provides an up-to-date summary on this complicated topic. Besides covering nephrogenic ascites, a common clinical presentation, this article covers some other common but sometimes overlooked issues, such as nephrogenic hepatic dysfunction, renal tubular disorders, and cholestasis, dialysis, and the liver.

Liver diseases and endocrine disorders may have a bidirectional and complex relationship. Drs Maheshwari and Thuluvath's article systematically reviews these issues.

Clin Liver Dis 15 (2011) xiii–xiv
doi:10.1016/j.cld.2010.09.009
liver.theclinics.com

The article concisely summarized the complicated relationship between metabolic syndrome and non-alcoholic fatty liver disease. It also reviews the hepatobiliary manifestation of other common endocrine disorders, such as thyroid dysfunction, adrenal insufficiency, and sex hormone-related disorders.

Drs Singh and Pockros provide a very detailed review on hepatobiliary manifestations of hematologic and oncologic diseases by dividing their article into two sections: nonmalignant hematologic disorders and malignant hematologic disorders.

Hepatobiliary manifestations of gastrointestinal and nutritional disorders can occur as part of the clinical spectrum of the underlying disease or as a consequence of the treatment of the disease. The article by Dr Samarasena and me provides a thorough review on a selection of gastrointestinal and nutritional disorders including inflammatory bowel disease, celiac disease, Whipple's disease, and parenteral nutrition associated disorders.

Infectious disease can present with a wide variety of hepatobiliary manifestations from asymptomatic elevations in aminotransaminases to acute liver failure, hepatic fibrosis, and cirrhosis. Drs Talwani, Gilliam, and Howell contribute an excellent review on this complicated topic. HIV infection can be associated with various hepatobiliary manifestations. Dr Merwat and Vierling's article well addresses two major and common issues: HIV and HCV coinfection and hepatotoxicity of HIV medications.

Rheumatologic diseases typically have multisystem involvement, including common hepatobiliary manifestations. Drs Schlenker, Halterman, and Kowdley's article provide an in-depth review on this complicated topic. Few publications have covered the topic "Dermatologic disorders and the liver" in the past. Drs Satapathy and Bernstein have done an excellent job. Their article provides a great review on primary dermatologic disorders affecting the liver.

Liver dysfunction is common in both critically ill and postoperative patients. Drs Aronsohn and Jensen's article addresses this important and complicated topic from hypoxic liver injury, liver dysfunction in sepsis, postoperative liver dysfunction, to parenteral nutrition-associated hepatobiliary manifestations.

Pregnancy may cause complex physiologic changes that may result in hepatobiliary manifestations and related liver disorders. Thus, we include this topic in this issue of *Clinics in Liver Disease*. We appreciate that Drs Pan and Perumalswami have contributed a thorough review on this topic.

I hope that you will enjoy this issue of *Clinics in Liver Disease*. I am indebted to all the authors for their outstanding contributions of this issue, and Dr Norman Gitlin, the Consulting Editor, for his invitation and support to my participation as Guest Editor for this issue. Also, I would like to thank Kerry Holland for her outstanding editorial support.

Finally, I would like to thank my wife Chang Hong Yu and my daughter Shirley X. Hu for their love, support, and inspiration.

Ke-Qin Hu, MD
Division of Gastroenterology and Hepatology
University of California, Irvine
School of Medicine
101 The City Drive
Orange, CA 92868, USA

E-mail address:
kqhu@uci.edu

Cardiovascular Diseases and the Liver

Ilan S. Weisberg, MD, MSc, Ira M. Jacobson, MD*

KEYWORDS

• Congestive hepatopathy • Ischemic hepatitis
• Cardiac cirrhosis

MACRO- AND MICROCIRCULATION OF THE LIVER

The liver has a rich dual blood supply derived from both the portal and systemic vascular compartments and is well protected against ischemic injury during brief periods of systemic hypotension. Two-thirds of total hepatic blood flow originates from the portal vein and the remainder from the hepatic artery.[1] Blood from these 2 tributaries subsequently mixes within a complex delta of hepatic sinusoids before draining into the hepatic veins, inferior vena cava (IVC), and, ultimately, the right side of the heart. Because portal blood originates from the mesenteric veins, it is nutrient rich with high concentrations of glucose, water-soluble vitamins, amino acids, and triglycerides, but is relatively oxygen deficient. By contrast, blood originating from the hepatic artery contains little nutritive value but provides more than half of the oxygen delivered to the liver.[1]

Although the hepatic lobule is the classic architectural unit of the liver, the acinus model (also known as the Rappaport classification) is a functional hepatic unit that helps to define the complex microcirculation of oxygen and nutrient delivery.[2,3] The hepatic lobule is a hexagonal structure of hepatocytes and sinusoids flanked by 6 portal triads with a single central vein (**Fig. 1**A). By contrast, the portal triad occupies the center of the acinus, with terminal branches of the hepatic vein situated at the periphery (see **Fig. 1**B). In the acinus model, a 3-tiered oxygen and nutrient gradient exists in the hepatic parenchyma with the highest P_{O_2} and nutrient concentration delivered to the periportal hepatocytes in zone 1. As blood percolates through the sinusoids toward the perivenular region of zone 3, oxygen is extracted and water-soluble nutrients are taken up by the zone 1 and 2 hepatocytes, resulting in the delivery of low-oxygen-tension blood to zone 3. Accordingly, zone 3 is the most susceptible to ischemic injury when hepatic blood flow is diminished.[2,3]

Division of Gastroenterology and Hepatology, Weill Cornell Medical Center, New York Presbyterian Hospital, 1305 York Avenue, 4th Floor, New York, NY 10021, USA
* Corresponding author.
E-mail address: imj2001@med.cornell.edu

Clin Liver Dis 15 (2011) 1–20
doi:10.1016/j.cld.2010.09.010
1089-3261/11/$ – see front matter © 2011 Elsevier Inc. All rights reserved.

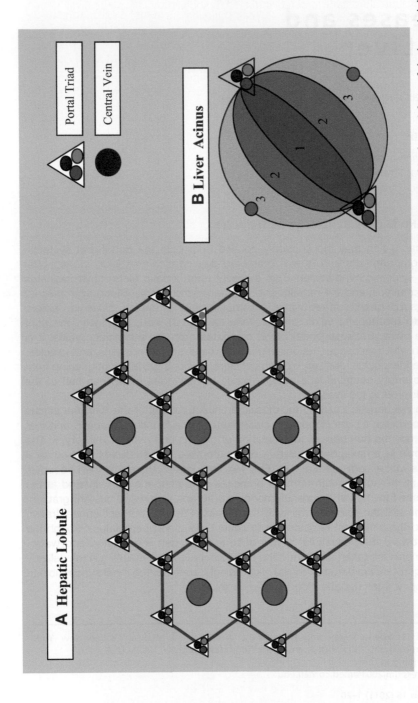

Fig. 1. The hepatic lobule (*A*) and the Rappaport classification of the liver acinus (*B*). The portal triad is situated in the periphery of the hepatic lobule, whereas the central vein is located in the middle of the hexagonal structure. By contrast, the portal triad brings oxygen- and nutrient-rich blood to the central area of the acinus (zone 1). As blood flows toward the periphery of the acinus to the central vein, hepatic extraction leads to a nutrient and oxygen tension gradient between zones 1, 2, and 3. (*Adapted from* Dancygier H. Clinical hepatology: principles and practice of hepatobiliary diseases. Berlin, Heidelberg: Springer-Verlag; 2010, Figs. 3.2 and 3.4; with permission.)

The acinar gradient additionally explains the subdivision of the parenchyma into 3 hepatic microenvironments for specific metabolic and enzymatic activities.[2,3] Zone 1 hepatocytes contain abundant large mitochondria and are responsible for gluconeogenesis, β-oxidation of fatty acids, amino acid and cholesterol synthesis, and bile acid secretion. Dominant processes in zone 3 include glycolysis and lipogenesis.[2]

Total hepatic blood flow is tightly autoregulated by the hepatic artery to maintain a near constant delivery of oxygen and nutrients to the liver.[4] When portal venous inflow is diminished, adenosine levels in the portal triad accumulate, leading to nitric oxide-mediated smooth-muscle relaxation of the hepatic arterioles and increased arterial flow.[5,6] At times of increased portal flow, adenosine concentration is diluted, hepatic arterioles constrict, and arterial flow appropriately decreases. In animal models, infusion of adenosine has been shown to reduce ischemia[7] and attenuate reperfusion injury after liver transplantation.[8] In addition, this hepatic artery buffer system is preserved in patients with advanced liver disease and cirrhosis.[9] Despite this complex system for maintaining adequate blood flow to the liver, in times of cardiovascular compromise these regulatory systems can be overwhelmed and lead to hepatic ischemia, infarction, and congestion.

ISCHEMIC HEPATITIS

Ischemic hepatitis, sometimes referred to as shock liver or hypoxic hepatitis, refers to the process of diffuse hepatocellular injury after impaired oxygen delivery to the liver. Most commonly, the condition arises in the context of profound systemic hypotension from acute cardiopulmonary collapse after myocardial infarction, exacerbation of congestive heart failure (CHF), or pulmonary embolism. In patients with chronic passive congestion or preexisting portal hypertension, even subclinical circulatory disturbances resulting in impaired hepatic perfusion can give rise to ischemic hepatitis.[10–12] Moreover, ischemic hepatitis in the absence of established hypotension has been shown in instances of severe hypoxemia, such as obstructive sleep apnea[12,13] or respiratory failure,[14,15] and in conditions of increased of metabolic activity and oxygen demand, as seen in toxic/septic shock.[12]

The central role of systemic hypotension in the pathogenesis of ischemic hepatitis was recognized more than half a century ago.[16–19] However, because decreased cardiac output, and the reduction of hepatic blood flow that ensues, is a central feature of both ischemic hepatitis and passive congestion, considerable overlap exists between these 2 conditions.[20] Moreover, it is evident that long-standing passive congestion augments the risk of hypoxic injury to zone 3 hepatocytes by promoting edema and fibrosis of the sinusoids to further impair diffusion of oxygen and nutrients. It has been proposed that profound hypotension alone is insufficient to result in the constellation of findings seen in ischemic liver injury without some element of hepatic venous congestion. Seeto and colleagues[21] compared 31 cases of documented ischemic hepatitis with 31 control patients with hemorrhagic shock after major trauma and free of primary liver disease or traumatic injury, many of whom had no recordable blood pressure for greater than 20 minutes. No patients in the traumatic shock group developed ischemic hepatitis although mild increases in the aspartate aminotransferase (AST) (78 ± 72 IU) and alanine aminotransferase (ALT) (51 ± 55 IU) levels were observed. More importantly, all cases of ischemic hepatitis had underlying cardiac disease, with 29 of 31 (94%) showing evidence of right heart failure. These data reinforce the protective dual blood supply of the liver and further the suggestion that passive congestion may predispose hepatocytes to hypoxic injury.[20,21]

Incidence

The term shock liver was first coined by Birgens and colleagues[22] in 1978 to describe just 5 cases accrued over 13 years from several Danish hospitals. Similarly, Bynum and colleagues[10] first used the term ischemic hepatitis in 1979 to describe only 7 cases identified in 5 years. These early reports created the false impression that this condition is a rare clinical entity. Contemporary studies have shown that the incidence of ischemic hepatitis approaches 0.3% of all inpatient admissions,[23,24] 1% to 2% of all intensive care unit admissions,[12,24,25] 3% of cardiac care unit admissions,[26] and 22% of cardiac care unit admissions with decreased cardiac output.[26] Recent evidence suggests that these numbers may be even higher in elderly patients.[27] Moreover, several studies evaluating the cause of massive increase in aminotransferase level in the inpatient setting have established ischemic hepatitis as the cause in more than 50% of cases.[28,29]

Clinical Features

The diagnosis of ischemic hepatitis is largely clinical and is defined by well-established criteria: (1) appropriate clinical setting of cardiac, circulatory, or pulmonary failure; (2) massive, transient increase in aminotransferase levels, usually to more than 20 times the upper limit of normal; and (3) exclusion of other known causes of liver damage. Liver biopsy is not required, nor is it advised, if these 3 conditions are met.

Patients with ischemic liver injury tend to be older (mean age 71 years), predominantly male, and acutely ill in the intensive care setting.[12] The hallmark finding of ischemic hepatitis is a massive increase in AST, ALT, and lactate dehydrogenase (LDH) levels 1 to 3 days after an episode of systemic hypotension. With return of hemodynamic stability, these values peak 1 to 3 days later and return to normal within 7 to 10 days. Increases in LDH level tend to be massive and an ALT/LDH ratio of less than 1.5 often distinguishes ischemic injury from other forms of acute hepatitis.[30,31] Total bilirubin level is usually increased as well, rarely more than 4 times the upper limit of normal, and tends to peak after the transaminases and LDH levels begin to decline. Alkaline phosphatase levels may be normal or mildly increased, but rarely more than 2 times the upper limit of normal. Increases in international normalized ratio (INR), a marker of hepatic synthetic function, are uncommon yet seen in cases of severe ischemic injury. The effects of systemic hypoperfusion are not isolated to the liver, and increases in creatinine level from acute tubular necrosis are nearly universal early in the clinical course.

Although there are no unique physical examination findings, some patients show tenderness to palpation in the right upper quadrant. Changes in mental status, when present, more often represent cerebral hypoperfusion and hypoxia rather than hepatic encephalopathy, although cases of hyperammonemia have been described. Recently, it has been suggested that a proportion of patients show transient intrapulmonary shunting, similar to hepatopulmonary syndrome, which may contribute to or exacerbate arterial hypoxemia.[32]

It is critical to consider and exclude other common and potentially treatable causes of acute hepatitis, most importantly viral hepatitis and toxin- or drug-induced liver injury.[10] A reasonable evaluation includes taking a careful medical history, serologic testing for hepatitis A, B, and C, a serum acetaminophen level, and when clinically indicated, evaluation for Wilson disease and autoimmune hepatitis. Doppler sonogram of the right upper quadrant is easily performed to evaluate patency of the portal and hepatic veins.

Histopathology

In the truest sense of the word, the term hepatitis is a misnomer because histologic evidence of inflammation is absent. Instead, the sine qua non of ischemic injury is centrolobular necrosis of zone 3 hepatocytes.[12,16-18,20-22] Simultaneous signs of sinusoidal congestion are common (see next section). In the absence of coexistent underlying liver disease or long-standing congestive hepatopathy, fibrosis is characteristically absent. The pattern of injury usually resolves spontaneously, with regeneration of hepatocytes and a return to normal histologic architecture in most patients.

Treatment

No specific therapy exists for ischemic hepatitis, as such. Treatment is directed toward correction of the underlying circulatory or respiratory disturbance. To improve hepatosplanchnic blood flow, infusion of renal-dose dopamine has been suggested,[33] but to date no proven clinical benefit has been shown. Adenosine infusion has been used in animal models but there are no human data to support its use in patients. Similarly, other investigators have suggested a role for administration of antioxidants[20] or N-acetylcysteine.[34] However, these findings are limited to case reports and need to be corroborated before any general recommendations can be made.

Prognosis

For most patients, ischemic hepatitis follows a benign and self-limited course, with complete resolution of the aminotransferase to normal values within 3 to 7 days of the inciting event.[21,30,35] However, because ischemic hepatitis mainly occurs in critically ill patients, survival in most series is expectedly poor. In the largest published series to date (142 episodes in 10 years of surveillance), the 1-month and 1-year survival was only 53% and 28%, respectively.[12] Similarly, in a recent survey of 31 historical case series published between 1956 and 2002, in-hospital mortality was 52%.[12] Recently, a report of 117 patients in Vienna documented a 72% overall mortality, with risk factors for death including underlying cause (sepsis), duration and severity of the ischemic event, and increased baseline sequential organ failure assessment scores.[36] Although increased values of aminotransferases, LDH, and INR were observed in nonsurvivors, nearly 80% of all deaths were attributed to septic shock, cardiogenic shock, or cardiac arrest, underscoring that survival is directly related to the severity of the underlying cardiopulmonary and circulatory disease.

Although fulminant hepatic failure has been reported after ischemic injury, it is rare and seems to be restricted to patients with long-standing CHF and cardiac cirrhosis[11] or other forms of chronic liver disease. In particular, patients with portal hypertensive bleeding after a variceal hemorrhage are at risk, and in this setting the mortality has been estimated to exceed 60%.[37,38]

CONGESTIVE HEPATOPATHY

Congestive hepatopathy refers to the spectrum of chronic liver injury attributed to passive hepatic congestion that arises in the setting of right-sided heart failure or any cardiopulmonary disease leading to increased central venous pressure (CVP).[39,40] Sherlock's seminal work on the topic published in 1951[39] still holds as the standard reference on the condition. Common causes include right ventricular infarction, biventricular failure from cardiomyopathy, severe pulmonary hypertension, cor pulmonale, constrictive pericarditis, and valvulopathies such as mitral stenosis and tricuspid regurgitation (TR). Incompetence of the tricuspid valve is particularly prone to result in passive congestion because pressure from the right ventricle is transmitted directly to the hepatic veins and sinusoids.[39] Untreated, long-standing congestion can lead to cardiac fibrosis and, ultimately, cardiac cirrhosis.

Incidence

The incidence of congestive hepatopathy, significant fibrosis, or cardiac cirrhosis is difficult to estimate because the condition is often subclinical and typically remains undiagnosed. However, depending on the definition and type of abnormality considered, range estimates of 15% to 65% in patients with significant heart failure have been reported.[41–44] The few available histologic studies evaluating the incidence of fibrosis after long-standing congestion are replete with selection bias because only those patients with clinically apparent disease (ascites, lower-extremity edema) and severe perturbations in liver function tests, or those undergoing evaluation for cardiac transplantation, are likely to be investigated.[41,45] Nonetheless, by today's accounts, cardiac cirrhosis is rare. Meyers and colleagues[41] investigated liver histology in a diverse population of 83 patients with heart failure and found that the presence of congestive changes was apparent in nearly all specimens; however, significant fibrosis associated with architectural distortion was present in 19% and only one individual had cirrhosis. In a series of 59 patients with severe heart failure awaiting cardiac transplant or left ventricular assist device (LVAD) placement, congestive changes and sinusoidal dilation were near universal.[45] In addition, most (~80%) had evidence of hepatic fibrosis with 26%, 17%, 28%, and 19% showing stage 1, 2, 3, and 4 (cirrhosis), respectively. The capacity to generalize from these values to better-compensated patients with CHF is not clear, and additional studies are warranted to ascertain the true incidence and prevalence of congestive liver damage.

Clinical Feature

Patients with congestive changes are typically asymptomatic and frequently identified only when routine laboratory analysis returns subtle abnormalities in liver function tests.[20] Occasionally, stretching of the hepatic capsule from congestion and hepatomegaly causes patients to report mild, dull pain in the right upper quadrant. Less frequently, patients present with signs of decompensation such as jaundice, ascites, and lower-extremity edema.

On physical examination, evidence of right heart failure is often evident, including jugular venous distension and a hepatojugular reflux. In addition, patients with constrictive pericarditis may display a pericardial knock or the classic Kussmaul sign. Abdominal palpation can reveal massive hepatomegaly with a firm, tender liver edge. In cases of TR, a pulsatile liver is sometimes appreciated and the loss of this pulsatility over time may suggest the progression from long-standing congestion to cardiac cirrhosis. Even in the presence of ascites and lower-extremity edema, splenomegaly is characteristically absent and varices are rarely identified on upper endoscopy.[41,46] This finding can be explained by the fact that varices typically form between the high-pressure portal system and the low-pressure systemic circulation, whereas in cardiac cirrhosis no pressure gradient exists because pressure is increased along the entire route of venous return to the right heart.[41]

Routine laboratory testing typically reveals mild, nonspecific increase in the serum aminotransferase level, rarely greater than 2 to 3 times the upper limit of normal.[39,40,47,48] The total bilirubin level is only mildly increased (<3 mg/dL) and predominantly unconjugated. Increases in bilirubin level have been shown to correlate with the severity of right atrial pressure and passive congestion[39,48] and in patients with severe right ventricular failure can become jaundice.[40] Even with jaundice, alkaline phosphatase level is normal or only mildly increased, which helps distinguish congestion from biliary tract disease. However, the investigators have seen exceptional cases in which more impressive increases in ALT or disproportionately increased alkaline phosphatase levels have been noted. Significant impairment of hepatic synthetic dysfunction is unusual. Although the INR is often increased to around 1.5, serum albumin level is usually normal or only slightly reduced. Although serum ammonia level is occasionally increased, hepatic encephalopathy is not a salient feature of congestive liver disease.[49]

Ascites, when present, should always be evaluated with a diagnostic paracentesis because its distinct profile can assist in the diagnosis of hepatic congestion. Like other conditions of portal hypertension, the serum ascites-albumin gradient (SAAG) is increased (>1.1). However, in cardiac ascites the total protein is characteristically increased to greater than 2.5 g/dL.[50,51] This situation is caused by preservation of hepatic synthetic function and the contribution of hepatic lymph to the peritoneal fluid. Sinusoidal congestion leads to the accumulation of protein-rich fluid in the space of Disse, which overwhelms the normal lymphatic drainage system of the liver and leaks into the peritoneal cavity.[1,40]

Congestive changes can readily be seen on cardiac and abdominal imaging.[52–54] Echocardiography often details evidence of right ventricular dysfunction, incompetence of the tricuspid valve, and increase of the right ventricular systolic pressure. Hepatic ultrasound typically shows hepatomegaly with a homogeneous increase in echogenicity throughout the liver and dilation of the suprahepatic veins and IVC. Routine findings on computed tomography (CT) and magnetic resonance (MR) abdominal cross-sectional imaging include hepatomegaly, distension of the IVC and hepatic veins, early reflux of contrast material from right atrium to the IVC, and a heterogeneous mottled-appearing liver parenchyma, often referred to as a mosaic pattern, which corresponds to the nutmeg liver seen on gross inspection (**Fig. 2**). In addition, large patchy areas of poor enhancement are often seen in the periphery of the liver as a result of stagnant blood flow. Additional nonspecific findings such as ascites and pleural and pericardial effusions are frequently reported.

Transjugular assessment of hepatic hemodynamics in patients with congestive liver disease shows an increase in the right-sided cardiac pressures that are transmitted

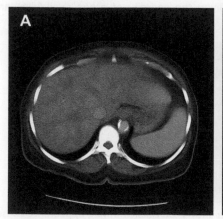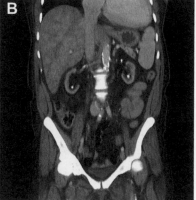

Fig. 2. Typical CT findings associated with congestive hepatopathy seen on axial (*A*) and coronal (*B*) cross-sectional imaging include hepatomegaly, distension of the IVC and hepatic veins, and a heterogeneous mottled hepatic parenchyma, resulting in a mosaic pattern of enhancement. (*Courtesy of* Dr Sophia Kung, Weill Cornell Medical Center, New York.)

caudad to the hepatic and portal venous circulations.[41] The free hepatic venous and wedged hepatic venous pressures are increased, but characteristically the hepatic to portal venous pressure gradient, which reflects the intraparenchymal contribution to portal hypertension, is normal ($\leq$4 mm Hg).[41]

Histopathology

On gross examination (**Fig. 3**A), the congested liver is enlarged, with a purple or reddish hue with prominent hepatic veins. The cut surface shows the classic nutmeg appearance, reflecting the alternating pattern of hemorrhage and necrosis of zone 3 (red in color) with the normal or slightly steatotic areas in zone 1 and 2 (yellow).

Microscopically (see **Fig. 3**B), the hallmark features of hepatic venous hypertension are prominence of the central veins, central vein hemorrhage, sinusoidal engorgement, and fibrosis of the terminal hepatic venules (phlebosclerosis).[39,55,56] Parenchymal fibrosis, when present, circumscribes the central veins and over time can form bridges with adjacent central veins to form discrete nodules (cardiac cirrhosis). Histologically, this is a unique form of cirrhosis because in all other causes of chronic liver disease, cirrhosis arises from portal-portal bridging fibrosis. In addition, the pattern of fibrosis is typically nonuniform, and it has been suggested from autopsy studies that the distribution of fibrosis may be influenced by thrombosis of the portal and hepatic vein branches.[57] Occasionally, discrete nodules can form in the absence of fibrosis as a result of regeneration of hepatocytes in zone 1 of the acinus, resulting in nodular regenerative hyperplasia (NRH).[56] Steatosis and zone 3 iron deposition from chronic hemorrhage[41] are commonly identified as well. Variable degrees of cholestasis are observed, with bile thrombi occasionally seen in cases associated with severe jaundice.[39]

The safety of liver biopsy in the evaluation of congestive hepatopathy has not been well studied and most of the histologic literature comes from older autopsy studies. However, 2 small reports suggest that tissue sampling, particularly when the transjugular route is used, can be performed effectively and safely. Parera and colleagues[58] successfully performed transjugular liver biopsy in 21 of 23 patients (91.3%) with advanced heart failure without any observed complications. Similarly, Gelow and colleagues[45] obtained adequate tissue for staging without any observed complications in all 35 patients in their series. Given the scarcity of organ availability and

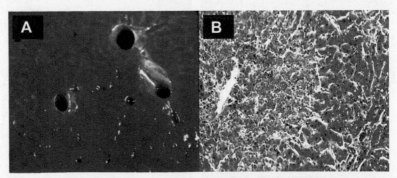

Fig. 3. The cut surface of the congested liver shows the classic nutmeg appearance caused by passive congestion of central veins with hemorrhage and necrosis in zone 3 (*A*). Congestive hepatopathy results in hepatocellular necrosis surrounding central venules (*left*) and preservation of hepatocytes in zones 1 and 2 (*B*) (original magnification ×200). (*Courtesy of* Dr Rhonda Yantiss, Weill Cornell Medical Center, New York.)

convincing data that cardiac patients with cirrhosis perform poorly after heart trans-plantation, preoperative tissue diagnosis is likely an important component of operative risk stratification and organ allocation.[59,60]

Diagnosis

The diagnosis of congestive liver disease should be suspected in any patient with abnormal liver tests and a clinical picture of CHF or increased CVP. Routine serologic evaluation for other causes of viral and metabolic liver disease should be performed to exclude primary hepatic disease, as clinically indicated. An additional important consideration is to exclude those liver diseases commonly associated with cardiomy-opathy, such as hemachromatosis, sarcoidosis, and infiltrative amyloidosis. Sources of additional supportive data include abdominal cross-sectional imaging and ascites fluid analysis. Liver histology and hepatic hemodynamic data can provide support in equivocal cases, establish the severity of fibrosis, and evaluate for concomitant hepatic disorders. The best support of the diagnosis is the improvement of liver func-tion with treatment of the underlying cardiac condition.

Treatment

The cornerstone of management is to treat the underlying cardiac disease and improve forward cardiac output, which leads to improvement in liver function tests and reduce ascites. Diuretics should be used with caution to avoid dehydration, hypo-tension, and hepatic ischemia.[61] Serial large-volume paracentesis can relieve symp-toms associated with tense ascites, but over time can lead to protein loss and exacerbate the protein malnutrition commonly seen in patients with advanced cardiac failure. Transjugular intrahepatic portosystemic shunts or peritoneal-venous shunts can worsen the underlying heart failure and are therefore contraindicated in this pop-ulation. Cautious use of anticoagulants, when indicated, is advised because patients often have a baseline mild increase in INR and are especially sensitive to warfarin and other related compounds.[62]

In patients refractory to medical therapy who are suitable operative candidates, both LVAD implantation[63,64] and cardiac transplantation[65] have been shown to improve and reverse the congestive liver injury associated with the failing heart. In select patients with established cirrhosis, combined heart and liver transplant is a feasible option.[60]

Prognosis

Over time, hepatic function typically remains stable. Even with the development of cardiac cirrhosis and ascites, patients with congestive hepatopathy rarely develop the sequela of liver disease[39,66] and long-term mortality is dictated by the underlying cardiac disease. Fulminant liver failure has been documented but seems to be restricted to those cases with superimposed ischemic liver injury[11,35,61,67] rather than passive congestion alone. The mortality in such patients is high (>90%) and is nearly always attributable to the underlying heart failure.[11,67]

Several studies have addressed the prognostic importance of liver function abnor-malities in predicting short- and long-term outcomes. Batin and colleagues[68] sug-gested that increases in bilirubin and AST levels correlate with increased mortality. Similarly, in a Japanese chronic heart failure study,[69] total bilirubin, alkaline phospha-tase, and γ-glutamyl transferase (GGT) levels were all associated with worsened outcomes. In the subanalysis of a large multinational heart failure study,[43] total bili-rubin level was independently associated with increased morbidity and mortality. However, only one study to date has evaluated the relationship between cardiac hemodynamic parameters, abnormal liver function testing, and clinical outcome.[44] Although, like other investigators, these investigators found increases in AST, alkaline phosphatase, GGT, and LDH levels correlated with increased patient mortality, after adjusting for cardiac index (CI) and CVP, no association between liver function tests and survival was observed. These data reinforce the idea that it is the primary cardiac disease, rather than hepatic dysfunction, that predicts patient morbidity and mortality.

CONGENITAL HEART DISEASE AND THE LIVER

With advances in pediatric cardiac surgery, many infants born with severe congenital heart defects are living into adulthood.[70] This is particularly the case for those children born with single ventricle malformations such as tricuspid or pulmonary atresia and the hypoplastic left heart syndrome, in which the Fontan procedure can result in near normal growth and development and good quality of life. This surgery diverts blood from the right atrium to the pulmonary arteries and is palliative but not curative because significant long-term complications are known to arise. The ensuing cavopulmonary anastamosis results in increased CVP 3 to 4 times normal, and passive hepatic congestion leading to fibrosis and cardiac cirrhosis is frequently observed. Moreover, reduction in CI and bradycardia leads to ischemic and hypoxic injury to the liver. As a result, these children often develop the same constellation of clinical findings, including abnormal liver function tests, ascites, and coagulopathy, as seen in adult patients with biventricular heart failure.[71–74] Management, as in adults, relies on restoration of cardiac output and relieving hepatic venous congestion and often requires cardiac transplantation. In addition, patients with cardiac cirrhosis should be surveyed at regular 6-month intervals with contrast-enhanced abdominal imaging of the liver and serum α-fetoprotein, similar to other causes of cirrhosis,[75] because at least 3 cases of hepatocellular carcinoma have recently been reported in this population.[70,76]

HEATSTROKE AND HEAT-RELATED DISORDERS OF THE LIVER

Heat stroke is the severe multisystem disorder that occurs with failure or overload of the thermoregulatory system of the body.[77] It is characterized by hyperthermia (core body temperature >40°C), neurologic impairment ranging from mild confusion to coma, and systemic hypotension. It represents the most serious of the heat-related disorders and without prompt and appropriate medical therapy can rapidly lead to multiorgan failure, disseminated intravascular coagulation (DIC), sepsis, and death.[77–79]

Broadly, heat stroke is classified into 2 categories that differ with regards to their cause and epidemiology, but are similar in terms of their clinical presentation and management.[78] Exertional heat stroke typically occurs in young, otherwise healthy individuals after intense exercise (ie, marathon runners, soldiers). The classic variety, by contrast, tends to involve elderly and chronically ill patients in times of extreme environmental heat exposure. Medications and illicit drugs that interfere with the thermoregulatory homeostasis of the body (eg, β-blockers, diuretics, cocaine) can augment the risk of heat stroke.[77,78]

Incidence

The reported incidence of heat stroke varies greatly by data source. Globally, outdoor laborers are the group most affected, but in the Unites States elderly inner-city residents with poor access to air conditioning and cognitive obstacles to self-care are at the greatest risk (10/100,000 individuals).[78] Each year, 240 deaths in the United States are attributed to heat stroke. In addition, epidemic heat stroke frequently arises with dramatic increases in rates of emergency room (ER) visits, hospital admissions, and patient mortality.[80,81] For example, during the Chicago heat wave in 1995, more than 3300 excess ER visits and an excess of 600 deaths were attributed to heat-related disorders.[81]

Clinical Features

In times of thermal stress, cardiac output and minute ventilation are markedly increased. However, to facilitate heat dissipation by the skin, splanchnic blood flow is reduced[82] and blood flow is shunted away from core vital organs to the peripheral vasculature, which leads to impaired visceral perfusion and hypotension. Ischemic injury to intestinal mucosa promotes bacterial translocation, leading to endotoxinemia and sepsis, and may account for many of the hematologic changes resembling DIC that are commonly identified.[83] Renal failure from massive rhabdomyolysis is frequently observed.

Mild to moderate hepatic injury is a common feature in nearly all patients with heat shock and is explained by 2 distinct mechanisms.[84,85] The severe systemic hypotension results in classic ischemic/hypoxic injury to zone 3 hepatocytes in the liver. In addition, excessive body temperature leads to direct thermal injury and hepatic necrosis.[84,85] The result is a profound increase in serum aminotransferase values and LDH levels. Although the ALT level is rarely increased more than 20 times the upper limit of normal, the AST level can be massively increased as a result of concomitant injury to skeletal and cardiac muscle, brain, and kidneys. Rarely, massive hepatocellular damage and acute liver failure are observed.[86–89] As in ischemic hepatitis, the aminotransferase levels peak 1 to 2 days after the inciting event. However, recovery takes a more protracted course, occurring over several weeks. Total bilirubin level is frequently normal or only mildly increased.

Physical examination findings are nonspecific, and a high index of suspicion is required to promptly make a diagnosis of heat shock and initiate appropriate therapy.[77,78] Affected patients present with hyperpyrexia, with core body temperatures ranging from 40 to 44°C (104–111.2°F) and signs of central nervous system (CNS) dysfunction (irritability, ataxia, confusion, seizure, coma). Additional findings may include hot dry skin, variable degrees of tenderness in the right upper quadrant, bleeding from sites of venipuncture, epistaxis, melena, or hematochezia. As a result of systemic endothelial damage, peripheral and pulmonary edema is commonly observed.

Histopathology

The pattern of liver injury suggests both direct thermal injury and hypoxic damage.[79,90,91] Evidence of ischemic hepatitis is apparent, with centrilobular dilatation of sinusoids and zone 3 necrosis, whereas heat-mediated degenerative changes to hepatocytes ranging from basophilia to necrosis are evident. Additional common features include steatosis, vacuolization, and cholangiolar proliferation. In survivors, these histologic features recover spontaneously without the formation of significant fibrosis.[90,92]

Treatment

The mainstay of therapy is rapidly reducing the body temperature to prevent thermal injury to vital organs.[78] External cooling by wetting the skin to promote evaporative heat loss, immersion in an ice bath, or applying ice packs to the axilla and groin should be initiated immediately. After transfer to an intensive care setting, internal cooling with gastric, bladder, or rectal cold-water lavage should be instituted. Hypotension should be treated with appropriate fluid resuscitation with the goal of improving end-organ perfusion. No pharmacologic therapies have shown any clinical benefit, including muscle relaxants, benzodiazepines, antipyretics, and dantrolene.[77,78]

Liver transplantation has been proposed for individuals with severe liver injury not responding to conservative medical therapy.[85] However, many of the features of acute liver failure are normal findings in heat shock (altered mental status, coagulopathy), making conventional prognostic algorithms such as the Kings College criteria difficult to apply in this clinical context. In addition, the long-term benefit of liver transplant has not been established. By way of example, 16 cases of fulminant liver failure after heat shock have been reported in the literature, only 3 of which were transplanted.[85,88,93,94] Amongst the 13 cases treated medically, 8 (61.5%) survived and 5 (31.5%) died, whereas all 3 of the transplanted patients died. Given these limited results and the fact that patients with massive hepatic necrosis have been shown to recover spontaneously,[92] caution should be applied before listing patients for liver transplant. Although further data are warranted, a single case report showing benefit with the molecular adsorbent recirculating system has been described, suggesting that, where available, liver assist devices may be a useful bridge to patient recovery.[95]

Prognosis

Heat shock is a true medical emergency, with mortality estimates of 10% to 25%. However, with early and aggressive therapy survival approaches 100%. Nonetheless, fulminant liver failure is observed in at least 5% of cases, and this may be an underestimate of the true risk.[93,96,97] In addition, permanent CNS dysfunction persists in up to 20% of survivors. Prognostic factors for morbidity and mortality have not been elucidated; however, some investigators have suggested that higher levels of aminotransferase and bilirubin,[84] extensive centrilobular necrosis, and persistent renal failure from rhabdomyolysis[85] portend increased risk of death and long-term morbidity. Prevention of heat-related injury is the most effective means to reduce the morbidity and mortality associated with this disorder.[81]

VASCULAR DISORDERS OF THE LIVER

With the exception of portal vein thrombosis in patients with cirrhosis, vascular disorders of the liver are rare.[98] However, 2 uncommon systemic conditions, hereditary hemorrhagic telangiectasia (HHT) and polyarteritis nodosa (PAN), can present with severe hepatic involvement and deserve mention.

HEREDITARY HEMORRHAGIC TELANGIECASIA

Also known as Osler-Weber-Rendu disease, HHT is a rare autosomal-dominant genetic disease characterized by diffuse mucocutaneous and visceral arteriovenous malformations (AVMs). A mutation in one of 2 genes, endoglin (ENG) and activin receptorlike kinase type 1 (ALK-1), is identified in most affected families. These genes encode for a vascular endothelial transmembrane protein involved in the transforming growth factor pathway.[99,100]

Incidence

HHT is said to affect only 10 to 20/100,000 individuals, with approximately 50,000 affected people in the United States. Although hepatic AVMs are observed in 75% of individuals with HHT, they are infrequently symptomatic (<10%)[101–104] and tend to be restricted to families and patients with ALK-1 mutations.[98,105] Fewer than 100 symptomatic cases of liver involvement by HHT have been documented in the English language literature.[102,103]

Clinical Manifestations

Symptomatic patients can present with one or more of 3 phenotypic expressions of the disease, including high-output heart failure, portal hypertension, or biliary ischemia. Three distinct types of vascular shunting in the liver help explain the variability in clinical presentation of this disorder: arteriovenous, portovenous, and arterioportal.[102,103]

The most common presentation is heart failure secondary to arteriovenous and portovenous shunting and the resultant hyperdynamic circulation.[98,102,103] Symptomatic patients display typical signs and symptoms of cardiac dysfunction, including fatigue, shortness of breath, reduced exercise capacity, ascites, and extremity edema. Noncirrhotic portal hypertension from arterioportal shunting or from NRH after variable blood flow to the liver leads to ascites, portal hypertensive gastropathy, and variceal formation. However, because hepatic synthetic function is preserved, hepatic encephalopathy is not a prominent feature. Shunting of hepatic artery blood flow can lead to complications of biliary ischemia, including cholestasis, strictures, and cholangitis. The term hepatic disintegration has been used to describe the extreme presentation of bile duct and liver necrosis that has rarely been documented.[106]

Diagnosis

International consensus criteria, the Curacao Diagnostic Criteria, are used to establish a diagnosis of HHT and are based on 4 findings: spontaneous and recurrent epistaxis, multiple mucocutaneous telangiectasias, visceral involvement (gastrointestinal, pulmonary, cerebral, or hepatic), and an affected first-degree relative.[107] When more than 3, 2, or one of the criteria are met the diagnosis is considered to be definite, suspected, or unlikely, respectively. Confirmatory genetic testing for mutations in the ENG or ALK-1 genes is commercially available and can help confirm the diagnosis. Patients with HHT with a typical clinical history should be evaluated for hepatic involvement.

Although angiography is the gold standard, the diagnosis is readily established with noninvasive testing such as Doppler ultrasound and contrast-enhanced CT.[98] Sonographic findings of intrahepatic hypervascularization and a markedly dilated common hepatic artery (>7 mm) have been shown to be highly sensitive and specific for the diagnosis of hepatic HHT.[108] Similar characteristic findings on CT include a dilated hepatic artery and heterogeneity of the hepatic parenchyma.[109] Nodularity secondary to NRH is often misinterpreted as cirrhosis. Liver biopsy is not required to make the diagnosis and should be avoided because of increased risk of complications related to bleeding.[98,102,103]

Treatment

No specific treatment is indicated for asymptomatic liver involvement by HHT and therefore screening for hepatic involvement in these individuals is not indicated. Symptoms of high-output cardiac failure should be managed like other patients with CHF from more typical causes (eg, salt restriction, diuretics, β-blockers). Similarly, complications from portal hypertension should be managed in accordance with guidelines for cirrhotic patients.[98,102,103] To avoid cholangitis, invasive biliary procedures should generally be avoided in patients with the biliary ischemic phenotype, and early initiation of antibiotics should be used for signs of biliary sepsis.

Case reports of surgical ligation and transarterial embolization of the hepatic artery have been described for control of medically refractory cases of high-output heart failure and portal hypertension. However, this approach is strongly unadvised because benefits are modest, transient at best, and associated with serious morbidity and mortality from the ensuing biliary ischemia and necrosis.[98,102,103] Garcia-Tsao[102] recently reported that more than one-third of patients undergoing this intervention developed serious complications leading to rescue liver transplantation or death.

The only definitive curative treatment of hepatic HHT is liver transplantation. A recent report from the European transplant registry of 40 patients with HHT documented excellent overall 5-year survival (80%), although patients with the portal hypertensive phenotype seem to perform slightly worse (63% survival at 47 months).[103,110] Symptomatic patients with hepatic HHT should be considered for Model for End-Stage Liver Disease exception points and given priority for liver transplantation because their laboratory parameters may inadequately represent their risk of morbidity and mortality from heart failure and other complications.[111]

Medical therapies with thalidomide and hormone-based therapies have had mixed results in the management of gastrointestinal bleeding from HHT. Recently, case reports using bevacizumab, an antibody to vascular endothelial growth factor with antioangiogenic properties, has been shown to reduce complications of portal hypertensive bleeding[112] and reduce the need for liver transplantation in a patient with heart failure.[113] Although these initial results are promising, more experience with this agent is needed before general recommendations can be made for its use in symptomatic patients with HHT.

POLYARTERITIS NODOSA

PAN is a systemic necrotizing vasculitis that results in immune complex deposition in small and medium-sized arteries, resulting in segmental necrotizing lesions, arterial stenoses and aneurysms, and tissue ischemia. The kidneys, muscles, skin, peripheral nervous system, and gastrointestinal tract are the most commonly involved, but any organ can be affected. Although rare, case reports of hepatic involvement have been described.[114–117]

Incidence

PAN is rare, affecting only about 2 to 33 cases per million individuals. The incidence increases with age and peaks in middle age. It is not possible to estimate the frequency of liver involvement because there are fewer than 20 reports in the literature of hepatic complications of PAN.[114–117] Although most cases of PAN are idiopathic, a clear association between chronic infection with hepatitis B virus (HBV) and hepatitis C virus exists, and universal HBV vaccination and improved blood donor screening have already led to a dramatic reduction in the frequency of this rare extrahepatic manifestation.[118]

Clinical Manifestations

Symptoms of PAN are nonspecific, with fever and lethargy being the most common presentation. Hepatic or gall bladder involvement is usually accompanied by abdominal pain, nausea, and vomiting. In more severe cases, patients can present with massive hepatic infarction,[115,116] hepatic abscess,[114] and cholecystitis.[115] In addition to laboratory values reflecting chronic hepatic ischemia, there is evidence of leukocytosis and the C-reactive protein and erythrocyte sedimentation rate are frequently increased. Diagnosis is confirmed when biopsy of affected tissues reveals necrotizing arteritis or when the typical pattern of arterial stenosis and aneurysmal dilation is seen on angiography. Noninvasive imaging with MR or CT arteriography may miss small vascular changes and may not be diagnostic.

Treatment

The goal of treatment is to rapidly suppress inflammation and end-organ damage.[118] Without appropriate therapy, 5-year survival is less than 15%. For systemic disease, treatment with corticosteroids plus cyclophosamide, methotrexate, or azathioprine is often used. In cases of HBV-associated PAN, plasma exchange to reduce antigenic excess and suppression of HBV viremia with antiviral agents facilitates induction and long-term maintenance of PAN remission [118]

SUMMARY

The dual blood supply of the liver provided by branches of the hepatic artery and the portal vein makes it relatively protected from ischemic injury. Nonetheless, minor or brief disruptions in cardiac output and hepatic perfusion, particularly in patients with underlying right or left heart failure, can result in ischemic liver damage. Similarly, conditions that lead to impaired venous return to the heart, when long-standing, may result in passive hepatic congestion, fibrosis, and rarely cardiac cirrhosis. Together, ischemic hepatitis and congestive hepatopathy represent 2 of the commonest indications for a hepatology consultation in the inpatient and outpatient setting and can serve as a framework to understand less common conditions such as heatstroke, congenital heart disease, and vascular disorders of the liver. Management is largely supportive, with care directed at correction of the inciting cardiac event. Although liver function typically resolves spontaneously in most cases, prognosis is dictated by the severity and reversibility of cardiac dysfunction.

REFERENCES

1. Lautt WW, Greenway CV. Conceptual review of the hepatic vascular bed. Hepatology 1987;7:952–63.
2. Rappaport AM. The microcirculatory hepatic unit. Microvasc Res 1973;6: 212–28.
3. Rappaport AM. Hepatic blood flow: morphologic aspects and physiologic regulation. Int Rev Physiol 1980;21:1–63.
4. Lautt WW. Mechanisms and role of intrinsic regulation of hepatic arterial blood flow: hepatic arterial buffer response. Am J Phys 1985;249:549–56.
5. Ezzat WR, Lautt WW. Hepatic arterial pressure flow autoregulation is adenosine mediated. Am J Phys 1987;252:836–45.
6. Smits P, Williams SB, Lipson DE, et al. Endothelial release of nitric oxide contributes to the vasodilator effect of adenosine in humans. Circulation 1995;92:2135–41.
7. Peralta C, Hotter G, Closa D, et al. The protective role of adenosine in inducing nitric oxide synthesis in rat liver ischemia preconditioning is mediated by activation of adenosine A2 receptors. Hepatology 1999;29:126–32.
8. Gao WS, Hijioka T, Lindert KA, et al. Evidence that adenosine is a key component in Carolina rinse responsible for reducing graft failure after orthotopic liver transplantation in the rat. Transplantation 1991;52:992–8.
9. Zipprich A, Steudel N, Behrmann C, et al. Functional significance of hepatic arterial flow reserve in patients with cirrhosis. Hepatology 2003;37:385–92.
10. Bynum TE, Boitnott JK, Maddrey WC. Ischemic hepatitis. Dig Dis Sci 1979;24: 129–35.
11. Nouel O, Henrion J, Bernuau J, et al. Fulminant hepatic failure due to transient circulatory failure in patients with chronic heart disease. Dig Dis Sci 1980;25: 49–52.

12. Henrion J, Schapira M, Luwaert R, et al. Hypoxic hepatitis: clinical and hemo-dynamic study in 142 consecutive cases. Medicine (Baltimore) 2003;82:
392–406.
13. Henrion J, Colin L, Schapira M, et al. Hypoxic hepatitis caused by severe hypox-emia from obstructive sleep apnea. J Clin Gastroenterol 1997;24:245–9.
14. Henrion J, Minette P, Colin L, et al. Hypoxic hepatitis caused by acute exacer-bation of chronic respiratory failure: a case-controlled, hemodynamic study of 17 consecutive cases. Hepatology 1999;29:427–33.
15. Mathurin P, Durand F, Ganne N, et al. Ischemic hepatitis due to obstructive sleep apnea. Gastroenterology 1995;109:1682–4.
16. Ellenberg M, Osserman KE. The role of shock in the production of central liver cell necrosis. Am J Med 1951;11:170–8.
17. Killip T, Payne MA. High serum transaminase in heart disease. Circulatory failure and hepatic necrosis. Circulation 1960;21:646–60.
18. Clarke WT. Centrilobular necrosis following cardiac infarction. Am J Pathol 1950;
26:249–55.
19. Cohen JA, Kaplan MM. Left-sided heart failure presenting as hepatitis. Gastro-enterology 1978;74:583–7.
20. Giallourakis CC, Rosenberg PM, Friedman LS. The liver in heart failure. Clin Liver Dis 2002;6:947–67.
21. Seeto RK, Fenn B, Rockey DC. Ischemic hepatitis: clinical presentation and pathogenesis. Am J Med 2000;109:109–13.
22. Birgens HS, Henriksen J, Matzen P, et al. The shock liver. Clinical and biochem-ical findings in patients with centrilobular necrosis following cardiogenic shock. Acta Med Scand 1978;204:417–21.
23. Hickman PE, Potter JM. Mortality associated with ischaemic hepatitis. Aust N Z J Med 1990;20:32–4.
24. Fuchs S, Bogomolski-Yahalom V, Paltiel O, et al. Ischemic hepatitis: clinical and laboratory observations of 34 patients. J Clin Gastroenterol 1998;26:183–6.
25. Birrer R, Takuda Y, Takara T. Hypoxic hepatopathy: pathophysiology and prog-nosis. Intern Med 2007;46:1063–70.
26. Henrion J, Descamps O, Luwaert R, et al. Hypoxic hepatitis in patients with cardiac failure. Incidence in a coronary care unit and measurement of hepatic blood flow. J Hepatol 1994;21:696–703.
27. Rashed KA, McNabb WR, Lewis RR. Ischaemic hepatitis in the elderly. Geron-tology 2002;48:245–9.
28. Johnson RD, O'Conner ML, Kerr RM. Extreme serum elevations of aspartate aminotransferase. Am J Gastroenterol 1995;90:1244–5.
29. Whitehead MW, Hawkes ND, Hainsworth I, et al. A prospective study of the causes of notably raised aspartate aminotransferase of liver origin. Gut 1999;
45:129–33.
30. Gitlin N, Serio KM. Ischemic hepatitis: widening horizons. Am J Gastroenterol 1992;87:831–6.
31. Cassidy WM, Reynolds TB. Serum lactate dehydrogenase in the differential diagnosis of acute hepatocellular injury. J Clin Gastroenterol 1994;19:118–21.
32. Fuhrmann V, Madl C, Mueller C, et al. Hepatopulmonary syndrome in patients with hypoxic hepatitis. Gastroenterology 2006;131:69–75.
33. Anghern W, Schmid E, Althaus F, et al. Effect of dopamine on hepatosplanchnic flow. J Cardiovasc Pharmacol 1980;2:257–65.
34. Desai A, Kadleck D, Hufford L, et al. N-Acetylcysteine use in ischemic hepatitis. Am J Ther 2006;13:80–3.

35. Logan RG, Mowry FM, Judge RD. Cardiac failure simulating viral hepatitis. Three cases with serum transaminase levels above 1,000. Ann Intern Med 1962;56:784–8.
36. Fuhrmann V, Kneidinger N, Herkner H, et al. Hypoxic hepatitis: underlying conditions and risk factors for mortality in critically ill patients. Intensive Care Med 2009;35:1397–405.
37. Henrion J, Colin L, Schmitz A, et al. Ischemic hepatitis in cirrhosis: rare but lethal. J Clin Gastroenterol 1993;16:35–9.
38. Pauwels A, Levy VG. Ischemic hepatitis in cirrhosis: not so rare, not always lethal. J Clin Gastroenterol 1993;17:88–9.
39. Sherlock S. The liver in heart failure. Relation of anatomical, functional, and circulatory changes. Br Heart J 1951;13:273–81.
40. Dunn GD, Hayes P, Breen KJ, et al. The liver in congestive heart failure: a review. Am J Med Sci 1973;265:174–89.
41. Meyers RP, Cerini R, Sayegh R, et al. Cardiac hepatopathy: clinical, hemodynamic and histologic characteristics and correlations. Hepatology 2003;37:393–400.
42. Lau GT, Tan HC, Kritharides L. Type of liver dysfunction in heart failure and its relation to severity of tricuspid regurgitation. Am J Cardiol 2002;90:1405–9.
43. Allen LA, Felker GM, Pocock, et al. Liver function abnormalities and outcomes in patients with chronic heart failure: results from the Candesartan in Heart Failure: Assessment of Reduction in Mortality and Morbidity (CHARM) program. Eur Heart J 2009;11:170–7.
44. Van Deursen VM, Damman K, Hillege HL, et al. Abnormal liver function in relation to hemodynamic profile in heart failure patients. J Card Fail 2010;16:84–90.
45. Gelow JM, Desai AS, Hochberg CP, et al. Clinical predictors of hepatic fibrosis in chronic advanced heart failure. Circ Heart Fail 2010;3:59–64.
46. Luna A, Meister HP, Szanto PB. Esophageal varices in the absence of cirrhosis. Incidence and characteristics in congestive heart failure and neoplasm of the liver. Am J Clin Pathol 1968;49:710–7.
47. Richman SM, Delman AJ, Grob D. Alterations in indices of liver function in congestive heart failure with particular reference to serum enzymes. Am J Med 1961;30:211–25.
48. Kubo SH, Walter BA, John DH, et al. Liver function abnormalities in chronic heart failure: influence of systemic hemodynamics. Arch Intern Med 1987;147: 1227–30.
49. Bessman AN, Evans JM. The blood ammonia in congestive heart failure. Am Heart J 1955;50:715–9.
50. Runyon BA. Cardiac ascites: a characterization. J Clin Gastroenterol 1988;10: 410–2.
51. Christou L, Economou M, Economou G, et al. Characteristics of ascitic fluid in cardiac ascites. Scand J Gastroenterol 2007;42:1102–5.
52. Moulton JS, Miller BL, Dodd GD, et al. Passive hepatic congestion in heart failure: CT abnormalities. AJR Am J Roentgenol 1988;151:939–42.
53. Holley HC, Koslin DB, Berland LL, et al. Inhomogeneous enhancement of liver parenchyma secondary to passive congestion: contrast-enhanced CT. Radiology 1989;170:795–800.
54. Gore RM, Mathieu DG, White EM, et al. Passive hepatic congestion: cross-sectional imaging features. Am J Roentgenol 1994;162:71–5.
55. Safran AP, Schaffner F. Chronic passive congestion of the liver in man. Electron microscopic study of cell atrophy and intralobular fibrosis. Am J Pathol 1967;50: 447–63.

56. Lefkowitch JH, Mendez L. Morphologic features of hepatic injury in cardiac disease and shock. J Hepatol 1986;2:313–27.
57. Wanless IR, Liu JJ, Butany J. Role of thrombosis in the pathogenesis of congestive hepatic fibrosis (cardiac cirrhosis). Hepatology 1995;21:1232–7.
58. Parera A, Banares R, Alvarez R, et al. The usefulness of transjugular hepatic biopsy in the evaluation of liver disease in candidates for heart transplantation. Gastroenterol Hepatol 1999;22:67–71.
59. Hsu RB, Lin FY, Chou NK, et al. Heart transplantation in patients with extreme right ventricular failure. Eur J Cardiothorac Surg 2007;32:457–61.
60. Raichlin E, Daly RC, Rosen CB, et al. Combined heart and liver transplantation: a single center experience. Transplantation 2009;88:219–25.
61. Kisloff B, Schaffer G. Fulminant hepatic failure secondary to congestive heart failure. Am J Dig Dis 1976;21:895–900.
62. Jafri SM. Hypercoagulability in heart failure. Semin Thromb Hemost 1997;23: 543–5.
63. Frazier OH, Rose EA, Oz MC, et al. Multicenter clinical evaluation of the Heart-Mate vented electric left ventricular assist system in patients awaiting heart transplantation. J Thorac Cardiovasc Surg 2001;122:1866–95.
64. Russell SD, Rogers JG, Milano CA, et al. Renal and hepatic function improve in advanced heart failure patients during continuous flow support with the Heart-Mate II left ventricular assist device. Circulation 2009;120:2352–7.
65. Dichtl W, Vogel W, Dunst KM, et al. Cardiac hepatopathy before and after heart transplantation. Transpl Int 2005;18:697–702.
66. Naschitz JE, Slobodin G, Lewis, et al. Heart disease affecting the liver and liver disease affecting the heart. Am Heart J 2000;140:111–20.
67. Saner FH, Heuer M, Meyer M, et al. When the heart kills the liver: acute liver failure in congestive heart failure. Eur J Med Res 2009;14:541–6.
68. Batin P, Wickens M, McEntegart D, et al. The importance of abnormalities of liver function tests in predicting mortality in chronic heart failure. Eur Heart J 1995;16: 1613–8.
69. Shinagawa H, Inomata T, Koitabashi T, et al. Prognostic significance of increased serum bilirubin levels coincident with cardiac decompensation in chronic heart failure. Circ J 2008;72:364–9.
70. Ghaferi AA, Hutchins GM. Progression of liver pathology in patients undergoing the Fontan procedure: chronic passive congestion, cardiac cirrhosis, hepatic adenoma, and hepatocellular carcinoma. J Thorac Cardiovasc Surg 2005; 129:1348–52.
71. Mace S, Borkat G, Liebman J. Hepatic dysfunction and cardiovascular abnormalities: occurrence in infants, children, and young adults. Am J Dis Child 1985;139:60–5.
72. Narkewicz MR, Sondheimer HM, Ziegler JW, et al. Hepatic dysfunction following the Fontan procedure. J Pediatr Gastroenterol Nutr 2003;36:352–7.
73. Miesewetter CH, Sheron N, Vettukattill JJ. Hepatic changes in the failing Fontan circulation. Heart 2007;93:579–84.
74. Camposilvan S, Milanesi O, Stellin G, et al. Liver and cardiac function in the long term after Fontan operation. Ann Thorac Surg 2008;86:177–82.
75. Bruix J, Sherman M. Management of hepatocellular carcinoma. Hepatology 2005;42:1208–36.
76. Saliba T, Dorkholm S, O'Reilly, et al. Hepatocellular carcinoma in two patients with cardiac cirrhosis. Eur J Gastroenterol Hepatol 2010;22:889–91.
77. Bouchama A, Knochel JP. Heat stroke. N Engl J Med 2002;346:1978–88.

78. Glazer JL. Management of heatstroke and heat exhaustion. Am Fam Physician 2005;71:2133–40.
79. Rubel LR, Ishak KG. The liver in fatal exertional heatstroke. Liver 1983;3: 249–60.
80. Hart GR, Anderson RJ, Crumpler CP, et al. Epidemic classical heat stroke: clinical characteristics and course in 28 patients. Medicine 1982;61:189–97.
81. Dematte JE, O'Mara K, Buescher J, et al. Near-fatal heat stroke during the 1995 heat wave in Chicago. Ann Intern Med 1998;129:173–81.
82. Roswell LB, Brengelmann GR, Blackmon JR, et al. Redistribution of blood flow during sustained high skin temperatures in resting man. J Appl Phys 1970;28: 415–20.
83. Bouchama A, Bridey F, Hammami MM, et al. Activation of coagulation and fibrinolysis in heatstroke. Thromb Haemost 1996;76:909–15.
84. Kew M, Bersohn I, Seftel H, et al. Liver damage in heat stroke. Am J Med 1970; 49:192–202.
85. Hassanein T, Razack A, Gavaler J, et al. Heatstroke: its clinical and pathological presentation with particular attention to the liver. Am J Gastroenterol 1992;87: 1382–9.
86. Feller RB, Wilson JS. Hepatic failure in fatal exertional heatstroke. Aust N Z J Med 1994;24:69.
87. Ichai C, Ciais JF, Hyvernat, et al. Fatal acute liver failure: a rare complication of exertion-induced heat stroke. Ann Fr Anesth Reanim 1997;16:64–7.
88. Berger J, Hart J, Millis M, et al. Fulminant hepatic failure from heatstroke requiring liver transplantation. J Clin Gastroenterol 2000;30:429–31.
89. Hadad E, Ben-Ari Z, Heled Y, et al. Liver transplantation in exertional heat stroke: a medical dilemma. Intensive Care Med 2004;30:1474–8.
90. Bianchi L, Ohnacker H, Beck K, et al. Liver damage in heatstroke and its regression. A biopsy study. Hum Pathol 1972;3:237–48.
91. Kew MC, Minick OT, Bahu RM, et al. Ultrastructural changes in the liver in heatstroke. Am J Pathol 1978;90:609–18.
92. Giercksky T, Boberg KM, Farstad IN, et al. Severe liver failure in exertional heatstroke. Scand J Gastroenterol 1999;8:824–7.
93. Hassanein T, Perper JA, Tepperman L, et al. Liver failure occurring as a component of exertional heatstroke. Gastroenterology 1991;100:1442–7.
94. Saissy JM. Liver transplantation in a case of fulminant liver failure after exertion. Intensive Care Med 1996;22:831.
95. Sein Anand J, Chodorowski Z, Korolkiewicz RP. Heat stroke complicated by liver failure and hyperbilirubinemia – case report. Przegl Lek 2007;64:344–5.
96. Weigand K, Riediger C, Stremmel W, et al. Are heat stroke and physical exhaustion underestimated causes of acute hepatic failure? World J Gastroenterol 2007;13:306–9.
97. Garcin JM, Bronstein JA, Cremades S, et al. Acute liver failure is frequent during heat stroke. World J Gastroenterol 2008;7:158–9.
98. DeLeve LD, Valla DC, Garcia-Tsao G. Vascular disorders of the liver. Hepatology 2009;49:1729–64.
99. McAllister KA, Grogg KM, Johnson DW, et al. Endoglin, a TGF-beta binding protein of endothelial cells, is the gene for hereditary haemorrhagic telangiectasia type 1. Nat Genet 1994;8:345–51.
100. Johnson DW, Berg JN, Baldwin MA, et al. Mutations in the activin receptor-like kinase 1 gene in hereditary haemorrhagic telangiectasia type 2. Nat Genet 1996;13:189–95.

101. Ianora AA, Memeo M, Sabba C, et al. Hereditary hemorrhagic telangiectasia: multidetector row helical CT assessment of hepatic involvement. Radiology 2004;230:250–9.
102. Garcia-Tsao G. Liver involvement in hereditary hemorrhagic telangiectasia (HHT). J Hepatol 2007;46:499–507.
103. Khalid SK, Garcia-Tsao G. Hepatic vascular malformations in hereditary hemorrhagic telangiectasia. Semin Liver Dis 2008;28:247–58.
104. Buonamico P, Suppressa P, Lenato GM, et al. Liver involvement in a large cohort of patients with hereditary hemorrhagic telangiectasia: echo-color-Doppler vs multislice computed tomography study. J Hepatol 2008;48:811–2.
105. Bayrak-Toydemir P, McDonald J, Markewitz B, et al. Genotype-phenotype correlation in hereditary hemorrhagic telangiectasia: mutations and manifestations. Am J Med Genet 2006;140:463–70.
106. Blewitt RW, Brown CM, Wyatt JI. The pathology of acute hepatic disintegration in hereditary haemorrhagic telangiectasia. Histopathology 2003;42:265–9.
107. Faughnan ME, Palda VA, Garcia-Tsao G, et al. International guidelines for the diagnosis and management of hereditary hemorrhagic telangiectasia. J Med Genet, in press, Epub 2009.
108. Caselitz M, Bahr MJ, Bleck JS, et al. Sonographic criteria for the diagnosis of hepatic involvement in hereditary hemorrhagic telangiectasia (HHT). Hepatology 2003;37:1139–46.
109. Wu JS, Saluja S, Garcia-Tsao G, et al. Liver involvement in hereditary hemorrhagic telangiectasia: CT and clinical findings do not correlate in symptomatic patients. AJR Am J Roentgenol 2006;187:399–405.
110. Lerut J, Orlando G, Adam R, et al. Liver transplantation registry for hereditary hemorrhagic telangiectasia: report of the European liver transplant registry. Ann Surg 2006;244:854–64.
111. Garcia-Tsao G, Gish RG, Punch J. MELD exception for hereditary hemorrhagic telangiectasia. Liver Transpl 2006;12:S108–9.
112. Bose P, Holter JL, Selby GB. Bevacizumab in hereditary hemorrhagic telangiectasia. N Engl J Med 2009;360:2143–4.
113. Mitchell A, Adams LA, MacQuillan G, et al. Bevacizumab reverses need for liver transplantation in hereditary hemorrhagic telangiectasia. Liver Transpl 2008;14:210–3.
114. Gilliland IC, Manning GC. Liver abscess and polyarteritis nodosa. Br Med J 1954;2:294.
115. Cowan RE, Mallinson CN, Thomas GE, et al. Polyarteritis nodosa of the liver: a report of two cases. Postgrad Med J 1977;53:89–93.
116. Haratake J, Horie A, Furuta A, et al. Massive hepatic infarction associated with polyarteritis nodosa. Acta Pathol Jpn 1988;38:89–93.
117. Takeshita S, Nakamura H, Kawakami A, et al. Hepatitis B-related polyarteritis nodosa presenting vasculitis in the hepatobiliary system successfully treated with lamivudine, plasmapheresis, and glucocorticoid. Intern Med 2006;45:145–9.
118. Guillevin L, Mahr A, Callard P, et al. Hepatitis B virus-associated polyarteritis nodosa: clinical characteristics, outcome, and impact of treatment in 115 patients. Medicine (Baltimore) 2005;84:313–22.

Pulmonary Diseases and the Liver

Rajan Kochar, MD, MPH, Michael B. Fallon, MD*

KEYWORDS

- Hypoxic hepatitis • Cystic fibrosis • α-1 Antitrypsin
- Hepatic sarcoidosis • Hepatic tuberculosis

Pulmonary complications of chronic liver disease such as hepatopulmonary syndrome, portopulmonary hypertension and hepatic hydrothorax are well known, and have been described extensively in the literature. Conversely, hepatobiliary manifestations of primary pulmonary disease also occur with high frequency, but have been less frequently reviewed. This article reviews the involvement of the liver and the biliary tract in selected primary pulmonary diseases including respiratory failure, cystic fibrosis, α-1 antitrypsin deficiency, sarcoidosis, and tuberculosis (TB).

RESPIRATORY FAILURE AND HEPATIC DYSFUNCTION

Hypoxic injury to the liver is a largely reversible condition occurring in at least 1% of critically ill patients and accounting for more than 50% of large increases in serum aminotransferases identified in hospital admissions.[1] Hepatic dysfunction caused by hypoxia was historically assumed to result from poor blood flow to the liver. The term ischemic hepatitis was coined in 1979 by Bynum and colleagues[2] to refer to centrilobular liver cell necrosis with an acute increase in serum transaminases in the setting of cardiac failure. A few years later, Arcidi and colleagues[3] published a study concluding that circulatory failure was required to make a diagnosis of ischemic hepatitis, giving rise to the term shock liver. For several years, it was widely agreed that ischemia was the sole cause of hypoxic liver injury. However, in recent years, other mechanisms of hypoxic liver injury have been identified, such as noncardiogenic shock and respiratory failure, giving rise to the more inclusive term hypoxic hepatitis (HH).

HH cases may be grouped based on primary pathophysiology: (1) decreased oxygen uptake (eg, respiratory failure), (2) reduced oxygen delivery (eg, hypotension), (3) decreased oxygen availability (eg, sepsis), and (4) increased oxygen consumption (eg, hyperthermia). Contrary to earlier theories, significant hypotension is observed as a contributory cause in only 50% of all patients with HH. However, congestive heart

Financial disclosure and conflict of interest: the authors have nothing to disclose.
Division of Gastroenterology, Hepatology and Nutrition, The University of Texas Health Science Center at Houston, 6431 Fannin Street, MSB 4.234, Houston, TX 77030, USA
* Corresponding author.
E-mail address: michael.b.fallon@uth.tmc.edu

failure (CHF) (chronic or acute) is present in most patients (80%). Both septic shock and respiratory failure are implicated as the primary insult in 15% to 20% of all patients with HH.[1,4] Henrion and colleagues[5] compared 17 episodes of HH associated with acute exacerbation of chronic respiratory failure with a control group of HH caused by CHF. They found that HH associated with respiratory failure showed low values of oxygen delivery resulting from extreme hypoxemia despite high cardiac output compared with HH cases caused by cardiac failure in which hypotension and low cardiac output resulted in low oxygen delivery. Another study comparing hemodynamics in different pathophysiologic groups of HH showed low oxygen delivery, marked hypoxemia, low systemic vascular resistance (SVR), increased cardiac output, increased central venous pressure (CVP), and normal arterial blood pressure in patients with respiratory failure (**Table 1**).[1] In patients with decreased oxygen delivery (eg, CHF) and decreased oxygen availability (eg, sepsis) as the primary cause of HH, the parameters were significantly different. In summary, HH in patients with respiratory failure seems to occur as a result of extreme arterial hypoxemia, whereas central venous congestion likely also plays a contributing role. Adaptive mechanisms tend to increase cardiac output and hepatic blood flow in these patients to improve tissue oxygenation, and the failure of these mechanisms leads to hepatocyte necrosis.

Several causes of respiratory failure have been reported to cause HH. In a recent study of 51 such patients, frequent causes included interstitial lung disease, chronic obstructive pulmonary disease, and pleural fibrosis.[1] In addition, other studies have reported coal mine pneumoconiosis and obstructive sleep apnea as underlying chronic lung disease in patients with respiratory failure–related HH.[4,6] The average age of patients with HH ranges from 60 to 70 years and it occurs 2 to 3 times more frequently in men. Similar demographic distribution has been observed in the subset of HH patients secondary to respiratory failure.[1,4]

The clinical features of HH include weakness, shortness of breath, and right upper quadrant abdominal pain from an enlarged and congested liver. Other constitutional symptoms common to hepatitides of all causes, such as anorexia, fatigue, and jaundice, are also encountered frequently. Laboratory testing shows characteristic increase of serum transaminases 10 to 100 times the upper limit of normal. Serum

Table 1
Hemodynamic parameters in different pathophysiologic groups of HH

Mean Values	Group 1: Decreased Oxygen Uptake (eg, Respiratory Failure)	Group 2: Decreased Oxygen Delivery (eg, CHF)	Group 3: Decreased Oxygen Availability (eg, Septic Shock)	Normal Range
Pao_2 (mm Hg)	32	67	84	>80
MAP (mm Hg)	95	86	44	>90
Sao_2 (%)	82	94	97	>95
CVP (cm H_2O)	16	20	2	1–12
CI (L/min/m²)	3.98	1.91	3.5	2.7–3.6
Do_2 (mL/min/m²)	382	325	477	530–730
SVR (dyn-s/cm⁵/m²)	1171	2283	1669	1750–2600

Abbreviations: CI, cardiac index; Do_2, measure of oxygen delivery; MAP, mean arterial pressure; Pao_2, partial pressure of oxygen in blood; Sao_2, oxygen saturation in arterial blood.

Data from Birrer R, Takuda Y, Takara T. Hypoxic hepatopathy: pathophysiology and prognosis. Intern Med 2007;46(14):1063–70.

lactate dehydrogenase (LDH) and lactic acid are significantly increased as well. Hyperbilirubinemia is characteristically mild and total bilirubin is rarely greater than 5 mg/dL. Coagulopathy is usually not significant and the serum prothrombin time peaks within the initial 24 to 48 hours of the insult with subsequent normalization.[1,4,7] Important distinguishing features of HH from toxin-induced liver injury and viral hepatitis include rapid reversal of increased serum transaminase levels, lower alanine aminotransferase (ALT)/LDH ratio, low degree of coagulopathy and bilirubinemia, and lower incidence of renal dysfunction. Imaging studies may show hypoechoic areas on ultrasonography and hypodensities on computed tomography (CT) that resolve completely in time.[7] Liver biopsy is usually not warranted to make a diagnosis, although the characteristic histopathologic feature is centrilobular necrosis. Multiple episodes of HH can lead to fibrosis around the central vein that may progress to bridging fibrosis and development of cirrhosis. Because the portal areas are spared, portal hypertension and its complications are rare.[7]

Although HH secondary to respiratory failure is a reversible condition, most studies have included patients in the critical care setting with other comorbidities and poor clinical status. Therefore, reported prognoses of these patients are poor with survival rates at 1 year between 18% to 26%.[1,4] Appropriate management includes treatment of underlying disease and supportive care.

GENETIC DISORDERS AND THE LIVER
α-1 Antitrypsin Deficiency

α-1 Antitrypsin (α-1 AT) deficiency is an autosomal recessive disorder affecting the lungs, liver, pancreas, and kidney. It is found in approximately 1 in 2000 to 5000 individuals and although most common in white populations, it has been described in all races.[8,9] α-1 AT is a serine protease inhibitor that is predominantly produced in the hepatocytes and, to a lesser extent, in other tissues such as renal tubular cells, macrophages, and small intestinal epithelial cells.[10] The disorder results from mutations in the coding sequence of α-1 AT that prevent its export from the hepatocyte, which in turn causes reduced circulating levels of α-1 AT, predisposing to early-onset panacinar emphysema. In addition, abnormal accumulation of the protein inside the hepatocytes leads to programmed cell death, inflammation, fibrosis, and cirrhosis.[11] In the last 4 to 5 decades, α-1 AT deficiency has been recognized as an important cause of cirrhosis and hepatocellular carcinoma (HCC), and is the leading metabolic cause for liver transplantation in children.[12]

α-1 AT is a glycoprotein encoded by a single gene, Pi, located on chromosome 14. The disorder is inherited in an autosomal recessive fashion with codominant expression, because each allele contributes 50% to the total circulating enzyme inhibitor. More than 100 alleles have been identified, only some of which are associated with liver disease.[13] The normal gene product is designated as PiMM. M is the most common allele, accounting for 95% of alleles among white people, whereas S and Z account for 2% to 3% and 1% of alleles respectively. The most prevalent carrier phenotypes are PiMZ and PiMS, and the most prevalent deficiency phenotypes are PiSS, PiSZ, and PiZZ.[14] In addition, the most common abnormal alleles, PiZZ, PiSS, and PiNull, produce approximately 15%, 60%, and 0% of the normal levels of α-1 AT, respectively.[15] The PiZZ phenotype is of the most clinical significance as it accounts for 95% of α-1 AT deficiency–induced pulmonary and liver disease.[16] A single amino acid substitution of lysine for glutamate at position 342 in the coding sequence produces the PiZ genotype. This mutation promotes polymerization of the α-1 AT protein, leading to accumulation of the polymers in the endoplasmic reticulum of the hepatocyte. These polymers are unable to complete the secretory pathway, resulting in retention of α-1 AT in the hepatocyte. The rate of polymerization of the S protein is much slower than the Z protein, favoring less hepatocyte retention and milder serum deficiency in patients with PiSS or PiSZ phenotypes.[17]

α-1 AT protects tissues from the proteolytic effect of serine proteases including neutrophil elastase. The mechanism of lung injury in α-1 AT deficiency is degradation of pulmonary elastic tissue by neutrophil elastase in the absence of α-1 AT, leading to panacinar emphysema. In contrast, the mechanism of liver injury is not related to increased activity of serine proteases but is likely caused by increased accumulation of α-1 AT polymers in the hepatocytes. However, only 10% to 30% of patients with the PiZZ phenotype develop liver disease, suggesting that other genetic and environmental factors also play a role in the pathogenesis.[18]

The diagnosis of α-1 AT deficiency is made from laboratory testing, including α-1 AT serum levels, phenotyping, and genotyping. Normal serum levels of α-1 AT range from 0.8 to 1.8 mg/dL, and patients with the PiZZ phenotype usually have levels of less than 0.6 mg/dL.[16] Because α-1 AT is also an acute phase reactant, test results may be falsely increased in inflammatory conditions. This finding may affect diagnosis in some heterozygous states. Although serum testing is readily available, α-1 AT levels are not sensitive or specific enough to be used alone for excluding α-1 AT deficiency. Phenotyping by isoelectric focusing and genotyping provides definitive diagnosis including identification of suspected new mutations.[15] On liver biopsy, the pathognomonic histologic feature is the presence of periodic acid-Schiff (PAS)–positive, diastase-resistant granules, located in periportal hepatocytes. These inclusion bodies are rare before 3 months of age and are found less frequently in heterozygous states.[15,16]

Patients with α-1 AT deficiency may present with abnormal liver enzymes without symptoms, clinical manifestations of cirrhosis and portal hypertension, or HCC. There is a characteristic bimodal distribution consisting of neonatal jaundice and neonatal hepatitis in infants and chronic liver disease in adults, with mean age of diagnosis in the fifth decade. About 10% of α-1 AT–deficient newborns develop neonatal hepatitis, and most of these patients recover. Only 2% to 3% of neonates with PiZZ phenotype progress to advanced cirrhosis and require liver transplantation in childhood.[19] Most patients have normal liver biochemistries and minimal or no clinical features of liver disease by adulthood.[20] However, autopsy studies have shown that more than a third of adults with PiZZ have cirrhosis and 30% of patients with cirrhosis have HCC at autopsy.[21] However, factors that predispose α-1 AT–deficient patients to liver disease are unclear; a recent retrospective study reported that male gender and increased body mass index were associated with more advanced liver disease.[22] A study from Sweden reported a strong correlation between α-1 AT deficiency and cirrhosis and HCC only for men.[21] It is unclear whether this gender predilection is a result of hormonal factors or other confounders such as alcohol use and presence of coexistent viral hepatitis.

The natural history of α-1 AT is variable and has been studied in both pediatric and adult populations. Sveger[8] prospectively screened 200,000 Swedish infants for α-1 AT deficiency between 1972 and 1974. Out of 122 infants with PiZ phenotype, cholestasis occurred in 11% and 6% had clinical manifestations of liver disease within the first 6 months. Among infants without clinical features of liver disease, approximately 50% had abnormal liver enzymes in the neonatal period. There were 5 infants who died from complications of cirrhosis or had cirrhosis at autopsy. Children were followed for clinical or biochemical signs of liver disease until age 16 or 18 years, none of the surviving patients had clinical manifestations of liver disease, and fewer than 10%

had abnormal liver enzymes, supporting the excellent prognosis of α-1 AT PiZ disease in childhood and adolescence. Another Swedish study examined the disease course in adult patients with α-1 AT deficiency by retrospective analysis after autopsy.[23] They confirmed cirrhosis in 35 of 94 patients, including 22 patients with clinical diagnosis of cirrhosis before death. They also found HCC in 14 patients at autopsy. There was higher incidence of both cirrhosis and HCC among men compared with women after controlling for alcohol use and hepatitis B infection, but hepatitis C testing was not developed at the time. Cirrhotic patients with α-1 AT deficiency outlived noncirrhotic patients with α-1 AT deficiency by 12 years; however, noncirrhotic patients died earlier because of advanced lung disease.

Cirrhosis from α-1 AT deficiency is a known risk factor for HCC; however, both HCC and cholangiocarcinoma have been found to have an increased incidence in patients with PiZ with varying stages of fibrosis and in those with heterozygous mutations without other concurrent liver diseases.[24,25] These findings suggest that α-1 AT deficiency might confer an increased risk of HCC because of features specific to the disease other than fibrosis and cirrhosis. Recent animal studies have shown that the fraction of proliferating hepatocytes is limited to normal areas in the liver that are devoid of PAS-positive globules, giving rise to the hypothesis that older cells with accumulated α-1 AT glycoprotein may be stimulating younger cells to proliferate.[26,27] This hypothesis is consistent with the clinical observation that HCCs in patients with α-1 AT deficiency typically arise in areas devoid of PAS-positive globules.

Currently, there is no approved treatment of liver disease associated with α-1 AT deficiency other than liver transplantation. Pulmonary disease can be treated with intravenous purified pooled human plasma α-1 AT, but this therapy has no effect on the hepatic manifestations of the disorder. In the pediatric population, α-1 AT deficiency is second only to biliary atresia as the most common indication for transplant,[28] and overall outcomes are excellent, with 3 year survival rates close to 85%.[29] In adult patients, α-1 AT deficiency is a rare indication for liver transplantation. However, adult transplant recipients acquire the donor phenotype and have normalization of α-1 AT levels,[30] and both graft and patient survival are similar to that of other indications for adult liver transplantation.[31]

Cystic Fibrosis

CF is one of the most common autosomal recessive disorders among white populations, affecting 1 in every 3000 live births.[32] It is a multiorgan disease with clinical manifestations primarily in the lungs and the gastrointestinal tract. The disease results from a mutation in the CF transmembrane regulator (CFTR), which is a cyclic AMP–regulated plasma membrane chloride channel. More than 1500 mutations of the CFTR can occur, and the most common mutation is a base pair deletion in position 508 of the protein product (ΔF508) leading to defective chloride transport. This deletion causes an inability to maintain the hydration of ducts, leading to thick and viscous secretions and obstruction of exocrine glands[33]; this is the primary mechanism that contributes to morbidity and mortality related to CF. Improved patient care has led to increased survival in CF, with a mean survival of more than 30 years, and more than 40% of the patient population reaching age 18 years or older.[34] This finding has led to the increased importance of later extrapulmonary manifestations of the disease, including hepatobiliary disease.

The CFTR protein, located on the apical surface of intrahepatic and extrahepatic cholangiocytes, functions with other chloride channels to create a relative chloride deficit inside the cell. This transmembrane chloride gradient drives the chloride-bicarbonate exchange that provides the correct ionic balance in the bile. Dysfunction of the CFTR protein results in a decrease in the water and sodium content and increased viscosity of bile, leading to thickened, inspissated secretions and biliary obstruction.[35–37] This condition leads to impaired bile flow and accumulation of hydrophobic bile acids, resulting in periductal inflammation, bile duct proliferation, and increased fibrosis in scattered portal tracts. Hepatic stellate cells play a key role in initiating fibrosis because they become activated to produce collagen and stimulate production of profibrogenic cytokines (TGF-β) by the bile duct epithelium.[36] Although less than one-third of patients with CF develop clinically significant liver disease, based on autopsy studies, most of the older patients have evidence of biliary cirrhosis.[38] Liver disease in CF occurs almost exclusively in patients with severe CFTR mutations; however, no specific mutations have been identified that are more likely associated with liver disease. Several factors have been found to be significantly associated with development of CF-related liver disease, including male sex, pancreatic insufficiency, history of meconium ileus, age at diagnosis, and severe genotype.[38–41]

Hepatobiliary involvement in CF includes a wide spectrum of manifestations with varying frequency of occurrence and underlying mechanisms (Table 2).[42–44] Transient increases in serum levels of ALT, aspartate aminotransferase (AST) or gamma-glutamyl transferase are common in CF but do not identify those with significant liver disease or predict development of end-stage liver disease.[45] In most patients with CF, liver disease is an early complication and manifests by the end of the first decade of life, and may develop earlier in those with a history of meconium ileus.[40] Rarely, CF may present with neonatal cholestasis caused by obstruction of extrahepatic bile ducts, mimicking biliary atresia, but usually resolves within a few months. The pathognomonic liver lesion in CF is focal biliary cirrhosis (FBC). FBC is present in about one-third of all patients with CF and results from biliary obstruction leading to chronic cholestasis, inflammation, bile duct proliferation, and periportal fibrosis. Over time, FBC can progress to multilobular biliary cirrhosis and clinically significant portal hypertension in 10% and 2% to 5% patients respectively. Postmortem studies have documented a progressive increase in the prevalence of mild FBC with age, from 11% in infants, 26% in those dying at 1 year, and in more than 70% of adults.[32,45,46]

CF-associated liver disease generally displays a slowly progressive course. A recent study on patients with CF surviving to more than 40 years of age reported a low prevalence of portal hypertension (0%–8%) on long-term follow-up.[47] In another study, portal hypertension was present in 6.5% (18/278) of patients with CF, and over a median follow-up duration of 7 years, only 5 patients developed decompensated

Table 2
Hepatobiliary manifestations in CF

Clinical Manifestation	Pathogenesis	Frequency (%)
Hepatic steatosis and steatohepatitis	Nutritional deficiencies	20–60
Focal biliary cirrhosis Multilobular biliary cirrhosis	Thickened bile duct secretions	20–30 10
Portal hypertension		2–5
Microgallbladder Cholelithiasis	Lithogenic bile	30 15
Sclerosing cholangitis	Thickened bile, inflammation	Rare
Neonatal cholestasis	Obstruction of extrahepatic bile ducts by thick biliary secretions	Rare
Common bile duct stenosis	Pancreatic fibrosis	Rare

liver disease (2 had variceal bleeding and 3 developed ascites).[48] A recent case control study by Gooding and colleagues[49] reported a median survival of greater than 8 years after episodes of variceal bleeding in a group of patients with CF (mean age at bleeding: 20 years). Therefore, although liver disease in CF is common and is becoming more important as patient survival improves, significant morbidity and mortality from portal hypertension is uncommon.

Diagnosing liver disease in CF is challenging because there is no single reliable test. Although diagnostic criteria have been used in clinical studies, including serum biochemistries, histology, and imaging, these are not standardized and are not used clinically.[40] Biochemical abnormalities can be transiently abnormal and therefore should not be relied on as the sole diagnostic measure. Imaging modalities including ultrasound and magnetic resonance cholangiopancreatography are sensitive, noninvasive methods for identifying abnormalities in the intrahepatic and extrahepatic biliary tract, fatty infiltration, cirrhosis, and portal hypertension. The usefulness of a liver biopsy is limited owing to the patchy distribution of liver disease in CF. However, a liver biopsy may provide important information on the type of the predominant lesion, extent of fibrosis, rate of progression of liver disease and response to treatment.

Because of decreasing mortality from extrahepatic causes, management of liver disease in patients with CF has become an important clinical issue. The mainstay of treatment of CF-related liver disease is ursodeoxycholic acid (UDCA). UDCA exerts beneficial effects through several mechanisms including improved bile flow, cytoprotective effect, displacement of toxic hydrophobic bile acids, and stimulation of biliary bicarbonate secretion.[50] The optimal daily dose of UDCA in patients with CF (20 mg/kg body weight/d) is higher than that used in other cholestatic conditions because of poor intestinal absorption. Therapy with UDCA has been shown to improve liver biochemistries, hepatic excretory function, liver histology, and nutritional and essential fatty acid status in adults with CF.[51,52] However, the effect of UDCA on the natural history of CF has not been evaluated, and therefore a definitive role in prevention of liver disease is not established. Several new therapeutic strategies are being studied, including pharmacologic correction of ionic imbalance in bile and liver-specific gene therapy; however, these approaches are still in experimental stages. Surgical intervention, transjugular intrahepatic portosystemic shunt (TIPS) placement, and endoscopic therapy may play a role in the management in patients with CF who have developed portal hypertension and progressed to end-stage liver disease. TIPS has been used successfully in patients with CF to manage portal hypertension and its complications.[53] Varices are treated with endoscopic variceal ligation or sclerotherapy because β-blockers are contraindicated in patients with CF with pulmonary disease because of the risk of bronchospasm. Traditionally, liver transplantation in patients with CF has been recommended for end-stage liver disease before worsening of pulmonary function, and studies have shown improved survival and improved pulmonary function and quality of life after a liver transplant.[54,55] However, whether liver transplantation provides any survival benefit is controversial, with some evidence suggesting no improvement.[56] Therefore, the decision to perform liver transplantation in patients with CF in the current environment should be made on a case-by-case basis.

GRANULOMATOUS DISEASES AND THE LIVER
Sarcoidosis

Sarcoidosis is a multisystem disease of unknown cause, characterized by presence of noncaseating granulomas in affected tissues.[57] The diagnosis of sarcoidosis is based on a compatible history, presence of noncaseating granulomas in at least 2 different organs, negative culture and staining for acid-fast bacilli, absence of history of occupational and/or domestic exposure to toxins, and lack of drug-induced disease. All races and age groups are affected, and the peak incidence is between 20 and 40 years of age. The prevalence of sarcoidosis in the United States is reported to be 40 per 100,000, and is 3 times higher in African Americans compared with whites.[58] In addition, African Americans tend to have more chronic and severe disease, with more frequent involvement of the liver, bone marrow, eyes, and the skin.[58,59]

The lung is the most commonly affected organ in sarcoidosis. Approximately 90% of patients with sarcoidosis will have an abnormal chest radiograph at some point in their disease course, and about 50% develop interstitial lung disease of variable severity.[60] The liver is the third most commonly affected organ, following the lung and lymph nodes. Studies on patients with sarcoidosis have reported 50% to 80% liver involvement by biopsy and ˜70% by autopsy.[61–63]

Hepatic involvement in sarcoidosis is highly variable. Patients may range from being asymptomatic to having chronic cholestasis or cirrhosis and portal hypertension. Although approximately 35% of patients with sarcoidosis have abnormal liver function tests, their presence does not correlate with the extent or severity of disease.[64] Symptoms related to liver disease are uncommon, but may include abdominal pain and pruritus. Hepatomegaly can be appreciated clinically in about 20% of patients, and in about 50% of patients on imaging.[65,66] Jaundice is rare and liver function tests are generally normal with the exception of increased ALP. About 75% of the patients have abnormal histology,[67] which may include noncaseating granulomas in different stages of maturation, loss of interlobular bile ducts, chronic cholestasis, periportal fibrosis, and biliary cirrhosis. The classic noncaseating granuloma of sarcoidosis consists of epitheloid cells surrounded by lymphocytes and scattered multinucleated giant cells. More mature granulomas may show fibrinoid necrosis, a fibrous rim, and formation of fibrinoid nodules. Schaumann bodies, which are calcium and protein cytoplasmic inclusions inside giant cells, are considered diagnostic of sarcoid granulomas, but are rarely seen in hepatic granulomas.

Some patients with hepatic sarcoidosis may present with chronic cholestasis, which may be intrahepatic or extrahepatic. Intrahepatic sarcoid cholestasis may mimic primary biliary cirrhosis (PBC) or primary sclerosing cholangitis (PSC). Extrahepatic cholestasis can be caused by compression of the hepatic hilum from adenopathy or by involvement of the common hepatic duct.

A recent review of the literature included 31 patients with sarcoid with intrahepatic cholestasis, and clinical and histologic features similar to PBC.[67] These patients were differentiated from PBC by virtue of negative antimitochondrial antibody, high rate of positive Kveim-Siltzbach test (80%, intradermal sarcoidosis test), male preponderance, increased serum angiotensin converting enzyme level, and histologic differences. The pathogenesis in hepatic sarcoid likely includes obliteration of interlobular bile ducts by noncaseating granulomas, compared with PBC in which chronic nonsuppurative inflammation causes destruction of bile ducts and triggers granuloma formation. In the same review, another 16 cases of hepatic sarcoid with features similar to PSC were studied.[67] These cases were differentiated from PSC by the absence of antineutrophil cytoplasm antibody autoantibodies and inflammatory bowel disease, and lack of characteristic histologic features of PSC such as concentric periductal fibrosis. Comparison between intrahepatic cholestasis of sarcoidosis, PBC, and PSC is shown in **Table 3**.

Hepatic sarcoidosis can rarely present acutely as a granulomatous hepatitis. These patients generally have systemic symptoms including fever, weight loss, and malaise. The diagnosis of sarcoidosis in such patients is supported by presence of

Table 3
Comparison of intrahepatic cholestasis caused by sarcoidosis, PBC, and PSC

Characteristic	Sarcoidosis	PBC	PSC
Gender prevalence	Male	Female	Male
Autoantibodies	–	AMA	ANCA
IgM level	Normal	Increased (~80%)	Increased (~50%)
Hepatic granulomas	+++	+	–
Extrahepatic granulomas	++	–	–
Bile duct histology/ destruction	Ductopenia/+	Ductopenia/+++	Concentric periductal fibrosis/ +++
ERCP	Normal/abnormal	Normal	Abnormal

Abbreviations: AMA, antimitochondrial antibody; ERCP, endoscopic retrograde cholangiopancrea-tography; +, weakly positive; ++, positive; +++, strongly positive.

noncaseating granulomas in other organs. In the absence of such granulomas else-where, the term idiopathic granulomatous hepatitis has been used. A retrospective analysis of 88 patients previously diagnosed with granulomatous hepatitis showed that 22% of patients met diagnostic criteria for sarcoidosis-related hepatitis, 50% of patients were diagnosed as having idiopathic granulomatous hepatitis, 9% had either TB or drug-induced hepatitis, and 19% were categorized as "other".[68] It is unknown whether these idiopathic patients have isolated hepatic sarcoidosis or are truly idio-pathic. Febrile patients with both sarcoid-related and idiopathic granulomatous hepa-titis respond well to steroids; prednisone is recommended at a starting dose of 0.5 to 1.0 mg/kg/d, tapered over a few weeks. Most patients resolve with steroid treatment and the relapse rate is low.[69]

A small proportion of patients with hepatic sarcoid may develop portal hypertension and cirrhosis. The first report of sarcoidosis and portal hypertension was published in 1949 by Mino and colleagues.[70] Since then, several series have been described in the literature. The cause of portal hypertension in sarcoidosis is not completely under-stood and different mechanisms have been proposed. It may be caused by biliary cirrhosis as a result of bile duct destruction by granulomas or from presinusoidal block caused by obstruction of bile flow by granulomas. Another theory suggests that ischemia secondary to granulomatous phlebitis of portal and hepatic veins causes focal fibrosis and cirrhosis, which increases both pre- and postsinusoidal resistance. Valla and colleagues[71] reviewed 47 patients with sarcoidosis and portal hypertension and found that 35 out of 47 patients did not have cirrhosis, supporting a presinusoidal mechanism. All patients with portal hypertension have hepatomegaly and about 75% have gastroesophageal varices,[72] but jaundice and severe liver dysfunction are uncommon. Another common complication of hepatic sarcoid is portal vein throm-bosis caused by stasis resulting from obliteration of portal veins by granulomas.[73] Budd-Chiari syndrome has also been reported in hepatic sarcoid as a result of extrinsic compression of hepatic veins by granulomas causing venous stasis and thrombosis.[74]

In general, corticosteroids are indicated in sarcoidosis when organ function is threatened, usually of the eyes, lungs, and the central nervous system. In addition, they may be used in persistent hypercalcemia, hypercalciuria, or extensive cutaneous lesions. The role for corticosteroids in hepatic sarcoidosis is unclear. Most studies on the subject have shown no overall benefit of steroid use because liver histology is either unchanged or worsened even though liver function tests may show improvement.[64,71,75] Other immunosuppressive agents, such as methotrexate, chloroquine, and azathioprine, may potentially reduce steroid requirements in selected patients. UDCA may be used in sarcoidosis based on data from patients with PBC. However, there is no direct evidence of benefit in hepatic sarcoidosis. Although organ transplantation in patients with sarcoidosis may result in recurrence of disease in the transplanted organ, it is an effective treatment modality for end-stage liver disease from hepatic sarcoidosis, with graft and patient survival comparable with transplantation for other diseases.[76,77] Therefore, these patients should be considered for a liver transplant if they are otherwise suitable candidates and do not have advanced lung disease.

TB

TB infection caused by *Mycobacterium tuberculosis* is a significant cause of morbidity and mortality in developing nations, and has gained importance in the developed world because of the human immunodeficiency virus (HIV) epidemic and the increasing migration of populations in recent years. Pulmonary TB is the most common form of infection, constituting about 70% of all cases in the United States. Extrapulmonary TB comprises ~20%, concurrent pulmonary and extrapulmonary TB ~7%, and disseminated TB ~2%.[78] Among extrapulmonary TB sites, gastrointestinal and hepatobiliary TB (HTB) ranks approximately sixth in frequency.[79]

HTB may be classified into different forms based on pattern of involvement and clinical manifestations (**Fig. 1**). Miliary TB is the most common form and may occur in 50% to 80% of patients with advanced pulmonary TB.[80] It is part of generalized TB and usually has no signs or symptoms related to the liver. In contrast, tuberculous hepatitis presents with constitutional symptoms such as fever and night sweats, and may result in jaundice and/or hepatomegaly. The third form, localized hepatic TB, has signs and symptoms relevant to the hepatobiliary tract, with or without biliary ductal involvement. Localized hepatic TB may present with hepatic abscess(es), solitary or multiple nodules, and obstructive jaundice, either caused by enlarged nodes surrounding the bile ducts or inflammatory strictures caused by tuberculous involvement of the ductal epithelium.[81] Primary HTB is rare, and almost always results from spread of tubercle bacilli from other sites, most commonly the lung. Usually the organisms reach the hepatobiliary tract through hematogenous spread via the hepatic artery; however, they may seed the liver via the portal vein or lymphatics, especially in concomitant

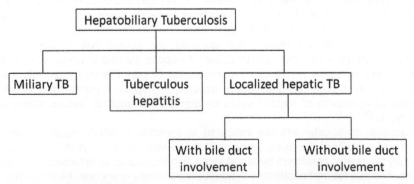

Fig. 1. Different forms of HTB.

gastrointestinal TB. Rupture of a tuberculous lymph node into the portal tract has also been reported as a possible route of infection.[82,83]

Globally, most patients with TB are between 15 and 49 years of age. Most of the patients with localized HTB reported in the literature are within the age group of 30 to 50 years with a 2:1 male preponderance and peak age of incidence in the second decade of life.[81,84] A recent study on the epidemiology of TB in the United States reported a mean age of patients with extrapulmonary TB as 44 years, compared with 47 years for pulmonary TB. Patients with extrapulmonary TB were also more likely to be Asian, foreign born, and health care workers.[84]

Frequent clinical manifestations of HTB include abdominal pain, fever, weight loss, jaundice, loss of appetite, and abdominal distension (**Table 4**).[79,85–88] Fever is the most common symptom reported, followed by weight loss and abdominal pain. Jaundice is present in 11% to 42% of patients with HTB and may result from biliary obstruction, hepatocellular damage, or both. Hepatomegaly is the most common physical examination finding and is present in more than 95% of cases of HTB. The liver may be tender in approximately half the cases, and splenomegaly is seen in 25% to 57% of patients. Laboratory features of HTB may include abnormally increased liver enzymes, more commonly alkaline phosphatase (ALP) and gamma-glutamyl transpeptidase, compared with aminotransferases (AST and ALT). A low albumin/globulin ratio, increased erythrocyte sedimentation rate, and increased total bilirubin are also common.[81] The presence of hepatic calcifications on abdominal radiography or CT scan is a characteristic finding, and may be seen in 50% to 64% of patients with HTB.[79,86] Ultrasonography of the liver may show complex masses and hypoechoic lesions in patients with tuberculous abscess. Intra- and extrahepatic dilation of bile ducts in obstructive jaundice and early detection of hepatic calcifications can be shown by liver ultrasound. CT scan of the liver can characterize solitary or multiple liver masses caused by tuberculous abscess or tuberculomas, and may be used to guide liver aspiration or biopsy for confirmation of diagnosis and treatment. In patients with HTB with obstructive jaundice, visualization of the biliary tract may be accomplished with either endoscopic retrograde cholangiopancreatography (ERCP) or percutaneous transhepatic cholangiography (PTC). The most common site of obstruction is at the porta hepatis and the bile ducts usually show an irregular stricture and proximal dilatation.[86,89] Biliary abnormalities in HTB are usually caused by external compression of bile ducts from enlarged tuberculous lymph nodes at the porta hepatis and the hepatoduodenal ligament, but can also result from direct involvement of the biliary epithelium by TB.[86,90]

Liver function tests are frequently abnormal in HTB, including increased ALP, AST, and ALT, and low serum albumin; however, these are not diagnostic and further testing is required to confirm the diagnosis. Histologically, the presence of caseating granulomas is considered diagnostic of TB. Liver biopsy may be performed as a blind

Table 4					
Frequent clinical manifestations of HTB					
Clinical Feature Occurrence	Chong,[79] 2008	Hersch,[85] 1964	Alvarez,[81] 1998	Essop et al,[87] 1984	Maharaj et al,[88] 1987
Fever (%)	50	90	65	70	63
Abdominal pain (%)	57	50	45	66	46
Weight loss (%)	64	75	55	–	61
Jaundice (%)	42	15	35	11	14
Hepatomegaly (%)	–	95	96	80	95

procedure or with ultrasound, CT, or laparoscopic guidance. The accuracy and success rate of guided liver biopsy specimens is high compared with blind biopsy. Caseating granulomas were found in biopsy specimens of 51% to 83% of cases with localized HTB.[86–88] In the absence of caseating granulomas, tissue specimens are stained and cultured for acid-fast bacilli. *M tuberculosis* bacilli are seen in less than 35% of tissue specimens from tuberculous granulomas, and the yield for a positive culture is much lower.[91] The polymerase chain reaction (PCR) assay for identification of *M tuberculosis* has a much higher sensitivity of 88%.[92] In the absence of tissue identification, the diagnosis of HTB may be made in the presence of hepatobiliary involvement and known extrahepatic TB.

Patients with HTB are treated similarly to those with pulmonary TB. The standard treatment consists of a 4-drug regimen because of the increasing incidence of drug-resistant TB. The duration of therapy is 1 year, with first-line drugs including isoniazid, rifampicin, ethambutol, and pyrazinamide. The most common side effects include mild drug-induced hepatitis and gastrointestinal symptoms. Patients with HTB with obstructive jaundice require biliary decompression in addition to drug therapy. Decompression may be achieved by ERCP with stent placement, PTC with external drainage or by surgical intervention. A recent study reported favorable outcomes up to 42 months follow-up in 5 patients with HTB requiring biliary stenting.[79] Tuberculous abscesses require a combination of aspiration of the abscess and antibiotics. Most patients with HTB respond well to standard antitubercular treatment with resolution of symptoms and the overall prognosis is good. However, poor outcomes have been reported in those with severe malnutrition, sepsis, and multiorgan failure.

SUMMARY

The liver is a complex organ and is frequently involved in systemic diseases. Several primary pulmonary disorders have hepatobiliary manifestations of clinical significance.

Ischemic or HH is the most common cause of a sharp, transient increase in serum transaminases in hospitalized patients, and 15% to 20% of these cases may have respiratory failure as the underlying cause. The overall prognosis is poor because of comorbidities and poor clinical condition, and management involves treatment of underlying conditions and supportive care.

The liver is also frequently affected in genetic disorders such as α-1 antitrypsin deficiency and CF. α-1 Antitrypsin deficiency results in panacinar emphysema caused by the unopposed action of neutrophil elastase in the lung. However, liver involvement in this condition results from an accumulation of α-1 antitrypsin precursor molecules inside hepatocytes causing toxic damage. Liver transplantation is curative for patients with α-1 antitrypsin deficiency. CF affects multiple organ systems as a result of a mutation in the CFTR gene causing defective chloride channel transport. The mechanism of hepatobiliary dysfunction in CF is defective composition and impaired excretion of bile. Patients with CF may have hepatobiliary involvement ranging from focal fibrosis and biochemical abnormalities to portal hypertension and decompensated cirrhosis. Management of liver disease in CF is symptomatic and the role of transplantation is unclear.

Sarcoidosis and TB are granulomatous diseases that primarily affect the lung and frequently have significant hepatobiliary involvement. Sarcoidosis is a multiorgan chronic inflammatory disease characterized by presence of noncaseating granulomas in affected tissues. Hepatic sarcoid may manifest as asymptomatic ALP increase, hepatomegaly, cirrhosis, and/or portal hypertension. The benefit of steroids and other immunosuppressive agents in hepatic sarcoid is unclear and management is largely symptomatic; however, liver transplantation outcomes in hepatic sarcoid are favorable in patients with preserved pulmonary function.

M tuberculosis most commonly spreads to the liver hematogenously and may lead to forms of localized TB such as tuberculoma and tubercular abscess, or may involve the liver in a more diffuse fashion causing miliary TB and tubercular hepatitis. In addition, TB may cause biliary tract obstruction because of granuloma formation and lymphadenopathy. Treatment of hepatic TB is with antibiotics and biliary drainage when required.

REFERENCES

1. Birrer R, Takuda Y, Takara T. Hypoxic hepatopathy: pathophysiology and prognosis. Intern Med 2007;46(14):1063–70.
2. Bynum TE, Boitnott JK, Maddrey WC. Ischemic hepatitis. Dig Dis Sci 1979;24(2): 129–35.
3. Arcidi JM Jr, Moore GW, Hutchins GM. Hepatic morphology in cardiac dysfunction: a clinicopathologic study of 1000 subjects at autopsy. Am J Pathol 1981; 104(2):159–66.
4. Henrion J, Schapira M, Luwaert R, et al. Hypoxic hepatitis: clinical and hemodynamic study in 142 consecutive cases. Medicine (Baltimore) 2003;82(6):392–406.
5. Henrion J, Minette P, Colin L, et al. Hypoxic hepatitis caused by acute exacerbation of chronic respiratory failure: a case-controlled, hemodynamic study of 17 consecutive cases. Hepatology 1999;29(2):427–33.
6. Henrion J, Colin L, Schapira M, et al. Hypoxic hepatitis caused by severe hypoxemia from obstructive sleep apnea. J Clin Gastroenterol 1997;24(4):245–9.
7. Ebert EC. Hypoxic liver injury. Mayo Clin Proc 2006;81(9):1232–6.
8. Sveger T. Liver disease in alpha1-antitrypsin deficiency detected by screening of 200,000 infants. N Engl J Med 1976;294(24):1316–21.
9. de Serres FJ. Worldwide racial and ethnic distribution of alpha1-antitrypsin deficiency: summary of an analysis of published genetic epidemiologic surveys. Chest 2002;122(5):1818–29.
10. Carlson JA, Rogers BB, Sifers RN, et al. Multiple tissues express alpha 1-antitrypsin in transgenic mice and man. J Clin Invest 1988;82(1):26–36.
11. Black LF, Kueppers F. Alpha1-antitrypsin deficiency in nonsmokers. Am Rev Respir Dis 1978;117(3):421–8.
12. Volpert D, Molleston JP, Perlmutter DH. Alpha1-antitrypsin deficiency-associated liver disease progresses slowly in some children. J Pediatr Gastroenterol Nutr 2000;31(3):258–63.
13. DeMeo DL, Silverman EK. Alpha1-antitrypsin deficiency. 2: genetic aspects of alpha(1)-antitrypsin deficiency: phenotypes and genetic modifiers of emphysema risk. Thorax 2004;59(3):259–64.
14. Cox DW, Billingsley GD. Rare deficiency types of alpha 1-antitrypsin: electrophoretic variation and DNA haplotypes. Am J Hum Genet 1989;44(6):844–54.
15. Vennarecci G, Gunson BK, Ismail T, et al. Transplantation for end stage liver disease related to alpha 1 antitrypsin. Transplantation 1996;61(10):1488–95.
16. Primhak RA, Tanner MS. Alpha-1 antitrypsin deficiency. Arch Dis Child 2001; 85(1):2–5.
17. Mahadeva R, Chang WS, Dafforn TR, et al. Heteropolymerization of S, I, and Z alpha1-antitrypsin and liver cirrhosis. J Clin Invest 1999;103(7):999–1006.
18. Perlmutter DH. Clinical manifestations of alpha-1-antitrypsin deficiency. Gastroenterol Clin North Am Part II 1995;24:27–43.

19. Sveger T. The natural history of liver disease in alpha 1-antitrypsin deficient children. Acta Paediatr Scand 1988;77(6):847–51.
20. Sveger T, Eriksson S. The liver in adolescents with alpha 1-antitrypsin deficiency. Hepatology 1995;22(2):514–7.
21. Eriksson S, Carlson J, Velez R. Risk of cirrhosis and primary liver cancer in alpha 1-antitrypsin deficiency. N Engl J Med 1986;314(12):736–9.
22. Bowlus CL, Willner I, Zern MA, et al. Factors associated with advanced liver disease in adults with alpha-1 antitrypsin deficiency. Clin Gastroenterol Hepatol 2005;3(4):390–6.
23. Eriksson S. Alpha 1-antitrypsin deficiency and liver cirrhosis in adults. An analysis of 35 Swedish autopsied cases. Acta Med Scand 1987;221(5):461–7.
24. Zhou H, Fischer HP. Liver carcinoma in PiZ alpha-1-antitrypsin deficiency. Am J Surg Pathol 1998;22(6):742–8.
25. Zhou H, Ortiz-Pallardó ME, Ko Y, et al. Is heterozygous alpha-1-antitrypsin deficiency type PIZ a risk factor for primary liver carcinoma? Cancer 2000;88(12): 2668–76.
26. Rudnick DA, Liao Y, An JK, et al. Analyses of hepatocellular proliferation in a mouse model of alpha-1-antitrypsin deficiency. Hepatology 2004;39(4):1048–55.
27. Rudnick DA, Perlmutter DH. Alpha-1-antitrypsin deficiency: a new paradigm for hepatocellular carcinoma in genetic liver disease. Hepatology 2005;42(3):514–21.
28. Gordon RD, Shaw BW Jr, Iwatsuki S, et al. Indications for liver transplantation in the cyclosporine era. Surg Clin North Am 1986;66(3):541–56.
29. Prachalias AA, Kalife M, Francavilla R, et al. Liver transplantation for alpha-1 antitrypsin deficiency in children. Transpl Int 2000;13(3):207–10.
30. Hood JM, Koep LJ, Peters RL, et al. Liver transplantation for advanced liver disease with alpha-1 antitrypsin deficiency. N Engl J Med 1980;302(5):272–5.
31. Zhang KY, Tung BY, Kowdley KV. Liver transplantation for metabolic liver diseases. Clin Liver Dis 2007;11(2):265–81.
32. Rowe SM, Miller S, Sorscher EJ. Cystic fibrosis. N Engl J Med 2005;352: 1992–2001.
33. Mehta A. CFTR: more than just a chloride channel. Pediatr Pulmonol 2005;39: 292–8.
34. Sokol RJ, Durie PR. Recommendations for management of liver and biliary tract disease in cystic fibrosis. Cystic Fibrosis Foundation Hepatobiliary Disease Consensus Group. J Pediatr Gastroenterol Nutr 1999;28:S1–13.
35. Feranchak AP, Sokol RJ. Cholangiocyte biology and cystic fibrosis liver disease. Semin Liver Dis 2001;21(4):471–88.
36. Lewindon PJ, Pereira TN, Hoskins AC, et al. The role of hepatic stellate cells and transforming growth factor-beta(1) in cystic fibrosis liver disease. Am J Pathol 2002;160(5):1705–15.
37. Nagel RA, Westaby D, Javaid A, et al. Liver disease and bile duct abnormalities in adults with cystic fibrosis. Lancet 1989;2(8677):1422–5.
38. Colombo C, Apostolo MG, Ferrari M, et al. Analysis of risk factors for the development of liver disease associated with cystic fibrosis. J Pediatr 1994;124:393–9.
39. Wilschanski M, Rivlin J, Cohen S, et al. Clinical and genetic risk factors for cystic fibrosis-related liver disease. Pediatrics 1999;103(1):52–7.
40. Colombo C, Battezzati PM, Crosignani A, et al. Liver disease in cystic fibrosis: a prospective study on incidence, risk factors, and outcome. Hepatology 2002; 36(6):1374–82.
41. Corbett K, Kelleher S, Rowland M, et al. Cystic fibrosis-associated liver disease: a population-based study. J Pediatr 2004;145(3):327–32.

42. Colombo C, Russo MC, Zazzeron L, et al. Liver disease in cystic fibrosis. J Pediatr Gastroenterol Nutr 2006;43(Suppl 1):S49–55.
43. Moyer K, Balistreri W. Hepatobiliary disease in patients with cystic fibrosis. Curr Opin Gastroenterol 2009;25(3):272–8.
44. Layden TJ, Kulik L. Hepatic manifestations of pulmonary diseases. Clin Liver Dis 2002;6(4):969–79, ix.
45. Wilschanski M. Patterns of gastrointestinal disease associated with mutations of CFTR. Curr Gastroenterol Rep 2008;10(3):316–23.
46. Colombo C, Battezzati PM, Podda M. Hepatobiliary disease in cystic fibrosis. Semin Liver Dis 1994;14:259–69.
47. Hodson ME, Simmonds NJ, Warwick WJ, et al. An international/multicentre report on patients with cystic fibrosis (CF) over the age of 40 years. J Cyst Fibros 2008; 7:537–42.
48. Desmond CP, Wilson J, Bailey M, et al. The benign course of liver disease in adults with cystic fibrosis and the effect of ursodeoxycholic acid. Liver Int 2007;27(10):1402–8.
49. Gooding I, Dondos V, Gyi KM, et al. Variceal hemorrhage and cystic fibrosis: outcomes and implications for liver transplantation. Liver Transpl 2005;11(12): 1522–6.
50. Paumgartner G, Beuers U. Mechanisms of action and therapeutic efficacy of ursodeoxycholic acid in cholestatic liver disease. Clin Liver Dis 2004;8(1):67–81, vi.
51. Lindblad A, Glaumann H, Strandvik B. A two-year prospective study of the effect of ursodeoxycholic acid on urinary bile acid excretion and liver morphology in cystic fibrosis-associated liver disease. Hepatology 1998;27(1):166–74.
52. Colombo C, Battezzati PM, Podda M, et al. Ursodeoxycholic acid for liver disease associated with cystic fibrosis: a double-blind multicenter trial. The Italian Group for the Study of Ursodeoxycholic Acid in Cystic Fibrosis. Hepatology 1996;23(6):1484–90.
53. Pozler O, Krajina A, Vanicek H, et al. Transjugular intrahepatic portosystemic shunt in five children with cystic fibrosis: long-term results. Hepatogastroenterology 2003;50(52):1111–4.
54. Mekeel KL, Langham MR Jr, Gonzalez-Perralta R, et al. Combined en bloc liver pancreas transplantation for children with CF. Liver Transpl 2007;13(3):406–9.
55. Milkiewicz P, Skiba G, Kelly D, et al. Transplantation for cystic fibrosis: outcome following early liver transplantation. J Gastroenterol Hepatol 2002;17(2):208–13.
56. Sharp HL. Cystic fibrosis liver disease and transplantation. J Pediatr 1995;127(6): 944–6.
57. Iannuzzi MC, Rybicki BA, Teirstein AS. Sarcoidosis. N Engl J Med 2007;357(21): 2153–65.
58. Rybicki BA, Major M, Popovich J Jr, et al. Racial differences in sarcoidosis incidence: a 5-year study in a health maintenance organization. Am J Epidemiol 1997;145(3):234–41.
59. Ebert EC, Kierson M, Hagspiel KD. Gastrointestinal and hepatic manifestations of sarcoidosis. Am J Gastroenterol 2008;103(12):3184–92; quiz 3193.
60. Fauci AS, Braunwald E, Kasper DL, et al. Harrison's principles of internal medicine. 17th edition. New York: McGraw-Hill; 2008.
61. Ricker W, Clark M. Sarcoidosis; a clinicopathologic review of 300 cases, including 22 autopsies. Am J Clin Pathol 1949;19(8):725–49.
62. Irani SK, Dobbins WO. Hepatic granulomas: review of 73 patients from one hospital and survey of the literature. Clin Gastroenterol 1979;1(2):131–43.
63. Iwai K, Oka H. Sarcoidosis. Report of ten autopsy cases in Japan. Am Rev Respir Dis 1964;90:612–22.

64. Kennedy PT, Zakaria N, Modawi SB, et al. Natural history of hepatic sarcoidosis and its response to treatment. Eur J Gastroenterol Hepatol 2006;18(7):721–6.
65. Branson JH, Park JH. Sarcoidosis hepatic involvement: presentation of a case with fatal liver involvement; including autopsy findings and review of the evidence for sarcoid involvement of the liver as found in the literature. Ann Intern Med 1954; 40(1):111–45.
66. Warshauer DM, Molina PL, Hamman SM, et al. Nodular sarcoidosis of the liver and spleen: analysis of 32 cases. Radiology 1995;195(3):757–62.
67. Blich M, Edoute Y. Clinical manifestations of sarcoid liver disease. J Gastroenterol Hepatol 2004;19(7):732–7.
68. Sartin JS, Walker RC. Granulomatous hepatitis: a retrospective review of 88 cases at the Mayo Clinic. Mayo Clin Proc 1991;66(9):914–8.
69. Zoutman DE, Ralph ED, Frei JV. Granulomatous hepatitis and fever of unknown origin. An 11 year experience of 23 cases with three years' follow-up. J Clin Gastroenterol 1991;13(1):69–75.
70. Mino RA, Murphy AI Jr, Livingstone RG. Sarcoidosis producing portal hypertension: treatment by splenectomy and splenorenal shunt. Ann Surg 1949;130(5): 951–7.
71. Valla D, Pessegueiro-Miranda H, Degott C, et al. Hepatic sarcoidosis with portal hypertension. A report of seven cases with a review of the literature. Q J Med 1987;63(242):531–44.
72. Rosenberg JC. Portal hypertension complicating hepatic sarcoidosis. Surgery 1971;69(2):294–9.
73. Moreno-Merlo F, Wanless IR, Shimamatsu K, et al. The role of granulomatous phlebitis and thrombosis in the pathogenesis of cirrhosis and portal hypertension in sarcoidosis. Hepatology 1997;26(3):554–60.
74. Russi EW, Bansky G, Pfaltz M, et al. Budd-Chiari syndrome in sarcoidosis. Am J Gastroenterol 1986;81(1):71–5.
75. Kelley ML Jr, McHardy RJ. An unusual case of fatal hepatic sarcoidosis. Am J Med 1955;18(5):842–50.
76. Casavilla FA, Gordon R, Wright HI, et al. Clinical course after liver transplantation in patients with sarcoidosis. Ann Intern Med 1993;118(11):865–6.
77. Barbers RG. Role of transplantation (lung, liver, and heart) in sarcoidosis. Clin Chest Med 1997;18(4):865–74.
78. Peto HM, Pratt RH, Harrington TA, et al. Epidemiology of extrapulmonary tuberculosis in the United States, 1993–2006. Clin Infect Dis 2009;49(9):1350–7.
79. Chong VH. Hepatobiliary tuberculosis: a review of presentations and outcomes. South Med J 2008;101(4):356–61.
80. Morris E. Tuberculosis of the liver. Am Rev Tuberc 1930;22:585–92.
81. Alvarez SZ. Hepatobiliary tuberculosis. J Gastroenterol Hepatol 1998;13(8): 833–9.
82. Rolleston HD, McNee JW. Diseases of the liver, gallbladder and bile ducts. 3rd edition. London: Macmillan; 1929. p. 370–81.
83. Feldman M, Friedman LS, Brandt LJ. Sleisenger and Fordtran's gastrointestinal and liver disease. 8th edition. Philadelphia: Saunders; 2006. p. 1731–55.
84. Frieden TR, Sterling TR, Munsiff SS, et al. Tuberculosis. Lancet 2003;362(9387): 887–99.
85. Hersch C. Tuberculosis of the liver. A study of 200 cases. S Afr Med J 1964; 38:857–63.
86. Alvarez SZ, Carpio R. Hepatobiliary tuberculosis. Dig Dis Sci 1983;28(3): 193–200.

87. Essop AR, Posen JA, Hodkinson JH, et al. Tuberculosis hepatitis: a clinical review of 96 cases. Q J Med 1984;53(212):465–77.
88. Maharaj B, Leary WP, Pudifin DJ. A prospective study of hepatic tuberculosis in 41 black patients. Q J Med 1987;63(242):517–22.
89. Maglinte DD, Alvarez SZ, Ng AC, et al. Patterns of calcifications and cholangiographic findings in hepatobiliary tuberculosis. Gastrointest Radiol 1988;13(4):331–5.
90. Fan ST, Ng IO, Choi TK, et al. Tuberculosis of the bile duct: a rare cause of biliary stricture. Am J Gastroenterol 1989;84(4):413–4.
91. Harrington PT, Gutiérrez JJ, Ramirez-Ronda CH, et al. Granulomatous hepatitis. Rev Infect Dis 1982;4(3):638–55.
92. Alcantara-Payawal DE, Matsumura M, Shiratori Y, et al. Direct detection of *Mycobacterium tuberculosis* using polymerase chain reaction assay among patients with hepatic granuloma. J Hepatol 1997;27(4):620–7.

Renal Diseases and the Liver

Florence Wong, MD, FRACP, FRCPC

KEYWORDS

• Renal disease • Liver complications • Viral hepatitis • Dialysis
• Cholestasis

Renal complications of liver disease are common. Examples include glomerulone-phritis related to viral hepatitis or renal sodium and water retention related to cirrhosis. In contrast, although there are many systemic diseases that can affect both the liver and the kidney, liver complications as a result of renal disease are infrequent. However, the presence of renal disease does pose diagnostic and treatment issues when concomitant liver problems arise. This article reviews both the liver complications of renal disease as well as the approach to liver conditions in the presence of renal disease.

THE PATIENT WITH RENAL DISEASE AND ABNORMAL LIVER TESTS

Asymptomatic abnormal liver tests are found in 1% to 6% of the general population.[1] Although there is no documented prevalence of abnormal liver tests in patients with renal disease, it is estimated to be higher than that in the general population for many reasons. For example, there are liver conditions such as viral hepatitis that are associated with glomerulonephritis, there are systemic conditions such as diabetes that cause chronic renal failure and are associated with a chronic liver condition such as nonalcoholic steatohepatitis, there are also many drugs used to treat patients with chronic renal disease that are known to be hepatotoxins (**Table 1**). Therefore, clinicians often have to assess a patient with renal disease who also has abnormal liver enzymes or function. The approach in this scenario is no different from that of a patient with abnormal liver tests but without renal disease.[2] A systematic approach is used to make the diagnosis, followed by various imaging procedures and special tests such as liver biopsy or endoscopy to characterize the stage of the liver disease and detect complications. Special attention needs to be paid to consider systemic diseases that affect both the liver and the kidney, and specific diagnoses that are prevalent in the population of patients with renal disease. **Fig. 1** describes the approach to abnormal liver tests in patients with chronic renal disease.

There is no financial support for this article.
Department of Medicine, Toronto General Hospital, University of Toronto, 9th floor, North Wing, Room 983, 200 Elizabeth Street, Toronto M5G 2C4, Ontario, Canada
E-mail address: florence.wong@utoronto.ca

Clin Liver Dis 15 (2011) 39–53
doi:10.1016/j.cld.2010.09.011
1089-3261/11/$ – see front matter © 2011 Published by Elsevier Inc.

Table 1
Renal conditions that could be associated with liver abnormalities

Renal Disease	Associated Liver Condition
Glomerulonephritis, membroproliferative	Viral hepatitis B Viral hepatitis C
IgA nephropathy	Alcoholic cirrhosis
Interstitial nephritis	Primary biliary cirrhosis
Renal tubular acidosis	Primary biliary cirrhosis Wilson disease
Diabetic nephropathy	Nonalcoholic fatty liver disease/steatohepatitis
Chronic renal failure: drug use	
ACE inhibitors	Cholestatic hepatitis
Angiotensin II receptor antagonists	Hepatitis

COMMON LIVER CONDITIONS IN PATIENTS WITH CHRONIC RENAL DISEASE

Patients with chronic renal disease usually have some degree of renal impairment, and a significant proportion of these patients are dialysis dependent. The latter form a special group of patients who are particularly susceptible to liver disease, especially hepatitis C viral (HCV) infection. The presence of chronic renal failure also reduces the clearance of drugs that are metabolized via the renal route, and the resultant increased plasma concentrations of any parent compound and metabolites with liver toxic potential makes the susceptible patient more likely to sustain liver injury.

Hepatitis B Viral Infection

Hepatitis B viral (HBV) infection is relatively common in patients with chronic renal failure (estimated to occur in 2.8% of predialysis patients[3]) related to their depressed immune system in the presence of chronic renal failure. The introduction of routine vaccination of noninfected patients and isolation of patients with HBV in dialysis units

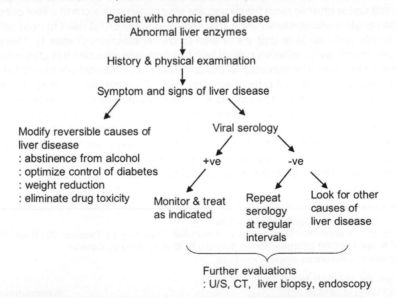

Fig. 1. Approach to abnormal liver tests in a patient with chronic renal disease.

has resulted in no further increase in HBV prevalence amongst patients who are undergoing hemodialysis. The natural history of HBV infection in patients with chronic renal failure before kidney transplant is similar to that in patients without chronic renal failure. That is, the patients may intermittently flare with their chronic HBV and this ultimately leads to the development of cirrhosis, or they may have low-grade chronic hepatitis with mildly abnormal liver enzymes, or their HBV infection may remain inactive for many years. Once diagnosed, regular 3- to 6-monthly monitoring is required to assess for progression of HBV-related liver disease, and for the development of hepatoma.

Antiviral treatment is indicated if active hepatitis is present,[4] although some have advocated treatment if HBV DNA is detectable, even at levels that do not meet current conventional indications for treatment,[5] especially in patients on dialysis. Agents with a high barrier to resistance should be used and dose adjustments according to the degree of renal dysfunction are necessary. Vigilance for the development of antiviral resistance is essential. To date, there are only scanty data on the outcome of antiviral therapy in patients with HBV infection and chronic renal failure,[6,7] and the long-term effects of treatment of HBV infection on patient outcome are not clear. There are also reports of HBV-related glomerulonephritis improving with antiviral therapy, with reduction in proteinuria.[8] It is not clear at present whether patients with chronic renal failure and viremia but inactive disease should be treated with antiviral therapy, as these patients are more likely to go on to develop chronic liver disease.

HCV Infection

HCV infection is more prevalent than HBV infection amongst patients with chronic renal failure, ranging from 4% to 17% among predialysis patients.[3,9] The prevalence has remained high despite routine screening of blood products, as nosocomial spread of HCV infection has continued.[10] Acute HCV infection in renal dialysis units may only be evident by a moderate but transient increase of transaminases, which return to within normal limits on seroconversion.[11] Patients with chronic renal failure and chronic HCV infection are more likely to present with grumbling low-grade hepatitis than those with HBV infection, but normal liver enzymes are not infrequent despite persistent viremia, associated with histologic progression of the liver disease.[12] Therefore, liver biopsy has been recommended as part of the management of patients with HCV infection and chronic renal disease. Hemodialysis seems to confer a protective effect on the HCV infection, with patients on hemodialysis having lower viral load and milder histologic abnormalities compared with patients with chronic renal failure not on dialysis[13] and to patients without renal disease.[14] It is unclear whether the dialysis process actually filters out the virus, resulting in a milder course of the infection.

The decision to treat the HCV infection has to be weighed against the likelihood of the patient succumbing to the chronic kidney disease or its associated comorbidities before developing significant liver complications. In general, patients with HCV infection and chronic renal failure who otherwise are suitable for antiviral therapy should be considered for such treatment. The current standard of care of interferon and ribavirin for the treatment of HCV infection in patients without renal impairment has been considered too intense for patients with chronic renal failure. The absorption and distribution of interferon alpha-2-a have been shown to be similar in predialysis patients with chronic renal failure versus patients with normal renal function,[15] but interferon degradation usually occurs in the kidneys, and the presence of renal dysfunction affects interferon pharmacokinetics. Therefore, when given together with ribavirin, which is renally excreted, the combination can cause excessive side effects, especially hemolytic anemia. The use of interferon monotherapy in reduced doses has been traditionally recommended in this population of patients, yielding a sustainable response rate in the range of 13% to 75%.[16] Several small trials have also used a combination of interferon and ribavirin in reduced doses, with close monitoring of the hemoglobin levels[17] with or without the preemptive use of erythropoietin. Ideally, treatment of HCV should be completed before renal transplant, as the presence of HCV infection has a negative effect on graft survival.[18]

Diabetes and Nonalcoholic Fatty Liver Disease or Steatohepatitis

Diabetes mellitus (DM) is a complex chronic metabolic disease characterized by hyperglycemia. Diabetes is also associated with vascular disease involving large and small vessels. Diabetic microangiopathy, affecting the capillaries of the kidney, is a leading cause of end-stage renal disease, accounting for 41% of all cases of chronic renal failure.[19] Poor glycemic control in type 2 DM with insulin resistance and hyperinsulinemia is associated with an increased risk for diabetic nephropathy. The hyperinsulinemic stages of type 2 DM are also associated with the development of nonalcoholic fatty liver disease (NAFLD)/nonalcoholic steatohepatitis (NASH), occurring in up to 75% of patients. NAFLD and NASH are considered the hepatic manifestations of the metabolic syndrome, which includes DM in its spectrum. Type 1 DM, on the other hand, is not often associated with liver abnormalities. In a population study involving more than 2000 patients with type 2 DM, there was a link between chronic renal disease as defined by a glomerular filtration rate (GFR) of less than 60 mL/min or overt proteinuria, and the presence of NAFLD, independent of any other risk factors for chronic renal disease.[19] Because most patients with NAFLD have normal liver enzymes,[20] diagnosis of NAFLD can be missed if assessment considers liver enzymes alone. Therefore, clinical examination searching for hepatomegaly and an ultrasound study to assess for fatty infiltration of the liver in patients with type 2 DM are needed. As NAFLD and NASH can progress to cirrhosis with all the attendant complications if the hepatic fatty infiltration is not reversed, it is imperative that patients with chronic renal disease related to type 2 DM undergo weight management to bring their body mass index to less than 25 kg/m^2.[21] Achieving stricter glycemic control can delay the progression of proteinuria, as well as reduce liver fatty infiltration, and therefore help to maintain an overall improved prognosis in these patients.

Drug Toxicity

Hypertensive nephrosclerosis and diabetic nephropathy are common causes of chronic renal disease. Therefore, these patients are commonly prescribed medications for control of their systemic hypertension, or for renal protection against proteinuria in DM. Several major classes of drugs are available, but the most popular include those that inhibit the renin-angiotensin pathway. These drugs are generally well tolerated, and liver injuries as a result of drug toxicity are rare. However, there are now several postmarketing reports of hepatotoxicity with these agents. Angiotensin-converting enzyme (ACE) inhibitors mainly cause a cholestatic injury, and several members of this class of drugs, including ramipril,[22] fosinopril,[23] lisinopril,[24] and enalapril,[25] have been implicated. Hepatotoxicity related to the use of angiotensin II receptor antagonists is less common. However, a clinical picture of acute hepatitis has been reported with losartan,[26] valsartan,[27] and candasartan.[28] With millions of prescriptions of ACE inhibitors and angiotensin II receptor antagonists written each year, it is not inconceivable that hepatotoxicity with these agents will be seen in patients with chronic renal disease. Therefore, physicians caring for patients with chronic renal disease need to be cognizant of these possible drug-related liver injuries, and promptly discontinue the potential liver toxin.

RENAL TUBULAR DISORDERS AND CHOLESTASIS

Patients with cholestasis with or without obstructive jaundice, whether it is from gall-stone disease, extrahepatic biliary obstruction, drug-induced intrahepatic cholestasis, or intrinsic biliary disease such as primary biliary cirrhosis or primary sclerosing cholangitis, have been shown to have renal tubular dysfunction, particularly involving the proximal renal tubule.[29] Such patients display uricosuria, phosphaturia, glucosuria, and increased urinary excretion of beta-2 microglobulin in the absence of any other causes of tubular defects despite a normal serum creatinine level. Patients with primary biliary cirrhosis are known to have defective post-secretory reabsorption of uric acid, believed to be related to excess copper from the cholestasis deposited in the proximal renal tubule, thereby causing tubular damage.[30] There does not seem to be a threshold of bilirubin level that is associated with the onset of tubular dysfunction. Recent data have indicated that this renal dysfunction may be partially reversible once the biliary obstruction is relieved,[29] suggesting that there is a functional component to the tubular dysfunction. Bomzon and colleagues[31] suggested that the increased levels of bile acids in cholestasis might alter the pH of the tubular milieu, thereby affecting proximal tubular reabsorption ability. In addition, bile acids can stimulate the generation of oxygen free radicals, causing oxidative stress with resultant renal tubular dysfunction.[32]

This tubular dysfunction associated with chronic cholestasis is to be distinguished from the renal failure that is observed in patients who have undergone surgical relief of obstructive jaundice during the post-operative period. In the latter scenario, acute renal failure with decreased glomerular filtration and rising serum creatinine level occurs within a few days of surgery in approximately 8% of patients undergoing biliary surgery, and is associated with high mortality once it develops.[33] Endotoxemia that is associated with bile duct obstruction has been proposed as the initiating mechanism that activates the endothelin[34] and thromboxane[35] systems. This, coupled with the direct hypotensive effects of jaundice and the impaired cardiac contractile performance associated with jaundice,[36] ultimately leads to renal vasoconstriction with consequent renal failure.

In the pediatric population, there is a syndrome of renal dysfunction and cholestasis associated with arthrogryposis, related to a genetic mutation that leads to the production of an abnormal protein involved in vesicular trafficking. Biopsies of the liver and the kidney usually show mislocalization of several apical membrane proteins. Clinically, these children have fluctuating conjugated hyperbilirubinemia, but a normal γ-glutamyl transferase level. Biliary isotope studies suggest biliary obstruction or severe intrahepatic cholestasis. The renal dysfunction involves leaky tubules, leading to aminoaciduria, occasional glycosuria, and renal tubular acidosis. These children usually present with failure to thrive and have recurrent infections. Only a small percentage of these children survive beyond the age of 1 year.[37]

NEPHROGENIC HEPATIC DYSFUNCTION

Renal cell carcinoma is associated with a paraneoplastic syndrome in up to 20% of cases. In 1961, Stauffer[38] first described 5 cases of nonmetastatic hepatic dysfunction in patients with renal cell carcinoma. Since then, there have been many more reports of Stauffer syndrome.[39–41] The incidence is approximately 10% to 15% of all patients with renal cell carcinoma.[42] Patients with Stauffer syndrome usually present with nonspecific constitutional symptoms, with anorexia and intermittent fever being the most common complaints. Anicteric intrahepatic cholestasis is the main hepatic finding, and jaundice is uncommon. Other laboratory abnormalities include an accelerated erythrocyte sedimentation rate, an increased levels of C-reactive protein and ferritin, thrombosis and anemia, all markers suggestive of an inflammatory process. Histologic examination of the liver only shows nonspecific changes including steatosis, mild focal hepatic necrosis, portal lymphocytic infiltration, and Kupffer cell hyperplasia.[43] The pathophysiology of Stauffer syndrome is unclear, although the production of various cytokines including interleukin 6 by the tumor has been implicated.[44]

Hepatic dysfunction may be the only manifestation of an otherwise occult renal cell carcinoma without the classic triad of hematuria, flank pain, and palpable abdominal mass.[45] Therefore, renal cell carcinoma should be considered in the differential diagnoses of hepatic dysfunction if no other causes are found. Nephrectomy can result in normalization of hepatic enzymes, although this is not always guaranteed.[46] Return of hepatic dysfunction suggests recurrence of renal cell carcinoma or the presence of liver metastasis.[47]

NEPHROGENIC ASCITES

Nephrogenic ascites is refractory ascites of unknown cause, seen in patients with end-stage renal disease in the absence of liver cirrhosis, cardiac failure, malignancy, or infection.[48] Its prevalence has been estimated to be between 0.7% to 20% of all patients with end-stage renal disease. Although most of the patients are on hemodialysis at the time ascites develops, it can also occur in patients who are on peritoneal dialysis alone. A small proportion of patients with nephrogenic ascites have received both hemodialysis and peritoneal dialysis, but others have never undergone either hemodialysis or peritoneal dialysis. The patient usually presents with massive ascites with little peripheral edema. Because of the gross abdominal distension, patients usually complain of early satiety, and it is not uncommon to see patients losing muscle bulk and fat weight rapidly. The cachexia that is observed in these patients is akin to the malnutrition found in patients with end-stage cirrhosis.

Ascitic fluid analysis reveals an average protein content of 4 g/dL, with the ascitic fluid albumin content usually half that of the protein. Total white cell count is usually approximately 500 cell/mm^3, although up to 1600 cells/mm^3 has been reported. The serum ascites albumin gradient (SAAG) is typically low, at approximately 0.9 g/dL. Ascitic fluid cultures for bacterial, fungal, and mycobacterial infections are always negative, as is the cytology of the ascitic fluid.[49] Laparoscopic inspection of the peritoneum can show a sugar coating appearance of the peritoneal surfaces. Biopsy of the peritoneum is normal in more than 50% of cases. The remainder usually show mild fibrosis, mild inflammation, or reactive changes (**Table 2**).

The pathogenesis of nephrogenic ascites is unclear. High levels of protein and albumin in the ascitic fluid, together with a low SAAG, suggest that there is leakage of protein into the peritoneal cavity. The usually low total white cell count of ascitic fluid supports the contention that it is not infection, inflammation, or malignancy that is responsible for the seeping of fluid into the peritoneal cavity. It has been proposed that there is increased permeability of the peritoneal membrane, the result of various vascular permeability factors being upregulated, leading to structural changes in the peritoneum in patients with end-stage renal disease.[50] Many patients with renal failure and nephrogenic ascites have low serum albumin concentrations compared with patients without ascites, suggesting that hypoalbuminemia with decreased oncotic pressure may contribute to the severity of the ascites. Other pathogenetic factors that have been implicated include hypoparathyroidism,[51] volume overload,[52] and circulating immune complexes causing uremic serositis.[53] However, none of these factors has been definitively proved to be involved in the pathogenesis of nephrogenic ascites.

Table 2
Diagnosis of nephrogenic ascites

Criterion	Diagnostic Features
Clinical	Ascites and minimal edema Early satiety and anorexia Cachexia End-stage renal disease
Ascitic fluid analysis	Straw color Low total white cell count 20–1600 cells/mm^3 High protein level of 4.0 g/dL High albumin level of 2.2 g/dL Low SAAG of 0.9 g/dL Negative culture and cytology
Other tests	Sugar coating of peritoneum Normal peritoneal biopsy
Exclusions	Congestive cardiac failure Pericardial disease Cirrhosis Budd-Chiari syndrome Peritoneal infection or malignancy Pancreatic pseudocyst Hypothyroidism

Abbreviation: SAAG, serum ascitic albumin gradient.

Treatment of nephrogenic ascites is unsatisfactory. Fluid and sodium restriction, albumin infusion, repeat large volume paracentesis, and hyperalimentation have all been tried but with limited success in the control of the ascites. Daily hemodialysis or continuous ambulatory peritoneal dialysis (CAPD) have been advocated as both can remove uremic toxins which are believed to be responsible for altering the permeability of the peritoneum. The use of daily hemodialysis has been reported to be successful in eliminating the ascites in 35% to 78% of patients.[48] The limiting factor is the systemic hypotension. Reinfusion of the ascitic fluid and isolated ultrafiltration can reduce the incidence of dialysis-induced hypotension. When successful, daily dialysis can eliminate the ascites in 1 to 2 weeks. The use of CAPD is effectively to perform a total paracentesis. The drawback is the removal of a large quantity of protein with the peritoneal dialysis with consequent reduction in serum protein levels. CAPD is not associated with hemodynamic changes and therefore obviates the concerns for hypotension. In general, the patients feel better with CAPD, as the total paracentesis allows room for increased meal size, and the increased caloric intake can partially offset the protein loss with the total paracentesis.[54]

Peritoneovenous shunting has been reported as a treatment option for nephrogenic ascites.[55] However, nowadays, it is difficult to find a manufacturer of the peritoneovenous shunt and a surgeon who is skilled enough to insert such a shunt. The insertion of a peritoneovenous shunt in patients with renal failure is associated with the same complications, such as dislodgement, kinking, and infection, as in patients with ascites caused by cirrhosis. The presence of the shunt precludes the use of CAPD. Kidney transplantation seems to be the most effective treatment of nephrogenic ascites.[56] Complete resolution of ascites within 2 to 6 weeks significantly improves the quality of life of these patients. Nephrogenic ascites will recur with graft failure from whatever reason. This can occur immediately on graft failure or up to 3 years after the onset of graft failure.

In patients who are awaiting a renal transplant, if ascites disappears with treatment, the prognosis is the same as that of a patient with chronic renal failure without nephrogenic ascites.[57] Therefore, nephrogenic ascites, if responsive to treatment, does not negatively affect the prognosis.[58] However, in those patients who do not respond to treatment, there is gradual worsening of the cachexia and progression to death within a year.

DIALYSIS AND THE LIVER

Many patients with end-stage renal disease requiring dialysis also have concomitant chronic liver disease. The exact prevalence of combined end-stage renal disease and chronic liver disease is unknown. The causes of the renal disease and the liver disease are usually unrelated. Diabetes and hypertension are the most common causes of the renal disease, and alcohol and viral hepatitis account for most cases of liver disease. The presence of liver disease, especially liver cirrhosis, poses challenges in decision regarding dialysis. The need for dialysis also makes treatment of common liver diseases such as viral hepatitis difficult.

Dialysis in Patients with Chronic Liver Disease

The 2 common problems in the management of chronic renal failure in patients with chronic liver disease, especially cirrhosis, are when to start dialysis and what form of dialysis to use. Patients with cirrhosis of the liver often have low serum creatinine levels, caused by reduced production of creatinine from creatine in the liver and significant muscle wasting. Therefore, estimation of renal function using serum creatinine in patients with cirrhosis is inaccurate as it can still be within the normal range despite significant renal dysfunction.[59] The use of creatinine clearance in cirrhosis to assess renal function is also unreliable because of the falsely low serum creatinine level in these patients. Furthermore, this requires a 24-hour urine collection, which is often incomplete especially in an outpatient setting.[60] Formulae such as the Cockcroft-Gault and Modification of Diet in Renal Disease, which are based on the serum creatinine concentration, also overestimate the GFR.[61] Using the inulin clearance technique, the gold standard for measuring GFR, cirrhotic patients with renal dysfunction and renal inulin clearance of 30 mL/min had a serum creatinine level of 133 μmol/L, whereas patients with chronic renal failure and the same renal inulin clearance but without cirrhosis had a serum creatinine level of 186 μmol/L.[62] Until better measurements of GFR can be found, serum creatinine measurement is still the most useful and widely accepted method for estimating renal function in clinical practice in patients with cirrhosis. Therefore, decisions regarding the timing of initiation of renal replacement therapy in patients with renal failure and cirrhosis should take into account the falsely low serum creatinine level in these patients. To compound the problem, symptoms of lethargy, loss of appetite, and weight loss which would normally favor the initiation of renal replacement therapy, may be related to cirrhosis rather than to uremia.

Once the decision for renal replacement therapy is made, the type of renal replacement therapy to be used is another issue. Patients with cirrhosis are vasodilated, and systemic hypotension is common in advanced cirrhosis.[63] They are also at risk for bleeding and infections. One of the major problems with hemodialysis is the occurrence of intradialysis hypotension, which limits the amount of ultrafiltration that can be done at each dialysis session. This is particularly challenging in patients with cirrhosis and ascites, as the inability to remove excess fluid results in little or no reduction in the ascites. The rapid osmotic shifts of intermittent dialysis can also lead to shifts in brain cell water, predisposing these patients to the development of hepatic encephalopathy.[64] The use of peritoneal dialysis obviates the issue with hypotension during dialysis. It has the additional advantage of draining the ascitic fluid with the dialysis and provides a caloric load with the glucose solution.[65] However, the presence of a foreign body such as the peritoneal dialysis catheter can increase the risk of peritonitis[66] with a potentially fatal outcome. The loss of protein from the dialysate can also exacerbate the protein malnutrition in these patients.

Because ascites in cirrhosis contributes to significant patient discomfort and predisposes the patient to potentially life-threatening complications such as bacterial peritonitis and development of various hernias, there have been suggestions to insert a transjugular intrahepatic portosystemic stent shunt (TIPS) as a treatment of ascites in patients with cirrhosis and chronic renal failure undergoing hemodialysis. Although TIPS has been used as a treatment of hepatorenal syndrome,[67] there are no reports in the literature on the use of TIPS as a treatment of ascites in patients with cirrhosis and chronic renal failure from organic renal disease. The return of a significant amount of splanchnic volume into the pulmonary circulation on opening of the TIPS shunt can potentially put the patient at risk for pulmonary edema. The proponents for such a procedure would argue that the excess fluid can be removed with ultrafiltration. However, the systemic hypotension that is commonly observed in cirrhosis usually worsens after TIPS insertion,[68] thus further limiting the amount of intravascular volume that can be removed. Furthermore, simply correcting one of the many pathogenetic factors of cirrhotic ascites, that is, removal of the portal hypertension, does not always lead to elimination of the ascites, especially because the peritoneum in patients with uremia seems to be more porous than the peritoneum in those without uremia, which will perpetuate the ascites. Therefore, the insertion of a TIPS as a treatment of ascites in patients with cirrhosis and chronic renal failure is to be discouraged.

Treatment of Chronic Liver Disease in Patients Undergoing Dialysis

The management of chronic liver diseases in patients with chronic renal disease on dialysis should follow the same principles as in patients without chronic renal failure. Patients with alcoholic liver disease should be encouraged to abstain from alcohol. Lifestyle changes to reduce cardiovascular risks also help to decrease the likelihood of NAFLD. Viral hepatitis, if present, should also be treated if possible. Adjustment of doses of antiviral therapy is required because of the renal failure. The use of dialysis is associated with lower transaminase levels and viral count.[69] Therefore, decisions regarding initiation of antiviral therapy should take this into consideration. Regular monitoring of liver enzymes, liver function, and screening abdominal ultrasound should be mandatory. Patients who have cirrhosis should also undergo regular surveillance gastroscopy to check for varices.

RENAL TRANSPLANT AND THE LIVER

Renal transplant is the treatment of choice for patients with end-stage renal disease, as this improves the quality of life and prolongs survival. Currently, all patients with chronic renal disease being assessed for renal transplant are screened for chronic liver disease including chronic HBV and HCV.[70] The presence of chronic liver disease is not a contraindication for kidney transplantation, but can negatively affect graft and patient survival after transplant.[71] Liver biopsy should be incorporated in the evaluation of renal transplant candidates with viral hepatitis because it is difficult, on clinical grounds alone, to estimate the severity of liver disease in uremic patients, especially because patients with chronic renal disease on dialysis tend to have normal enzyme levels (**Fig. 2**). Management of chronic liver disease in renal transplant candidates should follow that of patients who are undergoing dialysis.

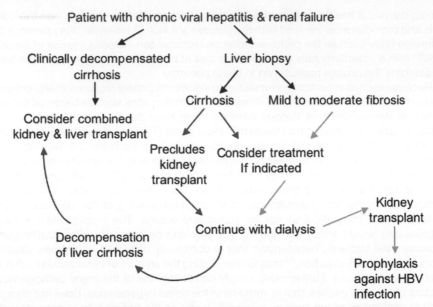

Fig. 2. Proposed algorithm for the management of viral hepatitis in patients with chronic renal failure. Red arrows: patients with cirrhosis and chronic renal failure; green arrows, patients with chronic renal failure but without cirrhosis.

In patients who have chronic HBV infection who have not required antiviral therapy before transplant, it is recommended that antiviral prophylaxis be given at the time of renal transplant.[72] The rationale is to prevent reactivation of HBV infection with immunosuppression, which was occurring at the rate of 50% to 94% before the introduction of lamivudine.[73,74] Since then, the use of lamivudine as antiviral prophylaxis has significantly improved the outcome of patients receiving renal transplant.[75] However, the duration of antiviral therapy in HBV-infected patients after transplant is unclear. The long-term benefit of such an approach is also unknown.

In renal transplant candidates who have chronic HCV infection and have failed previous treatment with interferon, it is recommended that repeat liver biopsy is done at 3-year intervals to assess progression of liver disease, especially for the detection of cirrhosis. Patients who are waiting for several years on the kidney transplant list may need retesting of HCV RNA to confirm the presence or absence of HCV infection.[76] In those who remain positive for HCV RNA, the options are to try retreatment or proceed with renal transplant with the HCV infection. Post-transplantation HCV therapy is generally not recommended because of concerns regarding risk for precipitating acute rejection.

The presence of cirrhosis is a relative contraindication for renal transplant alone, as the survival of graft and patient is dismal.[77] Therefore, combined renal and liver transplants have been advocated for patients with end-stage renal disease and advanced cirrhosis.[78] However, patients who have a less severe degree of cirrhosis, and who otherwise do not fulfill listing criteria for liver transplant, will have to continue with dialysis and have their cirrhosis managed expectantly. These patients can be considered for combined renal and liver transplants when the cirrhosis deteriorates.

In patients with chronic renal failure, defined as a GFR of less than 30 mL/min, and advanced cirrhosis, combined kidney and liver transplantation (CLKT) is indicated.[78] Since the introduction of Model for End Stage Liver Disease (MELD) criteria for

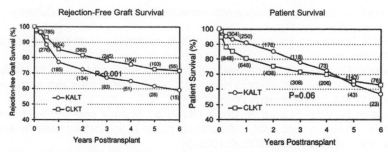

Fig. 3. Rejection-free graft survival and patient survival in patients undergoing combined liver and kidney transplantation (CLKT) versus those undergoing kidney after liver transplant (KALT). (*From* Simpson N, Cho YW, Cicciarelli JC, et al. Comparison of renal allograft outcomes in CLKT versus subsequent kidney transplantation in liver transplant recipients: analysis of UNOS database. Transplantation 2006;82:1298–303; with permission.)

selection of patients for liver transplant, there has been a dramatic increase in CLKT,[79] as an abnormal serum creatinine level weighs heavily in the MELD score calculation. That is, the use of MELD criteria has favored patients with chronic renal disease who also have advanced cirrhosis to receive CLKT. Although sequential kidney after liver transplant (KALT) is an acceptable treatment option for patients with chronic renal disease and advanced cirrhosis, this is inferior to simultaneous liver and kidney transplantation in terms of patient outcome. Patients with KALT have been shown to have shorter renal half-life, higher incidence of chronic rejection, and lower 1 and 3-year rejection-free renal graft survival compared with those who receive CLKT. Patient overall survival, however, is similar for the 2 treatment modalities (**Fig. 3**).[80]

SUMMARY

Patients with primary renal disease often have coexisting liver disease, because many conditions can affect both the liver and the kidney. There is also a potpourri of liver complications that are the direct result of the primary renal disease. Viral hepatitis is common amongst patients who undergo renal dialysis, and this adds to the dimension of problems faced by these chronically ill patients. Treatment of viral hepatitis in patients with chronic renal disease poses additional challenges, but these can be managed in specialized centers. Kidney transplant should only be performed either in conjunction with liver transplant or after liver transplant in patients with end-stage kidney disease and advanced cirrhosis, as this offers the best chance for patient and graft survival. For those patients with cirrhosis and chronic renal disease not suitable for CLKT, there is a need to develop better treatment options other than dialysis and monitoring for complications of cirrhosis.

REFERENCES

1. Giboney PT. Mildly elevated liver transaminase levels in the asymptomatic patient. Am Fam Physician 2005;71:1105–10.
2. Krier M, Ahmed A. The asymptomatic outpatient with abnormal liver function tests. Clin Liver Dis 2009;13:167–77.
3. Lopez-Alcorocho JM, Barril G, Ortiz-Movilla N, et al. Prevalence of hepatitis B, hepatitis C, GB virus C/hepatitis G and TT viruses in predialysis and hemodialysis patients. J Med Virol 2001;63:103–7.

4. Peters MG. Special populations with hepatitis B virus infection. Hepatology 2009; 49:S146–55.
5. Lok AS. Navigating the maze of hepatitis B treatments. Gastroenterology 2007; 132:1586–94.
6. Lapinski TW, Flisiak R, Jaroszewicz J, et al. Efficiency and safety of lamivudine therapy in patients with chronic HBV infection, dialysis or after kidney transplantation. World J Gastroenterol 2005;11:400–2.
7. Fontaine H, Vallet-Pichard A, Chaix ML, et al. Efficacy and safety of adefovir dipivoxil in kidney recipients, hemodialysis patients, and patients with renal insufficiency. Transplantation 2005;80:1086–92.
8. Fabrizi F, Dixit V, Martin P. Meta-analysis: anti-viral therapy of hepatitis B virus-associated glomerulonephritis. Aliment Pharmacol Ther 2006;24:781–8.
9. Lemos LB, Perez RM, Lemos MM, et al. Hepatitis C among predialysis patients: prevalence and characteristics in a large cohort of patients. Nephron Clin Pract 2008;108:135–40.
10. Fabrizi F, Poordad FF, Martin P. Hepatitis C infection and the patient with end-stage renal disease. Hepatology 2002;36:3–10.
11. Fabrizi F, Martin P, Dixit V, et al. Acquisition of hepatitis C virus in hemodialysis patients: a prospective study by branched DNA signal amplification assay. Am J Kidney Dis 1998;31:647–54.
12. Martin P, Carter D, Fabrizi F, et al. Histopathological features of hepatitis C in renal transplant candidates. Transplantation 2000;69:1479–84.
13. Fabrizi F, Messa P, Martin P. Impact of hemodialysis therapy on hepatitis C virus infection: a deeper insight. Int J Artif Organs 2009;32:1–11.
14. Trevizoli JE, de Paula Menezes R, Ribeiro Velasco LF, et al. Hepatitis C is less aggressive in hemodialysis patients than in non-uremic patients. Clin J Am Soc Nephrol 2008;3:1385–9.
15. Martin P, Mitra S, Farrington K, et al. Pegylated (40 KDA) interferon alfa-2a (PegasysTM) is unaffected by renal impairment [abstract]. Hepatology 2000; 32:842.
16. Fabrizi F, Dixit V, Messa P, et al. Interferon monotherapy of chronic hepatitis C in dialysis patients: meta-analysis of clinical trials. J Viral Hepat 2008;15:79–88.
17. Berenguer M. Treatment of chronic hepatitis C in hemodialysis patients. Hepatology 2008;48:1690–9.
18. Weclawiack H, Kamar N, Mehrenberger M, et al. Alpha-interferon therapy for chronic hepatitis C may induce acute allograft rejection in kidney transplant patients with failed allografts. Nephrol Dial Transplant 2008;23:1043–7.
19. Renal Data System. USRDS: 2006 annual data report: atlas of end-stage renal disease in the United States. Bethesda (MD): National Institute of Diabetes and Digestive and Kidney Disease; 2006.
20. Targher G, Bertolini L, Rodella S, et al. Non-alcoholic fatty liver disease is independently associated with an increased prevalence of chronic kidney disease and proliferative/laser-treated retinopathy in type 2 diabetic patients. Diabetologia 2008;51:444–50.
21. Rucker D, Tonelli M. Cardiovascular risk and management in chronic kidney disease. Nat Rev Nephrol 2009;5:287–96.
22. Yeung E, Wong FS, Wanless IR, et al. Ramipril-associated hepatotoxicity. Arch Pathol Lab Med 2003;127:1493–7.
23. Nunes AC, Amaro P, Macoas F, et al. Fosinopril-induced prolonged cholestatic jaundice and pruritis. A first case report. Eur J Gastroenterol Hepatol 2001;13: 279–82.

24. Droste HT, de Vries RA. Chronic hepatitis caused by lisinopril. Neth J Med 1995; 46:95–8.
25. Macías FM, Campos FR, Salguero TP, et al. Ductopenic hepatitis related to Enalapril. J Hepatol 2003;39:1091–2.
26. Kiykim A, Altintas E, Sezgin O, et al. Valsartan-induced hepatotoxicity in a HBs-Ag-positive patient. Am J Gastroenterol 2003;98:507.
27. Tabak F, Mert A, Ozaras R, et al. Losartan-induced hepatic injury. J Clin Gastroenterol 2002;34:585–6.
28. González-Jiménez D, Varela JM, Calderón E, et al. Candesartan and acute liver injury. Eur J Clin Pharmacol 2000;56:769–70.
29. Bairaktari E, Liamis G, Tsolas O, et al. Partially reversible renal tubular damage in patients with obstructive jaundice. Hepatology 2001;33:1365–9.
30. Izumi N, Hasumura Y, Takeuchi J. Hypouricemia and hyperuricosuria as expressions of renal tubular damage in primary biliary cirrhosis. Hepatology 1983;3:719–23.
31. Bomzon A, Holt S, Moore K. Bile acids, oxidative stress and renal function in biliary obstruction. Semin Nephrol 1997;17:549–62.
32. Sokol RJ, Devereaux M, Khandwala R, et al. Evidence for involvement of oxygen free radicals in bile acid toxicity to isolated rat hepatocytes. Hepatology 1993;17: 869–81.
33. Fogarty BJ, Parks RW, Rowlands BJ, et al. Renal dysfunction in obstructive jaundice. Br J Surg 1995;82:877–84.
34. Kramer HJ, Schwarting K, Backer A, et al. Renal endothelin system in obstructive jaundice: its role in impaired renal function in bile-duct ligated rats. Clin Sci 1997; 92:579–85.
35. Kramer HJ. Impaired renal function in obstructive jaundice: roles of the thromboxane and endothelin systems. Nephron 1997;77:1–12.
36. Green J, Better OS. Systemic hypotension and renal failure in obstructive jaundice - mechanistic and therapeutic aspects. J Am Soc Nephrol 1995;5:1853–71.
37. Gissen P, Tee L, Johnson CA, et al. Clinical and molecular genetic features of ARC syndrome. Hum Genet 2006;120:396–409.
38. Stauffer MH. Nephrogenic hepatomegaly. Gastroenterology 1961;40:694.
39. Dourakis SP, Sinani C, Deutsch M, et al. Cholestatic jaundice as a paraneoplastic manifestation of renal cell carcinoma. Eur J Gastroenterol Hepatol 1997;9:311–4.
40. Yong TL, Birks SE, Rudinski C. Stauffer's syndrome. ANZ J Surg 2008;78:1138–9.
41. Kranidiotis GP, Voidonikola PT, Dimopoulos MK, et al. Stauffer's syndrome as a prominent manifestation of renal cancer: a case report. Cases J 2009;2:49.
42. MoDougal WS, Garnick MB. Clinical signs and symptoms of renal cell carcinoma. In: Vogelzang NJ, Scardino PT, Shipley WV, et al, editors. Comprehensive textbook of genitourinary oncology. 2nd edition. Philadelphia: Lippincott, Williams & Wilkins; 2000. p. 112.
43. Strickland RC, Schenker S. The nephrogenic hepatic dysfunction syndrome: a review. Am J Dig Dis 1977;22:49–55.
44. Blay JY, Rossi JF, Wijdenes J, et al. Role of interleukin-6 in the paraneoplastic inflammatory syndrome associated with renal-cell carcinoma. Int J Cancer 1997;72:424–30.
45. Motzer RJ, Bander NH, Nanus DM. Renal-cell carcinoma. N Engl J Med 1996; 335:865–75.
46. Muñoz Vélez D, Rebasa Llull M, Hidalgo Pardo F, et al. Etiopathogenesis and management of paraneoplastic fever and Stauffer syndrome in renal carcinoma. Actas Urol Esp 1999;23:379–83.

47. Malnick S, Melzer E, Sokolowski N, et al. The involvement of the liver in systemic diseases. J Clin Gastroenterol 2008;42:69–80.

48. Han SH, Reynolds TB, Fong TL. Nephrogenic ascites. Analysis of 16 cases and review of the literature. Medicine 1998;77:233–45.

49. Hammond TC, Taylyyuddin MA. Nephrogenic ascites: a poorly understood syndrome. J Am Soc Nephrol 1994;5:1173–7.

50. Combet S, Ferrier ML, Van Landschoot M, et al. Chronic uremia induces permeability changes, increased nitric oxide synthase expression, and structural modifications in the peritoneum. J Am Soc Nephrol 2001;12:2146–57.

51. Nasr EM, Joubran NI. Is nephrogenic ascites related to secondary hyperparathyroidism? Am J Kidney Dis 2001;37:E16.

52. Gunal AI, Karaca I, Celiker H, et al. Strict volume control in the treatment of nephrogenic ascites. Nephrol Dial Transplant 2002;17:1248–51.

53. Twardowski ZJ, Alpert MA, Gupta RC, et al. Circulating immune complexes: possible toxins responsible for serositis (pericarditis, pleuritis, and peritonitis) in renal failure. Nephron 1983;35:190–5.

54. Ing TS, Daugirdas JT, Popli S, et al. Treatment of refractory hemodialysis ascites with maintenance peritoneal dialysis. Clin Nephrol 1981;15:198–202.

55. Holm A, Rutsky EA, Aldrete JS. Short- and long-term effectiveness, morbidity, and mortality of peritoneovenous shunt inserted to treat massive refractory ascites of nephrogenic origin. Analysis of 14 cases. Am Surg 1989;55:645–52.

56. Gluck Z, Nolph KD. Ascites associated with end-stage renal disease. Am J Kidney Dis 1987;10:9–18.

57. Mauk P, Schwartz JT, Lowe JE, et al. Diagnosis and course of nephrogenic ascites. Arch Intern Med 1988;148:1577–9.

58. Feingold LN, Gutman RA, Walsh FX, et al. Control of cachexia and ascites in hemodialysis patients by binephrectomy. Arch Intern Med 1974;134:989–97.

59. Sherman DS, Fish DN, Teitelbaum I. Assessing renal function in cirrhotic patients: problems and pitfalls. Am J Kidney Dis 2003;41:269–78.

60. Proulx NL, Akbari A, Garg AX, et al. Measured creatinine clearance from timed urine collections substantially overestimates glomerular filtration rate in patients with liver cirrhosis: a systematic review and individual patient meta-analysis. Nephrol Dial Transplant 2005;20:1617–22.

61. MacAulay J, Thompson K, Kiberd BA, et al. Serum creatinine in patients with advanced liver disease is of limited value for identification of moderate renal dysfunction: are the equations for estimating renal function better? Can J Gastroenterol 2006;20:521–6.

62. Roy L, Legault L, Pomier-Layrargues G. Glomerular filtration rate measurement in cirrhotic patients with renal failure. Clin Nephrol 1998;50:342–6.

63. La Villa G, Gentilini P. Hemodynamic alterations in liver cirrhosis. Mol Aspects Med 2008;29:112–8.

64. Winney RJ, Kean DM, Best JJ, et al. Changes in brain water with hemodialysis. Lancet 1986;2:1107–8.

65. Chaudhary K, Khanna R. Renal replacement therapy in end-stage renal disease patients with chronic liver disease and ascites: role of peritoneal dialysis. Perit Dial Int 2008;28:113–7.

66. Selgas R, Bajo MA, Jimenez C, et al. Peritoneal dialysis in liver disorders. Perit Dial Int 1996;16(Suppl 1):S215–9.

67. Wong F. Hepatorenal syndrome: current management. Curr Gastroenterol Rep 2008;10:22–9.

68. Wong F, Sniderman K, Liu P, et al. The mechanism of the initial natriuresis after transjugular intrahepatic portosystemic shunt. Gastroenterology 1997;112: 899–907.

69. Yasuda K, Okuda K, Endo N, et al. Hypoaminotransferasemia in patients undergoing long-term hemodialysis: clinical and biochemical appraisal. Gastroenterology 1995;109:1295–300.

70. Knoll G, Cockfield S, Blydt-Hansen T, et al, for the Kidney Transplant Working Group of the Canadian Society of Transplantation. Canadian Society of Transplantation consensus guidelines on eligibility for kidney transplantation. CMAJ 2005;173:1181–4.

71. Mathurin P, Mouquet C, Poynard T, et al. Impact of hepatitis B and C virus on kidney transplantation outcome. Hepatology 1999;29:257–63.

72. Hoofnagle JH. Reactivation of hepatitis B. Hepatology 2009;45:S156–65.

73. Marcellin P, Giostra E, Martinot-Peignoux M, et al. Redevelopment of hepatitis B surface antigen after renal transplantation. Gastroenterology 1991;100:1432–4.

74. Degos F, Lugassy C, Degott C, et al. Hepatitis B virus and hepatitis B-related viral infection in renal transplant recipients. A prospective study of 90 patients. Gastroenterology 1988;94:151–6.

75. Park SK, Yang WS, Lee YS, et al. Outcome of renal transplantation in hepatitis B surface antigen-positive patients after introduction of lamivudine. Nephrol Dial Transplant 2001;16:2222–8.

76. Terrault NA, Adey DB. The kidney transplant recipient with hepatitis C infection: pre- and posttransplantation treatment. Clin J Am Soc Nephrol 2007;2:563–75.

77. Mouquet C, Mathurin P, Sylla C, et al. Hepatic cirrhosis and kidney transplantation outcome. Transplant Proc 1997;29:2406.

78. Chava SP, Singh B, Zaman MB, et al. Current indications for combined liver and kidney transplantation in adults. Transplant Rev 2009;23:111–9.

79. Davis CL, Feng S, Sung R, et al. Simultaneous liver-kidney transplantation: evaluation to decision making. Am J Transplant 2007;7:1702–9.

80. Simpson N, Cho YW, Cicciarelli JC, et al. Comparison of renal allograft outcomes in combined liver-kidney transplantation versus subsequent kidney transplantation in liver transplant recipients: analysis of UNOS database. Transplantation 2006;82:1298–303.

Endocrine Diseases and the Liver

Anurag Maheshwari, MD[a], Paul J. Thuluvath, MD, FRCP[a,b],*

KEYWORDS

- Endocrine disorders • Fatty liver disease
- Abnormal liver function test result

Endocrine disorders and liver diseases are both common in the general population. It is therefore not uncommon to see both these disorders in the same individual. Certain chronic liver disorders, however, are commonly associated with endocrine disorders, including nonalcoholic fatty liver disease (NAFLD), autoimmune hepatitis (AIH), and primary biliary cirrhosis (PBC). In addition, there are increasing data to indicate an association between hepatitis C and type 2 diabetes mellitus (DM) as well as thyroid disorders. The effect of endocrine diseases on liver is examined in this article.

METABOLIC SYNDROME AND NAFLD

NAFLD is a spectrum of chronic liver diseases, ranging from benign steatosis (fat accumulation) to advanced cirrhosis and cancer. NAFLD is closely linked to type 2 DM, obesity, hyperlipidemia, or the metabolic syndrome (MS). Its incidence in the world is increasing, including the countries where malnutrition was more prevalent until recently. Current estimates indicate that the prevalence of steatosis in the general US population approaches 30%,[1] and it has been suggested that secondary to NAFLD, cirrhosis or hepatocellular carcinoma (HCC) may become the leading indication for liver transplant in the United States by 2025, replacing chronic hepatitis C infection.[2]

The hallmark of NAFLD is the MS, which is characterized by a cluster of metabolic abnormalities that include truncal obesity, glucose intolerance, hypertension, and dyslipidemia (with elevated triglyceride levels and low levels of high-density lipoprotein [HDL] cholesterol). Although various organizations have proposed different cutoff values for each of these variables in their diagnostic criteria for MS (**Table 1**), there is a general consensus that insulin resistance is the most important metabolic

The authors have nothing to disclose.

[a] Institute for Digestive Health & Liver Diseases, Mercy Medical Center, 301 Saint Paul Place, Physician Office Building 718, Baltimore, MD 21202, USA

[b] Georgetown University School of Medicine, Washington, DC, USA

* Corresponding author. Georgetown University School of Medicine & The Institute for Digestive Health & Liver Diseases, Mercy Medical Center, 301 Saint Paul Place, Physician Office Building, MD 21202.

E-mail address: thuluvath@gmail.com

Table 1
Proposed minimum criteria for MS

	WHO	EGIR	ATP III	AACE	IDF
Obesity	WHR >0.9 (M) >0.85 (F) BMI>30	WC >94 cm (M) >88 cm (F)	WC >102 cm (M) >88 cm (F)	WC >102 cm (M) >88 cm (F) BMI>25	WC >94 cm (M) >80 cm (F)
Lipid levels	TG>150 mg/dl HDL <35 mg/dl (M) <39 mg/dl (F)	TG>175 mg/dl HDL<39 mg/dl	TG>150 mg/dl HDL <40 mg/dl (M) <50 mg/dl (F)	TG>150 mg/dl HDL <40 mg/dl (M) <50 mg/dl (F)	TG>150 mg/dl HDL <40 mg/dl (M) <50 mg/dl (F)
Glucose	Any abnormality of glucose metabolism	BG>110 mg/dl	BG>110 mg/dl	BG 110–125 mg/dl or PP 140–200	BG>100 mg/dl
Hypertension	BP>140/90 mm Hg	BP>140/90 mm Hg	BP>130/85 mm Hg	BP>130/85 mm Hg	BP>130/85 mm Hg
Other criteria	Microalbuminuria	Elevated fasting insulin levels	—	Age >40 y, PCOS, CVD, FH of above factors	—
Diagnostic criteria	Altered glucose metabolism with 2 other factors	Hyperinsulinemia with 2 other factors	3 of 5 criteria	IFG or IGT with a combination of other factors	Obesity with 2 other factors

BMI, body mass index; calculated as the weight in kilograms divided by height in meters squared.

Abbreviations: AACE, American Association of Clinical Endocrinologists; ATP III, Adult Treatment Panel III from NCEP report 2001; BG, blood glucose; BP, blood pressure; CVD, cardiovascular disease; EGIR, European Group for Study of Insulin Resistance; F, female; FH, family history; IDF, International Diabetes Foundation; IFG, impaired fasting glucose; IGT, impaired glucose tolerance; M, male; PCOS, polycystic ovarian syndrome; PP, postprandial; TG, triglycerides; WC, waist circumference; WHO, World Health Organization; WHR, waist/hip ratio.

abnormality of this syndrome. Even in the absence of obesity and overt DM, insulin resistance seems to play an important role in the pathogenesis and progression of NAFLD.

A detailed discussion on the pathogenesis of NAFLD or the development of insulin resistance and type 2 DM in patients with hepatitis C[3] is beyond the scope of this section, but the role of insulin resistance and cytokines in the pathogenesis of NAFLD is briefly reviewed. Some interrelated pathways may also be involved in the pathogenesis of insulin resistance and type 2 DM in patients with hepatitis C.[4] Defective insulin signaling and obesity result in a cascade of events leading to increased delivery of free fatty acids (FFA) to the liver. When FFA uptake from plasma and de novo FFA synthesis exceed FFA oxidation and export from hepatocytes as triglycerides, excess triglycerides accumulate within hepatocytes leading to steatosis, the histologic hallmark of NAFLD. In the presence of steatosis, excessive intracellular concentrations of FFA may also cause oxidative stress leading to apoptosis of the hepatocytes and the activation of the stellate cells, with resultant fibrosis. Many other systemic and tissue (liver, adipose tissue) inflammatory cytokines play an important role in the pathogenesis of NAFLD. Increasing evidence suggests that NAFLD and MS are interrelated in a bidirectional and complex manner. Irrespective of body mass index, the presence of type 2 DM independently increased the risk of NAFLD when compared with subjects with normal glucose levels or impaired glucose tolerance.[5] Not all patients with insulin resistance, however, demonstrate evidence of MS,[6] NAFLD, or nonalcoholic steatohepatitis (NASH), indicating that hitherto unknown genetic or environmental factors are also involved in the pathogenesis of NAFLD and its progression.[7]

Cytokines play an important role in the development of insulin resistance and the pathogenesis of NAFLD. Several adipocytokines, including adiponectin, leptin, resistin, and tumor necrosis factor (TNF) α, have been linked to alterations in insulin sensitivity and development of NAFLD. Adiponectin decreases hepatic gluconeogenesis and increases peripheral use of glucose and FFA by the muscles. Low concentrations of this cytokine have been observed in obesity, insulin resistance, and NAFLD.[8,9] Adiponectin is also thought to have antiinflammatory properties, and in the mouse model, administration of exogenous adiponectin reduced steatosis as well as the markers of liver inflammation.[10] Leptin, another cytokine produced by the adipose tissue, is involved in the regulation of food intake. In animal models, leptin deficiency causes several metabolic and endocrine disorders including marked obesity, hypogonadism, hypothyroidism, insulin resistance, and diabetes, and administration of leptin has been shown to reverse most of these abnormalities. Limited data on humans on the use of recombinant leptin in patients with congenital leptin deficiency or leptin receptor mutation have also shown encouraging results.[11] In addition, the administration of leptin has also shown to decrease insulin resistance and hepatic steatosis in patients with severe lipodystrophy.[12] However, the long-term treatment with leptin in obese patients seems to be ineffective because of the rapid development of resistance.[13] Moreover, leptin and its functional receptors may play an important role in fibrogenesis of the liver, and this fibrogenic effect is perhaps mediated by the activation of hepatic stellate cells.[14] Therefore, leptin administration may not have a consistent therapeutic benefit because of its competing effects on the liver. Resistin, another cytokine, is a potent proinflammatory agent that causes hepatic insulin resistance among patients with type 2 DM, and high levels of resistin are observed in patients with significant NASH.[15] In the mouse model, administration of rosiglitazone lowers resistin levels as well as resistin gene expression.[16] Clinical trials with rosiglitazone in patients with NASH have shown improvement in liver enzymes but without an improvement in NASH-associated fibrosis.[17] Increased expression of TNF-α by the adipose tissue has been proposed to mediate peripheral insulin resistance in obesity and type 2 DM. TNF-α expression in the liver is also increased in the presence of NAFLD[18] and is thought to represent the link between insulin resistance and steatosis. TNF-α production is also linked to oxidative stress in the liver, promoting the development of fibrosis and progression of NASH. Currently available anti-TNF antibodies neither have shown to increase insulin sensitivity in diabetic patients nor have they proven to be effective therapeutic agents for NASH. To summarize these findings, it seems that despite the strong clinical association of insulin resistance with the development and progression of NAFLD, effective treatment strategies could not be developed because of an incomplete understanding of the pathogenesis of this common disorder.

The presence of DM has a negative effect on the outcome of patients with liver disease. The relationship between diabetes and vascular complications is well recognized, and therefore, it is not surprising to find a similar relationship in patients with NAFLD. In addition, it has been shown that DM has a negative effect on the survival of patients with NAFLD. In patients with NAFLD, it has been shown that the presence of MS increased the risk of cardiovascular diseases, type 2 DM, and more severe liver disease (NASH and severe fibrosis).[19,20] Other studies have also shown an increased 10-year probability of cardiovascular events among patients with NASH and advanced fibrosis.[21] In addition, studies have also demonstrated an increase in liver-related mortality among diabetic patients during a short follow-up of 5 years.[22] Irrespective of the cause of liver disease, it has been shown that the presence of pre- or posttransplant DM increased the risk of cardiovascular complications and mortality after a liver transplant.[23,24]

THYROID DYSFUNCTION AND LIVER DISEASE

Alterations in thyroid function can lead to liver dysfunction, and conversely, various liver diseases can have differing effects on thyroid hormone metabolism. In addition, a host of systemic conditions can result in altered liver and thyroid functions. Patients with cirrhosis often have biochemical profiles that resemble the sick euthyroid syndrome. In patients with acute hepatitis, total thyroxine (T_4) level is frequently elevated in the presence of a normal free T_4 level because of the elevation of thyroid-binding globulin levels, which is an acute phase reactant. Patients with auto-immune liver diseases such as PBC and AIH also have an increased prevalence of autoimmune thyroid disease. Hypothyroidism is seen in 10% to 25% of patients with PBC,[25] whereas both hypothyroidism and Graves disease have been associated with AIH.[26] Primary sclerosing cholangitis is associated with an increased incidence of Hashimoto thyroiditis, Graves disease, and Riedel thyroiditis.[27] A potential association between thyroid disorders and hepatitis C has been reported.[28]

Hyperthyroidism

Liver injury caused by thyrotoxicosis is common and is classified as hepatocellular or cholestatic injury. The mechanism of injury among patients is a relative hypoxia in the perivenular regions caused by the increased oxygen demand due to thyrotoxicosis.[29] Additional increases in bile acid production and oxidative stress induced by elevated thyroid hormonal levels may lead to a cholestatic pattern of injury. Elevations of aminotransferase levels may be observed in one-third of patients with Graves disease, but the changes are usually transient and asymptomatic. There are case reports describing patients with thyrotoxicosis who presented with fulminant liver failure as the initial manifestation of the disease.[30] Jaundice is an uncommon presentation and when present, it may be secondary to the systemic effects of thyrotoxicosis, such as heart failure or septic shock.[29]

The therapies for hyperthyroidism can also lead to alterations of liver function. Hepatotoxicity is observed more frequently with propylthiouracil than methimazole (27% vs 7%),[31] and in the United States, propylthiouracil is the second leading cause of non-acetaminophen–associated drug-induced liver injury requiring liver transplant.[32] Liver toxicity associated with carbimazole or methimazole is frequently cholestatic and may persist for months despite the discontinuation of drug use.[33] Therefore, routine liver function tests are recommended in all patients treated for hyperthyroidism.

Hypothyroidism

Hypothyroidism is common in patients (and often their relatives) with autoimmune liver diseases, and recently, an increased prevalence of hypothyroidism has been reported in patients with hepatitis C and NAFLD. Hypothyroidism also can cause liver and gallbladder abnormalities. Subclinical hypothyroidism can induce both hyperlipidemia and obesity, conditions that are also associated with gallstone disease and steatosis. A large study found an independent association between hypothyroidism and gallstones, particularly among men.[34] Subclinical hypothyroidism is more prevalent among patients with MS[35] and those with NASH (NASH vs controls; odds ratio 2.3; 95% confidence interval, 1.2–4.2).[36] Another study also suggested a potential association between hypothyroidism and HCC of unknown cause.[37] More controlled data are necessary before reliably suggesting an association between hypothyroidism and progressive liver disease or HCC.

Severe ascites is a rare manifestation of uncontrolled hypothyroidism in patients with cirrhosis. Hypothyroidism can also cause ascites (myxedema ascites) in the absence of cirrhosis. In this situation, analysis of the ascitic fluid shows a high protein content with low serum-ascites albumin gradient and a cell count that is predominantly lymphocytic. The mechanism of injury may be the development of central scarring in the liver because of chronic right-sided heart failure. This finding is supported by biopsy evidence of central congestive fibrosis in several patients with myxedema ascites.[38] Thyroid hormone replacement therapy results in regression of the ascites over a few months. Hypothyroidism should be considered in patients with portal hypertension when they present with diuretic resistant ascites, and hormone replacement therapy often makes them diuretic sensitive. The authors have occasionally encountered patients referred for a liver transplant or transjugular intrahepatic portosystemic shunt surgery for refractory ascites with undiagnosed hypothyroidism, and these patients have avoided these procedures just with thyroid hormone replacement, diuretics, and sodium restriction.

Thyrotoxic Effects of Drugs Used in Liver Disease

Interferon therapy for chronic hepatitis C has been a well-recognized cause of thyroid dysfunction and may cause both autoimmune and subacute thyroiditis. Hypothyroidism is observed more frequently than hyperthyroidism during interferon alfa therapy, and therefore, routine monitoring of thyroid function and antithyroid antibody levels is recommended during therapy. The risk factors for the development of thyroid dysfunction with interferon alfa therapy include female gender, hepatitis C, the presence of thyroid autoantibodies (before or during therapy), and longer duration of therapy.[39] Spontaneous resolution of thyroid dysfunction occurs in only a fraction of patients, necessitating continued monitoring after cessation of therapy. In contrast to hepatitis C, patients with hepatitis B are not thought to be at significant risk for thyroid dysfunction during interferon therapy,[40] and therefore, routine monitoring of thyroid function during therapy is not mandatory.[41]

Hypothyroidism has been reported rarely among patients treated with transarterial chemoembolization for HCC[42] and this low incidence may be due to the use of iodized contrast medium. The use of sorafenib in patients with metastatic renal cell carcinoma has been associated with the development of hypothyroidism.[43] Sorafenib has been recently approved for use in HCC therapy, and routine monitoring of thyroid function is recommended during therapy.[44]

Systemic Conditions Causing Concomitant Liver and Thyroid Dysfunction

Systemic pathologic conditions that cause organ infiltration may cause concomitant liver and thyroid dysfunction. These conditions include malignancies (such as non-Hodgkin lymphoma), amyloid deposition, or secondary hemochromatosis with diffuse iron deposition in both the organs. In addition, medications such as amiodarone, mefloquine, carbamazepine and anticancer chemotherapeutics can frequently cause concomitant liver and thyroid dysfunction; thyroid dysfunction is usually transient but may occasionally persist after withdrawal of drug use.

ADRENAL DYSFUNCTION AND LIVER DISEASE

The relationship between the adrenal gland and the liver is complex and bidirectional, that is, dysfunction in one organ tends to cause abnormalities of function in the other organ too. The mechanisms of interactions remain unclear and are largely speculative at this time.

Adrenal Insufficiency and Liver Disease

Addison's disease is a well-recognized cause of mildly elevated aminotransferase levels, usually up to 2 to 3 times the upper limit of normal.[45] Therefore, Addison disease should be a part of the differential diagnosis of unexplained aminotransferase level elevations.[46] The mechanisms of enzyme level elevations are unclear but may be related to changes in body weight, and liver enzyme levels return to normal with appropriate glucocorticoid replacement therapy.

Recent data have shown a higher prevalence of adrenal insufficiency (absolute or relative) in patients with septic shock. There are also reports of improved outcomes with the use of corticosteroid therapy. Relative adrenal insufficiency (RAI) is a term used to describe the inappropriate response of plasma cortisol levels to stimulation by adrenocorticotrophic hormone in patients with normal or elevated basal plasma cortisol levels. Because of the similarities in physiologic mechanisms of septic shock and cirrhosis, it has been speculated that there may be a higher prevalence of RAI in patients with cirrhosis. The prevalence of RAI may range from 33% in acute liver failure to 69% in acute-on-chronic liver failure.[47–49] The degree of adrenal dysfunction correlates with the severity of liver disease. RAI is also seen in patients immediately after a liver transplant, even in the absence of sepsis. These findings may suggest that RAI is a manifestation of underlying liver disease, prompting some investigators to propose the existence of hepatoadrenal syndrome.[50] An inverse correlation between RAI and high-density lipoprotein (HDL) levels has been found, and it has been proposed that low HDL levels could be used as a surrogate marker for the development of RAI.[51] Whether RAI in liver disease is a manifestation of the liver disease itself or occurs by pathways similar to sepsis physiology remains unknown and awaits further research.

Studies examining the effect of corticosteroid therapy in septic patients with cirrhosis have shown conflicting results. Although these studies have consistently demonstrated a reduction in the vasopressor use, the benefit on survival remains unclear. One study showed an increase in infection rates due to resistant organisms[52] that negated any survival benefit, whereas 2 other uncontrolled studies showed improved survival associated with corticosteroid therapy.[49,50] There have been no randomized controlled studies that had examined the survival benefits with corticosteroid therapy among patients with liver disease and RAI. Current recommendations suggest that the use of corticosteroids in liver disease should be reserved for patients with sepsis requiring vasopressors, whereas its use in other patients with liver failure should be based on further clinical trials.[53]

Adrenal Excess and Liver Disease

Cushing's syndrome is associated with features of MS, with accumulation of fat at specific sites including liver and omental tissues. It is also associated with the development of insulin resistance. The hypertension caused by the upregulation of the renin-angiotensin system also contributes to the development of NAFLD that is also observed among patients with adrenal excess because of exogenous corticosteroid administration. Some investigators have also proposed that patients with MS show hyperactivity of the hypothalamic-pituitary-adrenal axis, which leads to a state of functional hypercortisolism. Increased exposure to cortisol causes increased fat accumulation in visceral depots, such as the liver, where elevation of 11β-hydroxysteroid dehydrogenase type 1 activity could also contribute to the development of MS.[54] Although intriguing, this hypothesis remains unproven and further research is needed to determine the role of cortisol in the pathogenesis of NAFLD among patients without clinical adrenal excess.

SEX HORMONES AND LIVER DISEASE

A balanced estrogen to androgen ratio is necessary to maintain normal fat metabolism in the body. Polycystic ovarian syndrome (PCOS) in women is associated with virilization, irregular menses, and infertility. In addition, the hyperandrogenism caused by PCOS is also associated with increased central adiposity, insulin resistance, and NAFLD. Recent studies have found a higher prevalence of NAFLD (41% vs 19%) and insulin resistance (63% vs 35%) among patients with PCOS as compared with healthy controls.[55] This finding has been confirmed by other studies,[56] and it is therefore recommended that all patients with PCOS should be systematically screened for NAFLD.[41]

Estrogens

With the widespread use of oral contraceptives, a variety of hepatic disorders (**Table 2**) associated with estrogens have now been recognized. This incidence has shown a steady decline over the years and may be related to the use of lower doses of estrogen and progesterone in currently available contraceptive preparations.[57]

Estrogens can cause intrahepatic cholestasis and jaundice. Because these conditions have been primarily reported with the use of oral contraceptives, the use of concomitant progestins is considered to augment the development of cholestasis. Other predisposing factors are genetic susceptibility,[58] prior history of pregnancy-associated cholestasis,[59] or the presence of concomitant cholestatic syndromes, such as subclinical PBC, Dubin-Johnson syndrome, or familial intrahepatic cholestasis.[60] Jaundice usually presents within the first 6 months of therapy and is not associated with elevation of aminotransferase or alkaline phosphatase levels. It usually resolves with cessation of therapy, but full recovery may take weeks to months.[61]

Vascular disorders of the liver associated with estrogen use include thrombosis of the hepatic (Budd Chiari syndrome) or portal veins and peliosis hepatis. The development

Table 2
Liver diseases associated with sex hormones

	Estrogens	Androgens
Disorders of Hepatic Metabolism	Cholestatic jaundice	Abnormal liver function test results Cholestatic jaundice Secondary biliary cirrhosis
Vascular Disorders	Budd-Chiari syndrome Portal vein thrombosis Peliosis hepatis	Peliosis hepatis
Hepatic Tumors	Hepatic adenoma Focal nodular hyperplasia Hemangioma Hepatocellular cancer	Hepatic adenoma HCC

of hepatic or portal vein thrombosis may represent an extension of the thrombophilic effect of estrogen use, and the association of this effect with Budd-Chiari syndrome is well described.[62] A significant proportion of patients, however, may also have other concomitant disorders of coagulation, such as myeloproliferative syndromes, in which estrogens may serve to augment the preexisting disposition to venous or arterial thrombosis. Hepatic peliosis is a rare complication of oral contraceptive use and can present with hepatomegaly associated with elevations of aminotransferase levels. The pathogenesis of the lesion remains largely unknown, although investigators have claimed radiographically that the lesions resolve with cessation of therapy.[63]

Oral contraceptive use has also been associated with benign hepatic tumors, including adenomas, focal nodular hyperplasia (FNH), and hemangiomas. Regression of the adenoma after cessation of estrogen use remains unpredictable[64] but it is routinely recommended. Because of the potential risk of malignant transformation, it is recommended at present that large adenomas should be resected if technically feasible. Multiple and bilobar adenomatoses could be followed by serial imaging, but whether this strategy would lead to early recognition of malignant transformation remains unknown. The association between estrogen use and the development of FNH and hemangiomas in the liver is less convincing. Certainly, hemangiomas are known to enlarge or recur under the influence of estrogen therapy, but evidence of their role in causing either lesion remains lacking. Nonetheless, withdrawal of estrogen therapy after detection of FNH or hemangioma is recommended, if clinically feasible.

Androgens

The incidence of liver abnormalities among patients using androgenic hormones is significantly higher than in those using estrogens. These abnormalities range from simple elevations of aminotransferase levels to the development of cholestasis and hepatic tumors including adenomas, peliosis hepatis, as well as HCC. The cholestasis associated with androgenic preparations is frequently associated with elevations of aminotransferase levels and has been implicated in the development of chronic liver disease, including secondary biliary cirrhosis.[61]

GROWTH HORMONE AND LIVER DISEASE

The metabolic effects of growth hormone include hyperglycemia, hyperinsulinemia, and lipolysis. Yet patients with untreated growth hormone deficiency present with

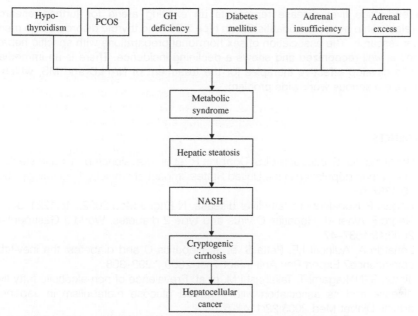

Fig. 1. Endocrine disorders associated with NAFLD. GH, growth hormone.

features that resemble MS. A retrospective study of patients with hypothalamic or pituitary disease showed a high prevalence of obesity, impaired glucose tolerance, and dyslipidemia with eventual development of NAFLD.[65] This cohort also demonstrated a large proportion of patients with NASH and cirrhosis, with significant liver-related morbidity and mortality on long-term follow-up. Other studies have also shown associations between NAFLD and NASH with adult-onset growth hormone deficiency,[66] and case reports have shown reversal of NAFLD with exogenous growth hormone replacement therapy.[67] These data highlight the role of growth hormone and insulinlike growth factor 1 in the pathogenesis of MS and oxidative stress within the liver. However, excess secretion of growth hormone, as seen in acromegaly, is associated with DM, insulin resistance (without increased visceral fat accumulations), elevated liver enzyme levels, and low adiponectin levels that are reversible after pituitary surgery.[68] Acromegaly has also been associated with an increased predisposition to gallstones.

SUMMARY

The endocrine pathways within the human body have a complex relationship with the liver. Many endocrine derangements are associated with NAFLD through changes in hepatic gluconeogenesis and shifts in body fat distribution, whereas other pathways may show transient asymptomatic elevations in aminotransferase levels (**Fig. 1**). Therefore, the clinician should have a high index of suspicion for the presence of liver disease among patients with endocrine disorders and vice versa. Autoimmune disorders affecting the endocrine organs and the liver may share common mechanisms, whereas the pathogenesis of certain disorders, such as myxedema ascites, remains unknown. The treatment modalities for thyrotoxicosis and chronic liver diseases can have undesirable effects on either organ system. The presence of RAI in patients with end-stage liver disease represents an exciting arena for further research. The relationship between hepatitis C with type 2 DM and thyroid disorders also merits further research. The association of sex hormonal preparations with specific hepatic lesions is well recognized and shows a declining incidence. There is an immediate need to develop effective therapies for the treatment of NAFLD and MS, which is becoming a serious worldwide problem.

REFERENCES

1. Browning JD, Szczepaniak LS, Dobbins R, et al. Prevalence of hepatic steatosis in an urban population in the United States: impact of ethnicity. Hepatology 2004; 40:1387–95.
2. Angulo P. Nonalcoholic fatty liver disease. N Engl J Med 2002;346:1221–31.
3. Negro F, Alaei M. Hepatitis C virus and type 2 diabetes. World J Gastroenterol 2009;15:1537–47.
4. Lonardo A, Adinolfi LE, Petta S, et al. Hepatitis C and diabetes: the inevitable coincidence? Expert Rev Anti Infect Ther 2009;7:293–308.
5. Jimba S, Nakagami T, Takahashi M, et al. Prevalence of non-alcoholic fatty liver disease and its association with impaired glucose metabolism in Japanese adults. Diabet Med 2005;22:1141–5.
6. McLaughlin T, Abbasi F, Cheal K, et al. Use of metabolic markers to identify overweight individuals who are insulin resistant. Ann Intern Med 2003;139:802–9.
7. Perlemuter G, Bigorgne A, Cassard-Doulcier AM, et al. Nonalcoholic fatty liver disease: from pathogenesis to patient care. Nat Clin Pract Endocrinol Metab 2007;3:458–69.
8. Pagano C, Soardo G, Esposito W, et al. Plasma adiponectin is decreased in nonalcoholic fatty liver disease. Eur J Endocrinol 2005;152:113–8.
9. Bugianesi E, Pagotto U, Manini R, et al. Plasma adiponectin in nonalcoholic fatty liver is related to hepatic insulin resistance and hepatic fat content, not to liver disease severity. J Clin Endocrinol Metab 2005;90:3498–504.
10. Xu A, Wang Y, Keshaw H, et al. The fat-derived hormone adiponectin alleviates alcoholic and nonalcoholic fatty liver diseases in mice. J Clin Invest 2003;112: 91–100.
11. Farooqi IS, Matarese G, Lord GM, et al. Beneficial effects of leptin on obesity, T cell hyporesponsiveness, and neuroendocrine/metabolic dysfunction of human congenital leptin deficiency. J Clin Invest 2002;110:1093–103.
12. Petersen KF, Oral EA, Dufour S, et al. Leptin reverses insulin resistance and hepatic steatosis in patients with severe lipodystrophy. J Clin Invest 2002;109: 1345–50.
13. Montez JM, Soukas A, Asilmaz E, et al. Acute leptin deficiency, leptin resistance, and the physiologic response to leptin withdrawal. Proc Natl Acad Sci U S A 2005;102:2537–42.
14. Saxena NK, Ikeda K, Rockey DC, et al. Leptin in hepatic fibrosis: evidence for increased collagen production in stellate cells and lean littermates of ob/ob mice. Hepatology 2002;35:762–71.
15. Pagano C, Soardo G, Pilon C, et al. Increased serum resistin in nonalcoholic fatty liver disease is related to liver disease severity and not to insulin resistance. J Clin Endocrinol Metab 2006;91:1081–6.
16. Steppan CM, Bailey ST, Bhat S, et al. The hormone resistin links obesity to diabetes. Nature 2001;409:307–12.

17. Ratziu V, Charlotte F, Bernhardt C, et al. Long-term efficacy of rosiglitazone in nonalcoholic steatohepatitis: results of the fatty liver improvement by rosiglitazone therapy (FLIRT 2) extension trial. Hepatology 2010;51:445–53.
18. Crespo J, Cayón A, Fernández-Gil P, et al. Gene expression of tumor necrosis factor alpha and TNF-receptors, p55 and p75, in nonalcoholic steatohepatitis patients. Hepatology 2001;34:1158–63.
19. Chitturi S, Abeygunasekera S, Farrell GC, et al. NASH and insulin resistance: insulin hypersecretion and specific association with the insulin resistance syndrome. Hepatology 2002;35:373–9.
20. Marchesini G, Bugianesi E, Forlani G, et al. Nonalcoholic fatty liver, steatohepatitis, and the metabolic syndrome. Hepatology 2003;37:917–23.
21. Villanova N, Moscatiello S, Ramilli S, et al. Endothelial dysfunction and cardiovascular risk profile in nonalcoholic fatty liver disease. Hepatology 2005;42:473–80.
22. de Marco R, Locatelli F, Zoppini G, et al. Cause-specific mortality in type 2 diabetes. The Verona Diabetes Study. Diabetes Care 1999;22:756–61.
23. John PR, Thuluvath PJ. Outcome of liver transplantation in patients with diabetes mellitus: a case-control study. Hepatology 2001;34:889–95.
24. Yoo HY, Thuluvath PJ. The effect of insulin-dependent diabetes mellitus on outcome of liver transplantation. Transplantation 2002;74:1007–12.
25. Sherlock S, Scheuer PJ. The presentation and diagnosis of 100 patients with primary biliary cirrhosis. N Engl J Med 1973;289:674–8.
26. Krawitt EL. Autoimmune hepatitis. N Engl J Med 1996;334:897–903.
27. Saarinen S, Olerup O, Broomé U. Increased frequency of autoimmune diseases in patients with primary sclerosing cholangitis. Am J Gastroenterol 2000;95:3195–9.
28. Antonelli A, Ferri C, Fallahi P, et al. Thyroid disorders in chronic hepatitis C virus infection. Thyroid 2006;16:563–72.
29. Malik R, Hodgson H. The relationship between the thyroid gland and the liver. QJM 2002;95:559–69.
30. Choudhary AM, Roberts I. Thyroid storm presenting with liver failure. J Clin Gastroenterol 1999;29:318–21.
31. Nakamura H, Noh JY, Itoh K, et al. Comparison of methimazole and propylthiouracil in patients with hyperthyroidism caused by Graves' disease. J Clin Endocrinol Metab 2007;92:2157–62.
32. Russo MW, Galanko JA, Shrestha R, et al. Liver transplantation for acute liver failure from drug induced liver injury in the United States. Liver Transpl 2004;10:1018–23.
33. Ayensa C, Diaz de Otazu R, Cia JM. Carbimazole-induced cholestatic hepatitis. Arch Intern Med 1986;146:1455.
34. Völzke H, Robinson DM, John U. Association between thyroid function and gallstone disease. World J Gastroenterol 2005;11:5530–4.
35. Uzunlulu M, Yorulmaz E, Oguz A. Prevalence of subclinical hypothyroidism in patients with metabolic syndrome. Endocr J 2007;54:71–6.
36. Liangpunsakul S, Chalasani N. Is hypothyroidism a risk factor for non-alcoholic steatohepatitis? J Clin Gastroenterol 2003;37:340–3.
37. Reddy A, Dash C, Leerapun A, et al. Hypothyroidism: a possible risk factor for liver cancer in patients with no known underlying cause of liver disease. Clin Gastroenterol Hepatol 2007;5:118–23.
38. Baker A, Kaplan M, Wolfe H. Central congestive fibrosis of the liver in myxedema ascites. Ann Intern Med 1972;77:927–9.

39. Koh LK, Greenspan FS, Yeo PP. Interferon-alpha induced thyroid dysfunction: three clinical presentations and a review of the literature. Thyroid 1997;7:891–6.
40. Fernandez-Soto L, Gonzalez A, Escobar-Jimenez F, et al. Increased risk of autoimmune thyroid disease in hepatitis C vs. hepatitis B before, during, and after discontinuing interferon therapy. Arch Intern Med 1998;158:1445–8.
41. Loria P, Carulli L, Bertolotti M, et al. Endocrine and liver interaction: the role of endocrine pathways in NASH. Nat Rev Gastroenterol Hepatol 2009;6:236–47.
42. Flohr F, Harder J, Seufert J, et al. Hypothyroidism in patients with hepatocellular carcinoma treated by transarterial chemoembolization. Hepatology 2008;47:2144.
43. Tamaskar I, Bukowski R, Elson P, et al. Thyroid function test abnormalities in patients with metastatic renal cell carcinoma treated with sorafenib. Ann Oncol 2008;19:265–8.
44. El-Serag HB, Marrero JA, Rudolph L, et al. Diagnosis and treatment of hepatocellular carcinoma. Gastroenterology 2008;134:1752–63.
45. Boulton R, Hamilton MI, Dhillon AP, et al. Subclinical Addison's disease: a cause of persistent abnormalities in transaminase values. Gastroenterology 1995;109:1324–7.
46. Milionis HJ, Dimos GA, Tsiara S, et al. Unexplained hypertransaminasaemia: clue to diagnosis of Addison's disease. Eur J Gastroenterol Hepatol 2002;14:1285–6.
47. Harry R, Auzinger G, Wendon J. The clinical importance of adrenal insufficiency in acute hepatic dysfunction. Hepatology 2002;36:395–402.
48. Tsai MH, Peng YS, Chen YC, et al. Adrenal insufficiency in patients with cirrhosis, severe sepsis and septic shock. Hepatology 2006;43:673–81.
49. Fernández J, Escorsell A, Zabalza M, et al. Adrenal insufficiency in patients with cirrhosis and septic shock: effect of treatment with hydrocortisone on survival. Hepatology 2006;44:1288–95.
50. Marik PE, Gayowski T, Starzl TE, et al. The hepatoadrenal syndrome: a common yet unrecognized clinical condition. Crit Care Med 2005;33:1254–9.
51. Marik PE. Adrenal-exhaustion syndrome in patients with liver disease. Int Care Med 2006;32:275–80.
52. Harry R, Auzinger G, Wendon J. The effects of supraphysiological doses of corticosteroids in hypotensive liver failure. Liver Int 2003;23:71–7.
53. O'Beirne J, Holmes M, Agarwal B, et al. Adrenal insufficiency in liver disease - what is the evidence? J Hepatol 2007;47:418–23.
54. Anagnostis P, Athyros VG, Tziomalos K, et al. Clinical review: the pathogenetic role of cortisol in the metabolic syndrome: a hypothesis. J Clin Endocrinol Metab 2009;94:2692–701.
55. Cerda C, Pérez-Ayuso RM, Riquelme A, et al. Nonalcoholic fatty liver disease in women with polycystic ovary syndrome. J Hepatol 2007;47:412–7.
56. Gambarin-Gelwan M, Kinkhabwala SV, Schiano TD, et al. Prevalence of nonalcoholic fatty liver disease in women with polycystic ovary syndrome. J Hepatol 2007;47:412–7.
57. Lindgren A, Olsson R. Liver damage from low-dose oral contraceptives. J Intern Med 1993;234:287–92.
58. Reyes H, Gonzalez MC, Ribalta J, et al. Prevalence of intrahepatic cholestasis of pregnancy in Chile. Ann Intern Med 1978;88:487–93.
59. Kreek MJ. Female sex steroids and cholestasis. Semin Liver Dis 1987;7:8–23.
60. Metreau JM, Dhumeaux D, Berthelot P. Oral contraceptives and the liver. Digestion 1972;7:318–35.

61. Dourakis SP, Tolis G. Sex hormonal preparations and the liver. Eur J Contracept Reprod Health Care 1998;3:7–16.
62. Maddrey WC. Hepatic vein thrombosis (Budd Chiari syndrome): possible association with the use of oral contraceptives. Semin Liver Dis 1987;7:32–9.
63. Weinberger M, Garty M, Cohen M, et al. Ultrasonography in the diagnosis and follow-up of hepatic sinusoidal dilatation. Arch Intern Med 1985;145:927–9.
64. Neuberger J, Portmann B, Nunnerley HB, et al. Oral-contraceptive-associated liver tumours: occurrence of malignancy and difficulties in diagnosis. Lancet 1980;1:273–6.
65. Adams LA, Feldstein A, Lindor KD, et al. Nonalcoholic fatty liver disease among patients with hypothalamic and pituitary dysfunction. Hepatology 2004;39: 909–14.
66. Ichikawa T, Hamasaki K, Ishikawa H, et al. Non-alcoholic steatohepatitis and hepatic steatosis in patients with adult onset growth hormone deficiency. Gut 2003;52:914.
67. Takahashi Y, Iida K, Takahashi K, et al. Growth hormone reverses nonalcoholic steatohepatitis in a patient with adult growth hormone deficiency. Gastroenterology 2007;132:938–43.
68. Wiesli P, Bernays R, Brändle M, et al. Effect of pituitary surgery in patients with acromegaly on adiponectin serum concentrations and alanine aminotransferase activity. Clin Chim Acta 2005;352:175–81.

Hematologic and Oncologic Diseases and the Liver

Marvin M. Singh, MD, Paul J. Pockros, MD*

KEYWORDS

- Hemolytic anemias • Malaria • Banti syndrome • Porphyrias
- Leukemias • Hepatic metastases

Both malignant and nonmalignant disorders may affect the liver, causing signs and symptoms ranging from mild increases of liver tests to fulminant hepatic failure (FHF). These disorders may sometimes present as primary hepatic diseases and thus be confusing to the clinician. This article outlines the most common hematologic disorders and discusses their effect on the liver in detail. The article is divided into 2 sections: nonmalignant hematologic disorders, including the anemias, paroxysmal nocturnal hemoglobinuria (PNH), disseminated intravascular coagulation (DIC), malaria, Banti syndrome, the porphyrias, thrombotic thrombocytopenic purpura (TTP), and hemolytic uremic syndrome (HUS); and malignant hematologic disorders, including leukemias, lymphomas, and myeloproliferative disorders (MPD). Other conditions causing portal hypertension are included under the nonmalignant disorders section and hepatic metastases are included in the malignant disorders section. Although not meant to be a comprehensive review, this article includes the most commonly encountered hepatic manifestations of hematologic and oncologic disorders.

NONMALIGNANT HEMATOLOGIC DISORDERS AND THE LIVER
Hemolytic Anemias

Background
The normal erythrocyte usually has a lifespan of approximately 120 days. When this length of survival is decreased to less than 100 days secondary to an increase in the rate of destruction, hemolytic anemia results. Hemolysis can be caused by either abnormalities of the erythrocyte, its membranes, or environmental (extrinsic) factors. There are many different causes of hemolytic anemia, including enzyme deficiencies, hemoglobinopathies, membrane defects, liver disease, hypersplenism, infections, and autoimmune causes, and several of these may affect the liver.

The authors have nothing to disclose.
Division of Gastroenterology and Hepatology, Scripps Clinic Torrey Pines, and The Scripps Research Institute, 10666 North Torrey Pines Road, N 203 La Jolla, CA 92037, USA
* Corresponding author.
E-mail address: pockros.paul@scrippshealth.org

Clin Liver Dis 15 (2011) 69–87
doi:10.1016/j.cld.2010.09.013
1089-3261/11/$ – see front matter © 2011 Elsevier Inc. All rights reserved.

Paroxysmal nocturnal hemoglobinuria

PNH is caused by an acquired defect of the erythrocyte membrane that results in complement-mediated hemolysis. The disease usually occurs in middle-aged adults and affects men and women equally. Patients usually present with complaints of red or dark-brown urine, often seen in the mornings. Mild hepatosplenomegaly and jaundice can occur in these patients, as it does in other hemolytic anemias.[1,2] One of the more serious complications of PNH is the development of a hypercoagulable state and the formation of thrombosis as a result of thrombogenic material released into the bloodstream after hemolysis.[1,3] Thromboses in PNH typically occur in the intracranial, hepatic, or portal vessels and thus may have devastating effects. PNH is one of the more common causes of a de novo presentation of portal vein thrombosis[1] and a rare cause of Budd-Chiari syndrome (BCS).[1] The diagnosis is suggested by the sucrose lysis test and confirmed with the acid Ham test.[1] Supportive care, treating the underlying process, and prevention of thrombotic events with anticoagulants are the mainstays of management.

Sickle cell anemia

Sickle cell anemia is a common hemoglobinopathy that affects 1 in 600 African Americans.[4] The erythrocytes form their classically described crescent shape because of homozygosity for hemoglobin S, which distorts the shape of the cells. These erythrocytes are then prone to hemolysis because of their fragility and often form clumps in the vasculature, which disrupts blood flow, causing vasoocclusive crises and injury to organs. The most common hepatic complications of sickle cell include secondary iron overload from multiple blood transfusions, and pigment cholelithiasis caused by red cell breakdown. Unlike thalassemia, ineffective erythropoiesis causing excess iron deposition in the liver does not seem to be a factor in sickle cell disease.[5]

Hyperbilirubinemia from hemolysis, infection, or intrahepatic sickling (sickle cell hepatopathy) is associated with mild to severe liver dysfunction.[6] Symptoms range from pain in the right upper quadrant, which is self-limited, to intrahepatic cholestasis and acute hepatic failure.[4] Hepatic complications affect 10% of patients who are hospitalized. Hepatomegaly may occur in up to 91% of patients with sickle cell anemia, sickle thalassemia, and sickle C disease.[4] Those who present with hepatic vasoocclusive crises typically have pain in the right upper quadrant, fever, jaundice, increase in liver tests, and hepatomegaly.

A more dreaded complication called intrahepatic cholestasis may present in a similar fashion with fever, pain in the right upper quadrant, encephalopathy, jaundice, leukocytosis, increased liver function tests, renal failure, and coagulopathy. This condition is caused by sickle cells that cause blockage in the hepatic sinusoids, vascular stasis, and hypoxia to the liver, which results in hypertrophy of the Kupffer cells and cholestasis secondary to plugging of the canaliculi.[4] Once this condition develops, liver transplantation is the only option for survival. The outcome of liver transplantation in these patients is often poor because of the risk of posttransplant hepatic artery thrombosis.[7] Other causes of hepatic failure in sickle cell disease include multiple blood transfusions, cocaine use, and intravascular hemolysis. As well, sickling may cause hepatic infarction.[4] A combination of clinical, laboratory, and imaging data (preferably computerized tomography [CT] with contrast when allowable) is used to diagnose hepatic complications of sickle cell anemia. Treatment includes hydration, analgesics, partial red blood cell exchanges, transfusions, and hydroxyurea.[4]

Malaria

Malaria is an infectious disease caused by *Plasmodium falciparum* or less commonly *Plasmodium vivax* that causes hemolysis and frequently involves the liver, a key organ in the life cycle of the parasite. After a victim is bitten by the *Anopheles* mosquito, the sporozoites travel to the liver and invade the hepatocytes. After an 8- to 12-day incubation period, merozoites are released into the circulation and invade erythrocytes, which eventually rupture, allowing the life cycle of the parasite to continue.[8]

Although the liver stage of the *Plasmodium falciparum* life cycle does not cause hepatic dysfunction, the blood stage often does. The mechanisms of liver injury are likely multifactorial, including sequestration of red cells in sinusoids and inflammation of hepatocytes.[9] In addition, hypoglycemia can occur as a result of reduced gluconeogenesis by the liver coupled with the increased glucose consumption of the parasites.[8] Malaria in pregnancy is a major cause of fetal and maternal mortality. The disease may present in pregnancy with thrombocytopenia, increase in liver tests, and/or hemolysis and can be indistinguishable from HELLP (hemolytic anemia; increased liver enzymes; low platelet count) syndrome.[9] A blood smear is key to the diagnosis of malaria and quinine sulfate is the major medication used to treat this infection worldwide.

TTP-HUS

TTP and HUS result from platelet aggregation in the microvasculature either systemically or in the renal circulation, respectively. In pregnancy, it can be difficult to distinguish preeclampsia and HELLP from TTP or HUS, because all of these conditions can be associated with microangiopathic hemolytic anemia. It is important to make the appropriate diagnosis in pregnancy because there have been reports of TTP-HUS being associated with BCS.[10] Although this hemolytic disorder is associated with thromboses in the microvasculature, there may be a common pathway by which thrombosis of the hepatic vein can occur, resulting in worsening jaundice, hepatosplenomegaly, and liver dysfunction. Diagnosis is made by imaging the hepatic vasculature, and treatment may include plasma exchange therapy for TTP and anticoagulation for BCS.[10]

Disseminated Intravascular Coagulation

Background

DIC is characterized by fibrin formation, fibrinolysis, depletion of clotting factors, thrombocytopenia, and organ damage.[11] The diagnosis of DIC may be established by a decreased fibrinogen level, increased fibrin-split products, decreased platelet count, and coagulopathy in the appropriate clinical setting. Treatment is directed at correcting the underlying process driving DIC and supportive care with blood products and factor replacement. Heparin, antithrombin III concentrates, and activated protein C have been used in certain settings as well.[12]

DIC and the liver

Those patients with severe DIC can have microvascular fibrin deposition, which causes multiorgan dysfunction. Severe hemorrhage may occur. The bleeding is caused by consumption of coagulation factors and platelets as a result of continued activation of the coagulation system.[11,13] Furthermore, research experiments with bacteremia and endotoxemia in this setting have shown that intravascular and extravascular fibrin deposition in the kidneys, lungs, brain, liver, and other organs occurs.[13] Fibrin deposition and subsequent ischemia and necrosis usually occur in small to midsized vessels.[14] This is one explanation for the liver dysfunction seen in DIC. Jaundice may occur as well and is more frequent in patients with infection, possibly for the reasons already explained.[15]

The interpretation of clotting abnormalities in cirrhotic patients is difficult. Some experts believe that DIC routinely accompanies cirrhosis, as a result of a shortened half-life of fibrinogen and the failure of factor replacement to significantly increase hemostatic factors, suggesting continuous consumption. Alternatively, some support the view that liver disease is not associated with DIC because of the low incidence of microthrombosis observed in the tissues of those who die from liver disease and because coagulopathy in patients with liver disease may be the result of causes other than DIC. An alternative hypothesis is that those with liver disease do not present with DIC but are sensitive to triggers of DIC because of the decreased ability to remove procoagulants and produce pertinent factors related to coagulation and fibrinolysis.[16] This observation might explain why patients with cirrhosis often develop worsening coagulopathy and liver failure in the setting of DIC.

Hypersplenism

Background
The spleen is considered a hematopoietic organ, which can support components of the reticuloendothelial system and, under certain conditions, can be a site of extramedullary hematopoiesis. The spleen has several other functions, including providing immune protection via its lymphoid elements (containing almost 25% of the lymphoid mass of the body), removing aging erythrocytes, and clearance of microorganisms from the circulation through the monocyte-macrophage system. Because of the role of the spleen in the hematopoietic system, cytopenias often develop when the spleen is enlarged. Some hypersplenic conditions have already been discussed in this article and include hemolytic anemias and sickle cell disease. A few other special causes of hypersplenism are discussed below.

Banti syndrome and noncirrhotic portal hypertension
Idiopathic portal hypertension or Banti syndrome is characterized by hypersplenism with resultant cytopenias and portal hypertension without portal vein obstruction or significant liver disease.[17–19] This condition is also known as hepatoportal sclerosis and noncirrhotic portal fibrosis.[18,19] The condition is characterized by an obliterative portovenopathy that leads to splenomegaly, portal hypertension, anemia, and variceal bleeding.[20] Intrasplenic and portal vein pressures and splenic and portal vein flow are significantly increased, suggesting a hyperdynamic circulatory state.[20] Most patients present solely with massive splenomegaly and complications of increased portal pressure; however, ascites, jaundice, and portosystemic encephalopathy can be seen in the setting of gastrointestinal bleeding.[20] The exact cause of idiopathic portal hypertension is not entirely clear but patients tend to have immunologic abnormalities and circulating autoantibodies.[19]

Noncirrhotic portal hypertension refers to conditions that have an increase in portal pressure as a result of intrahepatic or prehepatic lesions without underlying cirrhosis. Usually the lesions are vascular, involving the portal vein, its branches, or the presinusoidal sinusoids. The cause of this condition is unclear but one favored hypothesis is thrombosis of small and medium-sized portal veins secondary to local infection. Causes of noncirrhotic portal hypertension beside noncirrhotic portal fibrosis (Banti syndrome) include extrahepatic portal vein thrombosis, schistosomiasis, hepatic venous outflow tract obstruction, venoocclusive disease, and congenital hepatic fibrosis.[19]

One of the most significant complications of noncirrhotic portal hypertension is life-threatening gastrointestinal hemorrhage from varices. Management of bleeding should be endoscopic band ligation initially and transjugular intrahepatic

portosystemic shunt (TIPS) placement if band ligation fails. Improvement in hematological counts and reduction of portal pressure after splenectomy in Banti syndrome
have been described.[20–22]

Left-sided portal hypertension

Left-sided portal hypertension or sinistral hypertension is a presinusoidal form of
portal hypertension. The condition typically presents after splenic vein thrombosis
and presents with gastric varices (most commonly), esophageal varices, splenomegaly, normal liver function tests, and less often, ascites.[23–25] Variceal bleeding
may occur in these patients as well and, if so, treatment should be focused on the
splenic side of the portal circulation. TIPS can be hazardous in this setting and does
not address the underlying disease process. In acute gastrointestinal bleeding,
patients should be treated initially as they normally would endoscopically, but if this
is not successful, transcatheter splenic artery embolization and/or splenectomy
should be considered because this decreases the venous outflow through collateral
circulation and decompresses bleeding varices.[23]

Porphyrias

Background

Porphyrias are deficiencies, either acquired or genetic, in enzyme activity involving the
heme biosynthetic pathway. There are a total of 8 enzymes in the pathway and a deficiency in any of these may cause a form of porphyria. The syndromes result from an
accumulation of metabolic products of hemoglobin breakdown (porphyrins) and may
cause abdominal pain, psychiatric disorders, neurologic symptoms, liver abnormalities, and/or dermatologic problems. Historically, this group of disorders is classified
as being hepatic or erythroid, depending on which is the major site of production or
accumulation of metabolites[26] (**Fig. 1**).[27]

5-Aminolevulinate dehydratase-deficient porphyria (ADP), acute intermittent
porphyria (AIP), hereditary coproporphyria (HCP), and variegate porphyria (VP) make
up the acute porphyrias.[28] Porphyria cutanea tarda (PCT), congenital erythropoietic
porphyria (CEP), and hepatoerythropoietic porphyria (HEP) are the nonacute
porphyrias. PCT, CEP, and HEP may present with dermatologic findings, typically blis-
ters, ulcers, and skin fragility associated with sunlight.[28] Erythropoietic protoporphyria
(EPP), AIP and PCT are the most common types of porphyria[26] and have thus been
selected for discussion in this focused review.

Erythropoietic protoporphyria

EPP is a predominantly autosomal-dominant disorder that is associated with a partial
deficiency of ferrochelatase activity, which causes significant accumulation of protoporphyrin (PP) in erythrocytes, plasma, liver, and feces; autosomal-recessive inheri-
tance occurs but is rare.[26,27,29] The prevalence worldwide is between 1/75,000 and
1/200,000.[30] EPP appears during the childhood years and usually with dermatologic
manifestations and mild hypochromic microcytic anemia. Liver injury is common and
is associated with formation of bile cytotoxic to the biliary epithelium.[26,28] Progressive
deposition and accumulation of insoluble PP IX in hepatocytes and bile canaliculi lead to
chronic liver disease, which can be serious.[31] Mild hepatic abnormalities occur in 20%
of affected individuals, severe disease occurs in 10%, and fatal disease occurs in less
than 5%.[28] Increase in urinary coproporphyrin excretion is an early and sensitive indi-
cator of liver involvement. A decrease in fecal PP excretion is frequently seen in those
patients with decompensated cirrhosis and carries a poor prognosis.[26]

Cholelithiasis secondary to PP crystallizing in bile has been described.[31] Minor
abnormalities in aminotransferase levels are common and liver biopsy often shows

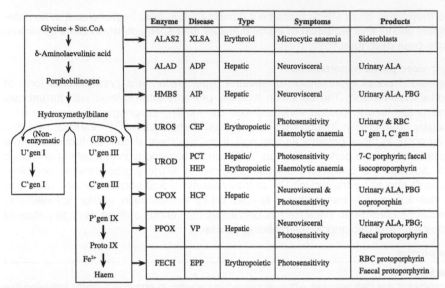

Enzyme	Disease	Type	Symptoms	Products
ALAS2	XLSA	Erythroid	Microcytic anaemia	Sideroblasts
ALAD	ADP	Hepatic	Neurovisceral	Urinary ALA
HMBS	AIP	Hepatic	Neurovisceral	Urinary ALA, PBG
UROS	CEP	Erythropoietic	Photosensitivity Haemolytic anaemia	Urinary & RBC U' gen I, C' gen I
UROD	PCT HEP	Hepatic/ Erythropoietic	Photosensitivity Haemolytic anaemia	7-C porphyrin; faecal isocoproporphyrin
CPOX	HCP	Hepatic	Neurovisceral & Photosensitivity	Urinary ALA, PBG coproporphin
PPOX	VP	Hepatic	Neurovisceral Photosensitivity	Urinary ALA, PBG; faecal protoporphyrin
FECH	EPP	Erythropoietic	Photosensitivity	RBC protoporphyrin Faecal protoporphyrin

Flow diagram (left side):
Glycine + Suc.CoA → δ-Aminolaevulinic acid → Porphobilinogen → Hydroxymethylbilane → (Non-enzymatic) U'gen I → C'gen I; (UROS) U'gen III → C'gen III → P'gen IX → Proto IX → Fe²⁺ → Haem

Fig. 1. Classification of the enzymatic defects, associated diseases, major symptoms, and principal accumulation products of porphyria are shown. ALAS2 defect is responsible for X-linked sideroblastic anemia (XLSA) but is not associated with any porphyria, because the enzymatic defect blocks production of ALA, the obligatory precursor for porphyrin formation. ALA dehydratase porphyria (ADP) and AIP are accompanied by acute hepatic porphyria but not by photocutaneous porphyria, because their enzymatic defects do not result in an increase in porphyrin synthesis. Enzymatic defects beyond uroporphyrinogen synthase (UROS) are all associated with photocutaneous porphyrias, because they produce excessive amounts of various porphyrins. HCP and VP are additionally associated with acute hepatic porphyria. Suc.CoA, succinyl coenzyme A; P'gen, rotoporphyrinogen; Proto, protoporphyrin; U'gen, uroporphyrinogen; C'gen, coproporphyrinogen. (*From* Sassa S. Modern diagnosis and management of the porphyrias. Br J Haematol 2006;135:281–92; with permission.)

some evidence of damage as an early feature of disease.[31] Histology may show cholestasis and fibrosis, and in more severe cases, micro- or macronodular cirrhosis with extensive deposits of dark pigment in hepatocytes, Kupffer cells, macrophages, and bile canaliculi. The pigmented deposits are birefringent and have a distinctive Maltese-cross appearance under polarized microscopy. In end-stage liver disease, the liver may contain so much PP that it appears black.[28]

When it progresses to decompensated cirrhosis, EPP can be fatal in the absence of liver transplantation. However, transplantation does not correct the underlying metabolic disorder, and PP damage can recur in the allograft. Therapies that may serve as a bridge to transplant include ursodeoxycholic acid (to increase excretion of PP into the bile); iron, red blood cell transfusions, or hematin infusions (to reduce the drive for heme synthesis); plasmapheresis, hemodialysis, and exchange transfusions (to reduce circulating PP); cholestyramine and activated charcoal (to reduce PP levels by interrupting the enterohepatic circulation); and intravenous vitamin E (to reverse oxidative stress).[31] Decompensation of the liver presents in the usual fashion in EPP; however, rapidly worsening photosensitivity may signify the onset of fulminant liver failure. Some patients are diagnosed with EPP initially when they present with acute liver failure.

Patients with progressive EPP liver disease may present with crises caused by various triggers. When this process progresses to cirrhosis, liver transplantation has been shown to effectively treat these patients.[32,33] Because there is a significant likelihood of recurrent liver disease in EPP after transplantation, some have proposed and successfully shown that bone-marrow transplant after liver transplant can be curative because it corrects the deficiency of ferrochelatase activity.[32,34] Sequential liver and bone-marrow transplant has been performed with success in a few cases.[30] Patient and graft survival rates after liver transplant have been reported to be 85% at 1 year, 69% at 5 years, and 47% at 10 years, with recurrence rate of EPP liver disease in 65% for those surviving more than 2 months.[32]

Acute intermittent porphyria

AIP is a multisystem disease with a prevalence of 1 to 2 per 100,000, and presents with a wide range of clinical features, most notably abdominal pain with neuropsychiatric features.[35] This condition is an autosomal-dominant disorder secondary to a partial deficiency of porphobilinogen (PBG)-deaminase activity.[26] The diagnosis is confirmed by excess urinary excretion of aminolevulinic acid (ALA) and PBG. Triggers include certain drugs, hormonal factors, fasting, alcohol, infections, and tobacco.[35] Mild abnormalities in liver function occur in acute porphyria, although these are usually not clinically significant.[36]

Patients with acute hepatic failure caused by AIP and VP have been successfully treated with liver transplantation.[36] Also, because acute attacks in AIP are associated with increased hepatic production of 5-ALA and PBG, restoring normal hepatic PBG-deaminase activity should prevent future attacks. One such case of resolution of AIP attacks by liver transplant has been reported.[37]

There is a strong association between AIP and the development of primary hepatocellular carcinoma (HCC), even in the absence of cirrhosis.[27,37] Reduced heme synthesis and oxidative damage to DNA may induce carcinogenic mutations in the hepatocyte.[26] Twenty-seven percent of patients who carry the mutation W198X in the PBG-D gene eventually develop HCC.[38] A French study showed this risk of HCC to be 36 times higher than in a nonporphyric population of comparable age and sex.[27]

Porphyria cutanea tarda

PCT is associated with diminished activity of uroporphyrinogen decarboxylase (UROD).[39] In PCT, the liver disease leads to the onset of porphyria, which presents with blistering, hirsutism, and skin fragility. Hemochromatosis, alcoholic liver disease, and hepatitis C are some of the liver diseases that are associated with PCT.[31] Approximately 50% of US patients with PCT are infected with chronic hepatitis C (CHC).[40] Treatment of the underlying infection resolves the skin disorder in most cases associated with CHC. Management is otherwise directed at skin protection from ultraviolet light (sunblock, long sleeves, cloth gloves), abstinence, and phlebotomy to achieve a reduction in heme synthesis.[41] These patients are often diagnosed by a dermatologist and referred to a hepatologist for abnormal liver panel tests. A liver biopsy is seldom necessary to confirm diagnosis because the urine test for UROD is easy to perform and is inexpensive.[29]

MALIGNANT HEMATOLOGIC DISORDERS AND THE LIVER
Leukemia

Background
Leukemia is a myeloproliferative disorder (MPD) that is caused by an acquired clonal abnormality of the hematopoietic stem cell of myeloid precursors. In some of these

disorders, there are specific chromosomal abnormalities, which have been identified. In this section, we review some instances in which leukemia can affect the liver.

Hairy cell leukemia

Hairy cell leukemia (HCL) is a rare, chronic leukemia that usually has an indolent course, caused by B cells in the circulation that have characteristic filamentous projections. Patients present with cytopenias and splenomegaly.[42] The abnormal cells also infiltrate the portal tracts and sinusoids of the liver, resulting in hepatomegaly in approximately 40% of patients.[5] Involvement in the liver can be diffuse infiltration, discrete nodular masses, or angiomatous lesions, with leukemic cells and blood cells filling the sinusoids. Patients rarely may be jaundiced and often have increased levels in liver function tests.[42] The difference in disease course and prognosis of a patient with diffuse liver infiltration versus nodular involvement is not clear, nor is the mechanism by which nodular lesions are produced.[42] Treatment is directed at the HCL and has been successful with oral outpatient therapies including cladribine.[43]

Chronic lymphoid leukemia

Patients with chronic lymphoid leukemia (CLL) may show mild to moderate hepatomegaly and extensive lymphocytic infiltration in the portal tracts, resulting in hepatic dysfunction in the later stages of disease.[5] The development of portal hypertension is uncommon. However, there is evidence in the literature that it is feasible to develop splenomegaly, portal hypertension, and bleeding esophageal varices in the absence of regenerative nodular hyperplasia or significant liver infiltration, favoring the role of increased splenic-portal blood flow.[44] This is a similar mechanism of portal hypertension to that described earlier in Banti syndrome.

CLL is generally indolent and most patients are symptom-free for years.[45] However, in 3.3% to 10.6% of patients with CLL, Richter transformation can occur, in which a high-grade non-Hodgkin lymphoma (NHL) or Hodgkin lymphoma (HL) develops. This situation may be triggered by a viral infection such as Epstein-Barr virus (EBV) and/or be related to chromosomal abnormalities.[46] Most of these patients have weight loss, fever, increasing lymphadenopathy, and hepatosplenomegaly; acute liver failure has been described as well. Prognosis is poor and the median survival after this condition occurs can be approximately 6 months.[45] The key to treating acute liver failure as a result of Richter transformation is making the appropriate tissue diagnosis and initiating chemotherapy rapidly, because success has been reported in treating patients in this manner.

Acute leukemia

Although hepatic involvement is usually silent at the time of diagnosis, greater than 95% of patients with acute lymphocytic leukemia (ALL) and 75% of patients with acute myeloid leukemia (AML) have hepatic infiltration at autopsy.[47] In ALL, the infiltration is in the portal tracts, while in AML it is in both the portal tracts and sinusoids.[5] When patients have overwhelming leukemic infiltration, FHF may result.[5]

ALL is a common acute leukemia in the pediatric population, and FHF caused by ALL has been described in children. The pathogenesis is not clear but may be related to comorbid viral infections, sepsis, or ischemic hepatopathy with submassive necrosis resulting from obstruction of hepatic blood flow by infiltrating leukemic cells.[48] In any child who presents with FHF, acute leukemia should be considered in the differential diagnosis, especially if there is hepatosplenomegaly, pancytopenia, and an increased lactate dehydrogenase.[49]

AML usually does not cause liver injury as a presenting feature; however, there have been reported cases of obstructive jaundice and cholestatic hepatitis secondary to sinusoidal infiltration, which improved with chemotherapy.[50] Acute megakaryoblastic leukemia is a rare type of AML that occurs in 3% to 5% of cases and may present with thrombocytopenia, liver failure, and ascites secondary to massive infiltration of hepatic sinusoids by leukemic cells.[51]

An important condition is venoocclusive disease of the liver or sinusoidal obstruction syndrome. This is an established complication of high-dose cytoreductive chemotherapy before bone-marrow transplantation, which is often the treatment chosen for the aforementioned leukemias. Although it is not common, significant vasoocclusive disease may also occur with less intense induction therapy for ALL.[52]

Lymphoma

Hodgkin's lymphoma
Background Hodgkin's lymphoma (HL) or Hodgkin's disease is a group of malignancies that arise in lymphoid tissue and spread in a contiguous fashion via the lymph system. HL is characterized by identification of the Reed-Sternberg cell, giant lymphocytes derived from B cells, within the appropriate cellular background. There is a bimodal age distribution of the disorder. Patients may have a variable presentation and liver involvement is possible.[53]

Hepatic manifestations of HL Lymphomatous cells may infiltrate the liver in up to 15% of patients with hepatomegaly and 45% in the later stages of disease. Cholestasis can occur as a result of direct infiltration, extrahepatic biliary obstruction, hemolysis, viral hepatitis, or drug hepatotoxicity.[5,54] In approximately 3% to 13% of patients jaundice is the presenting symptom in HL.[54] Acute liver failure can occur in the setting of hepatic infiltration and is usually preceded by a prodrome including malaise, weight loss, pain in the right upper quadrant, fever, and jaundice.[55] One of the mechanisms by which malignant infiltration may cause liver failure is ischemia secondary to the compression of the hepatic sinusoids by the infiltrating cells.[45] Cholestasis in zone 3 has been described as the result of vanishing bile duct syndrome associated with HL, a syndrome that causes irreversible destruction of the small intrahepatic bile ducts and leads to significant liver damage.[5] The mechanism by which this syndrome occurs is poorly understood but may be a paraneoplastic effect, a defect in liver microsomal function, or a toxic effect of cytokines released from lymphoma cells.[56] Other causes of this vanishing bile duct syndrome should be considered in the differential diagnosis before attributing it to HL.[54] Even with adequate treatment of lymphoma, most of these patients die of liver failure. Also, they often experience lymphoma progression because of the difficulty in giving them potentially hepatotoxic agents.[57]

Non-Hodgkin's lymphoma
Background The NHLs are a large and diffuse group of malignancies involving mutations of B and T cells that essentially include all lymphomas other than HL. Compared with HL, this type of lymphoma is more common, it spreads in a less-contiguous fashion, and it usually affects patients over the age of 60 years. Treatment, survival, and presenting symptoms differ between NHL and HL but discussion in this article focuses on hepatic involvement only.

Hepatic manifestations of NHL Lymphomatous infiltration and extrahepatic obstruction occur more commonly in NHL than in HL; 16% to 43% of patients with NHL have liver involvement. Infiltrating disease is found more often in low-grade lymphomas than in those that are high-grade. Mild to moderate increases in alkaline phosphatase level and hepatomegaly commonly occur in NHL whether or not there is lymphomatous hepatic involvement.[5]

As described earlier with HL, acute liver failure can also occur in NHL. The mechanism by which this occurs is likely similar to that in HL, with sudden ischemia related to massive infiltration of the sinusoids or replacement of liver parenchyma by malignant cells.[58] This condition should be suspected when a patient presents with new-onset hepatomegaly and lactic acidosis, and prompt evaluation including liver biopsy should ensue.[5] Submassive necrosis has been described in those patients with the cytotoxic phenotype of peripheral T-cell lymphoma and is often fatal.[59] Although the prognosis is poor, there have been reports of successful treatment with immediate initiation of chemotherapy.[58]

Primary hepatic NHL Primary NHL of the liver encompasses less than 1% of all extranodal lymphomas and occurs primarily in men (two-thirds of cases) around the age of 50 years. Although the cause is unclear, some hypothesize the involvement of viral hepatitis or EBV. Patients typically present with right-upper-quadrant or epigastric pain, fever, anorexia, nausea, hepatomegaly, and abnormal liver tests with a greater increase of lactate dehydrogenase than alanine aminotransferase.[60,61] The most common type of primary hepatic NHL is diffuse large B-cell lymphoma, comprising 80% to 90% of the cases. This disease may present with nodules in the liver or diffuse portal infiltration and sinusoidal spread.[62] Rapid identification of this type of lymphoma is critical so that appropriate chemotherapy can be initiated in a timely manner. Because this condition is uniformly fatal, patients with FHF from primary hepatic lymphoma have been treated with liver transplantation and subsequent chemotherapy.[63] The long-term success of this approach has not been substantiated and is probably poor.

Hepatosplenic T-cell lymphoma (HSTCL) is a rare and aggressive form of NHL associated with patients using antitumor necrosis factor α (anti-TNF) therapy and purine analogues together to treat inflammatory bowel disease (IBD).[64] Patients typically have hepatosplenomegaly, increased levels in liver-function tests, fever, weight loss, night sweats, pancytopenia, and peripheral lymphocytosis. Thiopurines are involved in the induction of apoptosis, possibly leading to the development of malignancy. This situation, together with the effect that anti-TNF therapy can have on T cells (complement-mediated lysis and apoptosis), may partially explain why patients treated with these agents are at risk.[65] Histology can resemble that seen in autoimmune hepatitis and may lead to misdiagnosis. If HSTCL is suspected, a bone-marrow biopsy should be performed to confirm the diagnosis.[64]

Hemophagocytic syndrome Hemophagocytic syndrome (HPS) is a severe hyperinflammatory condition that can clinically mimic sepsis and presents with prolonged fever, significant cytopenias, hepatosplenomegaly, and hemophagocytosis in bone marrow, spleen, and lymph nodes.[66,67] Essentially, HPS is a result of hypercytokinemia, which is triggered by highly stimulated natural killer (NK) and cytotoxic T cells. HPS has been described in patients with lymphomas, immunodeficiency syndromes, rheumatic disorders, and viral infections (usually EBV).[68] The diagnosis of HPS should be suspected if the patient has at least 5 of the following 8 criteria: fever, splenomegaly, cytopenia, hypertriglyceridemia (>3.0 mmol/L fasting value), low fibrinogen level (<1.5 g/L), hemophagocytosis on bone-marrow biopsy, low or absent NK-cell activity, increased ferritin level (>500 μg/L), or soluble CD-25 level greater than 2400 IU/mL.[66]

Significant hepatic manifestations of HPS have been described, including hepatomegaly, jaundice with cholestasis, moderate transaminitis, hyperferritinemia, decreased hepatic synthetic function, and FHF. Injury to the liver is attributed to the hemophagocytosis in the hepatic sinusoids and portal tracts or focal hepatocellular necrosis.[68] Although this uncontrolled immune response can cause significant hepatic dysfunction, death usually occurs as a result of multiorgan failure. Prognosis is generally poor, with treatment limited to corticosteroids, rituximab, and/or immunoglobulin infusions.[68,69]

Chronic Myeloproliferative Disorders

Background

The major MPDs include polycythemia vera (PV), essential thrombocythemia (ET), and agnogenic myeloid metaplasia (also known as idiopathic myelofibrosis [IMF]). These disorders are classified as being Philadelphia chromosome negative and are characterized by an overproduction of certain cell types: PV is caused by an overproduction of red blood cells; ET is caused by an overproduction of platelets; and IMF is caused by red blood cells and granulocytes that do not mature properly. The hepatic manifestations in this group of hematologic disorders are similar.

Hepatic manifestations of MPD

The hepatic circulatory system is most affected by MPD, causing BCS, portal vein thrombosis, and/or nodular regenerative hyperplasia (NRH).[70] Patients may present with acute or chronic BCS as a result of the prothrombotic and hyperviscous state seen in PV.[5,71] When BCS occurs, the liver becomes hypoxic acutely, causing injury and necrosis. It is possible that the surge in erythropoietin (Epo) levels that occurs in this setting is related to spillage from necrotic liver tissue, because small amounts of Epo are produced in the adult liver. This situation may confuse the diagnosis of PV in a patient with BCS, which is usually associated with a low Epo level, but other diagnostic tools such as analysis for the V617F point mutation of the Janus 2 tyrosine kinase (JAK2), have helped to make the diagnosis easier.[71] Testing for JAK2 secures a diagnosis of occult MPD in those who previously were believed to have BCS of unclear cause. After PV, ET is also commonly associated with BCS.[70,72] On rare occasions, when a patient has PV and factor V Leiden mutation, they can present with fulminant BCS. Liver transplantation has been performed successfully in these patients using hydroxyurea with aspirin after transplant to prevent hepatic artery thrombosis. If the prothrombotic state is not corrected by transplant, the other complications of thrombosis and bleeding should be anticipated.[70,73]

Portal vein thrombosis may also occur in MPD, more commonly in PV and ET.[74] After the thrombosis occurs, collaterals often develop, resulting in cavernous transformation of the portal vein. Patients usually present with variceal hemorrhage, but may be seen with abdominal pain related to mesenteric ischemia.[70] Many of these patients can also have the JAK2 mutation, and screening for this in patients with portal vein thrombosis may prove useful to recognize patients with occult MPD or those at risk of developing MPD.[74]

NRH is described as the development of micronodules in the liver parenchyma that do not communicate via fibrotic septa. IMF and PV are a few of the conditions associated with NRH. The hypercoagulable state in MPD predisposes the patient to developing thromboses in the small portal venules. It is believed that NRH occurs when there is a differential perfusion of the liver with focal or segmental impairment of the circulation at the portal venule or sinusoid level, resulting in ischemia, apoptosis, and atrophy in the areas of the liver that do not have optimal perfusion. This situation, in turn, results in reactive hyperplasia, which is the cardinal histologic feature of NRH.[70] In patients with IMF, NRH following obstruction of the intrahepatic portal

Table 1
Summary of hematologic and oncologic diseases and the liver

	Category	Manifestations	Management	Key Point(s)
Paroxysmal nocturnal hemoglubinuria	Hemolytic anemia	Dark urine in morning, HSM, J, T	SC, treat underlying process	Diagnosed by sucrose lysis and acid Ham tests
Sickle cell anemia	Hemolytic anemia	Fever, T, AP, HM, J, LFT	Hydration, analgesics, transfusion, hydroxyurea	Affects 1:600 African Americans; OLT for intrahepatic cholestasis
Malaria	Hemolytic anemia	Fever, hypoglycemia, LFT	Quinine sulfate	Blood smear for Dx; *Plasmodium falciparum or vivax*
TTP-HUS	Hemolytic anemia	T, J, HSM, LFT	Plasma exchange, anticoagulation	Important to identify in pregnancy
DIC	DIC	Bleeding, T, J, LFT	Treat underlying process, supportive care	Heparin, antithrombin III, activated protein C may be useful
Banti syndrome	Hypersplenism	SM, anemia, bleeding, ascites, J, T	Manage bleeding, splenectomy	No underlying liver disorder
Left-sided portal hypertension	Hypersplenism	T, varices, SM, LFT, ascites	Manage bleeding, splenic artery embolization, splenectomy	TIPS is contraindicated
EPP	Porphyria	LFT, cholelithiasis, liver failure	Ursodeoxycholic acid, transfusion, hematin, plasma exchange, dialysis, cholestyramine, vitamin E, OLT	Autosomal-dominant, partial deficiency of ferrochelatase activity
AIP	Porphyria	AP, neuropsychiatric features, LFT, liver failure, HCC	OLT, eliminate triggers	Autosomal-dominant, partial deficiency of PBG-deaminase activity
PCT	Porphyria	Blistering, hirsutism, skin fragility	Treat underlying process, skin protection, phlebotomy	Caused by liver disease
HCL	Leukemia	HSM, cytopenia, diffuse infiltration, J, LFT	Chemotherapy (cladribine)	B cells with filamentous projections

Chronic lymphocytic leukemia	Leukemia	HSM, lymphocytic infiltration, LFT, varices	Chemotherapy	Richter transformation may cause liver failure
Acute leukemia	Leukemia	Liver infiltration, fulminant liver failure, HSM, cytopenias, J, LFT, ascites	Chemotherapy	Consider vasoocclusive disease as a complication of chemotherapy
HL	Lymphoma	Lymphomatous infiltration, HM, cholestasis, AP, fever, J	Chemotherapy	Reed-Sternberg cell; vanishing bile duct syndrome
NHL	Lymphoma	Lymphomatous infiltration, LFT, HM	Chemotherapy	More common than HL
Primary hepatic NHL	Lymphoma	AP, fever, nausea, HM, LFT, diffuse portal infiltration	Chemotherapy	Most commonly in men; <1% of extranodal lymphomas; HSTCL with anti-TNF therapy in IBD
HPS	Lymphoma	Fever, cytopenia, HSM, J, LFT, hemophagocytosis	Steroids, rituximab, immunoglobulin infusion	Severe hyperinflammatory condition (hypercytokinemia)
MPDs	MPDs	T, liver failure, variceal bleeding, AP	Treat thrombotic complications, OLT, hydroxyurea, aspirin	Diagnosed with JAK2 assay
Hepatic metastases	Solid tumors with hepatic metastases	Malaise, AP, HM, J, ascites, acute liver failure	Surgical resection, chemotherapy, chemoembolization, interferon, radiofrequency ablation	Usually from GI tract, pancreas, breast, lung, bladder, head/neck, prostate, or ocular melanoma

Abbreviations: AP, abdominal pain; Dx, diagnosis; GI, gastrointestinal; HM, hepatomegaly; HSM, hepatosplenomegaly; J, jaundice; LFT, abnormal LFTs; OLT, orthotopic liver transplant; SC, supportive care; SM, splenomegaly; T, thromboses.

vein branches has been associated with augmentation of portal hypertension.[5] This condition can lead to variceal hemorrhage, splenomegaly, and ascites.[70]

Other liver involvement frequently seen in MPDs are caused by extramedullary hematopoiesis, increased hepatic blood flow, or secondary hemosiderosis from multiple blood transfusions. Portal hypertension is found in up to 7% of patients.[5] Portopulmonary hypertension has also been described when the diagnosis of latent or atypical MPD is made.[75] Occasionally, MPD transforms to leukemia and causes extensive infiltration in the liver, resulting in hepatic decompensation, as described earlier.[72,76]

MALIGNANT SOLID TUMORS WITH HEPATIC METASTASES
Background

The liver is frequently involved as a site of metastasis from malignant solid tumors. Multiple liver lesions seen in a normal liver by imaging usually indicate this diagnosis. Liver metastases generally involve both lobes of the liver, occurring as a solitary lesion only 20% of the time.[77] Liver metastases are most commonly associated with malignancy from the gastrointestinal tract (commonly the colon, esophagus, and stomach), pancreas (including neuroendocrine tumors), breast, lung, bladder, head and neck, ocular melanoma, and prostate.[77,78]

The reason why the liver is a common site for metastases is because of its large blood supply, originating from portal and systemic circulation.[79] This discussion excludes HCC, because it usually involves cirrhotic patients and those with chronic hepatitis B, and other primary liver tumors, because they are beyond the scope of this topic.

Hepatic Metastases

Patients with hepatic metastases can present with malaise, epigastric or right-upper-quadrant abdominal pain, hepatomegaly, jaundice, or ascites. Increased levels in liver function tests are also often noted, as are coagulopathy and hypoalbuminemia. Acute liver failure has been described with diffuse infiltrating malignant tumors. Liver failure is attributed to hypoxic hepatocellular necrosis secondary to diffuse sinusoidal infiltration and invasion of the vasculature by metastases.[80]

Various imaging modalities can be used to further investigate hepatic metastases. CT typically shows metastases from colorectal cancer to have a characteristic appearance with irregular margins and necrotic centers. During the early arterial phase of CT, metastases have increased enhancement and the sensitivity of this imaging modality can be increased with CT arterial portography.[77] Magnetic resonance imaging (MRI) can be used to better evaluate hypervascular lesions and is equally effective at diagnosis of hepatic metastases. Most hepatic metastases, even those that are hypovascular, show arterial hypervascularity on contrast-enhanced ultrasound that would not be appreciated on CT or MRI.[81,82] Positron emission tomography/CT is helpful in staging colon, lung, and breast cancers. Intraoperative ultrasound has high sensitivity and specificity for metastatic disease from colorectal adenocarcinoma.[77] Somatostatin receptor scintigraphy can be used to localize 90% of neuroendocrine tumor hepatic metastases.[77] Once the lesion is identified, one can pursue an ultrasound- or CT-guided liver biopsy or fine-needle aspiration to confirm the diagnosis, but this may not always be necessary.

Treatment of hepatic metastases may include surgical resection. Approximately 10% to 25% of cases are suitable for surgery and much of this depends on the extent and location of the metastases in addition to the patient's overall health and baseline liver function.[83] For hepatic colorectal cancer metastases, performing laparoscopic liver resections has been reported to be safe, with disease-free survivals at 1 and 3 years being 74% and 51%, respectively.[84] Advantages of laparoscopic resection can include minimal scarring, fewer adhesions, and increased feasibility of performing a repeat resection in the future.[85] Neuroendocrine tumors of the pancreas are often metastatic to the liver as well, and surgical resection in this setting may also offer the patient some benefit. However, much of the time the liver metastases are bilateral and curative resection or tumor debulking is not possible. Management could include chemotherapy, chemoembolization, or interferon. If the patient has unresectable tumors and untreatable symptoms from hepatic metastases caused by a pancreatic neuroendocrine tumor, liver transplantation can be performed, but has not been shown to change long-term prognosis.[86,87]

As stated earlier, although resection is a favorable approach to hepatic metastases, often this is not possible. Therefore, managing these patients requires a multidisciplinary approach. Radiofrequency ablation can be effective and safe, especially with lesions less than 3 cm in those with metastases from unknown primary.[79] Chemotherapy, either systemic or via hepatic artery infusion, can be used and can increase survival, particularly in colorectal cancer. Multiagent chemotherapy, including FOLFOX, FOLFIRI, and FOLFOXIRI, has shown improved outcomes in patients with hepatic metastases from colorectal cancer. Chemotherapy can also provide patients who initially have unresectable hepatic metastases with the opportunity to undergo a resection.[88]

SUMMARY

This article outlines in some detail the most common hematologic and oncologic disorders that affect the liver. Both nonmalignant hematologic disorders, including the anemias, PNH, DIC, malaria, Banti syndrome, the porphyries, TTP, HUS, and malignant hematologic disorders, including leukemias, lymphomas and myeloproliferative disorders, may cause liver injury. Liver injury ranging from mild increases of aminotransferase levels to conditions causing portal hypertension, acute liver failure, and often death are discussed. Although not meant to be a comprehensive review, this article includes the most commonly encountered hepatic manifestations of hematologic and oncologic disorders (**Table 1**) that a hepatologist is likely to encounter in any tertiary practice.

REFERENCES

1. Shah A. Acquired hemolytic anemia. Indian J Med Sci 2004;58(12):533–6.
2. Gehrs BC, Friedberg RC. Autoimmune hemolytic anemia. Am J Hematol 2002; 69(4):258–71.
3. Muncie HL, Campbell JS. Alpha and beta thalassemia. Am Fam Physician 2009; 80(4):339–44.
4. Norris WE. Acute hepatic sequestration in sickle cell disease. J Natl Med Assoc 2004;96(9):1235–9.
5. Shimizu Y. Liver in systemic disease. World J Gastroenterol 2008;14(26):4111–9.
6. Bandyopadhyay R, Bandyopadhyay SK, Dutta A. Sickle cell hepatopathy. Indian J Pathol Microbiol 2008;51:284–5.
7. Emre S, Kitibayashi K, Schwartz ME, et al. Liver transplantation in a patient with acute liver failure due to sickle cell intrahepatic cholestasis. Transplantation 2000; 69(4):675–7.
8. Beeson JG, Brown GV. Pathogenesis of *Plasmodium falciparum* malaria: the roles of parasite adhesion and antigenic variation. Cell Mol Life Sci 2002;59:258–71.

9. Ducarme G, Thuillier C, Wernet A, et al. Malaria in pregnant woman masquerading as HELLP syndrome. Am J Perinatol 2010;27(2):171–2.
10. Hsu HW, Belfort MA, Vernino S, et al. Postpartum thrombotic thrombocytopenic purpura complicated by Budd-Chiari syndrome. Obstet Gynecol 1995;85 (5 Pt 2):839–43.
11. Mammen EF. Disseminated intravascular coagulation (DIC). Clin Lab Sci 2000; 13(4):239–45.
12. Levi M. Current understanding of disseminated intravascular coagulation. Br J Haematol 2004;124(5):567–76.
13. Levi M, de Jonge E, van der Poll T. New treatment strategies for disseminated intravascular coagulation based on current understanding of the pathophysiology. Ann Med 2004;36(1):41–9.
14. Levi M, de Jonge E, van der Poll T. Sepsis and disseminated intravascular coagulation. J Thromb Thrombolysis 2003;16(1–2):43–7.
15. Siegal T, Seligsohn U, Aghai E, et al. Clinical and laboratory aspects of disseminated intravascular coagulation (DIC): a study of 118 cases. Thromb Haemost 1978;39(1):122–34.
16. Levi M, de Jonge E, van der Poll T, et al. Advances in the understanding of the pathogenetic pathways of disseminated intravascular coagulation result in more insight in the clinical picture and better management strategies. Semin Thromb Hemost 2001;27(6):569–75.
17. Turner JD. Banti's disease: evolution of thought. McGill Med J 1956;25(4):187–99.
18. Cordeau M, Prosmanne O, Robillard P. Cases of the day. Noncirrhotic idiopathic portal hypertension (Banti syndrome). Radiographics 1990;10(1):114–6.
19. Okuda K. Non-cirrhotic portal hypertension versus idiopathic portal hypertension. J Gastroenterol Hepatol 2002;17(Suppl 3):S204–13.
20. Sarin SK. Non-cirrhotic portal fibrosis. J Gastroenterol Hepatol 2002;17(Suppl): S214–23.
21. Sato T, Suda Y, Watanabe S, et al. Mechanism of hematological disorders in Banti's syndrome. Tohoku J Exp Med 1967;93(2):163–78.
22. Spaander VM, van Buuren HR, Janssen HL. Review article: the management of non-cirrhotic non-malignant portal vein thrombosis and concurrent portal hypertension in adults. Aliment Pharmacol Ther 2007;26(Suppl 2):203–9.
23. Köklü S, Coban S, Yüksel O, et al. Left-sided portal hypertension. Dig Dis Sci 2007;52(5):1141–9.
24. Cichoz-Lach H, Celiński K, Słomka M, et al. Pathophysiology of portal hypertension. J Physiol Pharmacol 2008;59(Suppl 2):231–8.
25. Evans GR, Yellin AE, Weaver FA, et al. Sinistral (left-sided) portal hypertension. Am Surg 1990;56(12):758–63.
26. Gross U, Hoffmann GF, Doss MO. Erythropoietic and hepatic porphyrias. J Inherit Metab Dis 2000;23(7):641–61.
27. Sassa S. Modern diagnosis and management of the porphysis. Br J Haematol 2006;135(3):281–92.
28. Schneider-Yin X, Harms J, Minder EI. Porphyria in Switzerland, 15 years experience. Swiss Med Wkly 2009;139(13–14):198–206.
29. Meerman L. Erythropoietic protoporphyria. An overview with emphasis on the liver. Scand J Gastroenterol Suppl 2000;232:79–85.
30. Lecha M, Puy H, Deybach JC. Erythropoietic protoporphyria. Orphanet J Rare Dis 2009;4:19.
31. Anstey AV, Hift RJ. Liver disease in erythropoietic protoporphyria: insights and implications for management. Gut 2007;56(7):1009–18.

32. McGuire BM, Bonkovsky HL, Carithers RL Jr, et al. Liver transplantation for erythropoietic protoporphyria liver disease. Liver Transpl 2005;11(12):1590–6.

33. Zhang F, Lu L, Qian X, et al. Liver transplantation for erythropoietic protoporphyria with hepatic failure: a case report. Transplant Proc 2008;40(5):1774–6.

34. Rand EB, Bunin N, Cochran W, et al. Sequential liver and bone marrow transplantation for treatment of erythropoietic protoporphyria. Pediatrics 2006;118(6): e1896–9.

35. Herrick AL, McColl KE. Acute intermittent porphyria. Best Pract Res Clin Gastroenterol 2005;19(2):235–49.

36. Seth AK, Badminton MN, Mirza D, et al. Liver transplantation for porphyria: who, when, and how? Liver Transpl 2007;13(9):1219–27.

37. Soonawalla ZF, Orug T, Badminton MN, et al. Liver transplantation as a cure for acute intermittent porphyria. Lancet 2004;363(9410):705–6.

38. Ventura P, Cappellini MD, Rocchi E. The acute porphyrias: a diagnostic and therapeutic challenge in internal and emergency medicine. Intern Emerg Med 2009; 4(4):297–308.

39. Pimstone NR. Hematologic and hepatic manifestations of the cutaneous porphyrias. Clin Dermatol 1985;3(2):83–102.

40. Sterling RK, Bralow S. Extrahepatic manifestations of hepatitis C virus. Curr Gastroenterol Rep 2006;8(1):53–9.

41. Yachimski P, Shah N, Chung RT. Porphyria cutanea tarda. Clin Gastroenterol Hepatol 2007;5(2):e6.

42. Sahar N, Schiby G, Davidson T, et al. Hairy cell leukemia presenting as multiple discrete hepatic lesions. World J Gastroenterol 2009;15(35):4453–6.

43. Huynh E, Sigal D, Saven A. Cladribine in the treatment of hairy cell leukemia: initial and subsequent results. Leuk Lymphoma 2009;50(Suppl 1):12–7.

44. Wilputte JY, Martinet JP, Nguyen P, et al. Chronic lymphocytic leukemia with portal hypertension and without liver involvement: a case report underlining the roles of increased spleno-portal blood flow and "protective" sinusoidal vasoconstriction. Acta Gastroenterol Belg 2003;66(4):303–6.

45. Shehab TM, Kaminski MS, Lok AS. Acute liver failure due to hepatic involvement by hematologic malignancy. Dig Dis Sci 1997;42(7):1400–5.

46. Omoti CE, Omoti AE. Richter syndrome: a review of clinical, ocular, neurological and other manifestations. Br J Haematol 2008;142(5):709–16.

47. Sharma Poudel B, Karki L. Abnormal hepatic function and splenomegaly on the newly diagnosed acute leukemia patients. JNMA J Nepal Med Assoc 2007; 46(168):165–9.

48. Litten JB, Rodríguez MM, Maniaci V. Acute lymphoblastic leukemia presenting in fulminant hepatic failure. Pediatr Blood Cancer 2006;47(6):842–5.

49. Kader A, Vara R, Egberongbe Y, et al. Leukaemia presenting with fulminant hepatic failure in a child. Eur J Pediatr 2004;163(10):628–9.

50. Wandroo FA, Murray J, Mutimer D, et al. Acute myeloid leukaemia presenting as cholestatic hepatitis. J Clin Pathol 2004;57(5):544–5.

51. Lewis MS, Kaicker S, Strauchen JA, et al. Hepatic involvement in congenital acute megakaryoblastic leukemia: a case report with emphasis on the liver pathology findings. Pediatr Dev Pathol 2008;11(1):55–8.

52. Papadopoulos A, Ntaios G, Kaiafa G, et al. Veno-occlusive disease of the liver during induction therapy for acute lymphoblastic leukemia. Int J Hematol 2008; 88(4):441–2.

53. Punnett A, Tsang RW, Hodgson DC. Hodgkin lymphoma across the age spectrum: epidemiology, therapy, and late effects. Semin Radiat Oncol 2010;20(1):30–44.

54. Guliter S, Erdem O, Isik M, et al. Cholestatic liver disease with ductopenia (vanishing bile duct syndrome) in Hodgkin's disease: report of a case. Tumori 2004;90(5):517–20.

55. Rowbotham D, Wendon J, Williams R. Acute liver failure secondary to hepatic infiltration: a single centre experience of 18 cases. Gut 1998;42(4):576–80.

56. Hubscher SG, Lumley MA, Elias E. Vanishing bile duct syndrome: a possible mechanism for intrahepatic cholestasis in Hodgkin's lymphoma. Hepatology 1993;17(1):70–7.

57. Leeuwenburgh I, Lugtenburg EP, van Buuren HR, et al. Severe jaundice, due to vanishing bile duct syndrome, as presenting symptom of Hodgkin's lymphoma, fully reversible after chemotherapy. Eur J Gastroenterol Hepatol 2008;20(2): 145–7.

58. Saló J, Nomdedeu B, Bruguera M, et al. Acute liver failure due to non-Hodgkin's lymphoma. Am J Gastroenterol 1993;88(5):774–6.

59. Ohtani H, Komeno T, Koizumi M, et al. Submassive hepatocellular necrosis associated with infiltration by peripheral T-cell lymphoma of cytotoxic phenotype: report of two cases. Pathol Int 2008;58(2):133–7.

60. Masood A, Kairouz S, Hudhud KH, et al. Primary non-Hodgkin lymphoma of liver. Curr Oncol 2009;16(4):74–7.

61. Haider FS, Smith R, Khan S. Primary hepatic lymphoma presenting as fulminant hepatic failure with hyperferritinemia: a case report. J Med Case Reports 2008; 2:279.

62. Baumhoer D, Tzankov A, Dirnhofer S, et al. Patterns of liver infiltration in lymphoproliferative disease. Histopathology 2008;53(1):81–90.

63. Cameron AM, Truty J, Truell J, et al. Fulminant hepatic failure from primary hepatic lymphoma: successful treatment with orthotopic liver transplantation and chemotherapy. Transplantation 2005;80(7):993–6.

64. Rosh JR, Gross T, Mamula P, et al. Hepatosplenic T-cell lymphoma in adolescents and young adults with Crohn's disease: a cautionary tale? Inflamm Bowel Dis 2007;13(8):1024–30.

65. Beigel F, Jürgens M, Tillack C, et al. Hepatosplenic T-cell lymphoma in a patient with Crohn's disease. Nat Rev Gastroenterol Hepatol 2009;6(7):433–6.

66. Créput C, Galicier L, Buyse S, et al. Understanding organ dysfunction in hemophagocytic lymphohistiocytosis. Intensive Care Med 2008;34(7):1177–87.

67. Janka GE. Hemophagocytic syndromes. Blood Rev 2007;21(5):245–53.

68. de Kerguenec C, Hillaire S, Molinié V. Hepatic manifestations of hemophagocytic syndrome: a study of 30 cases. Am J Gastroenterol 2001;96(3):852–7.

69. Rouphael NG, Talati NJ, Vaughan C, et al. Infections associated with haemophagocytic syndrome. Lancet Infect Dis 2007;7(12):814–22.

70. Poreddy V, DeLeve LD. Hepatic circulatory diseases associated with chronic myeloid disorders. Clin Liver Dis 2002;6(4):909–31.

71. Thurmes PJ, Steensma DP. Elevated serum erythropoietin levels in patients with Budd-Chiari syndrome secondary to polycythemia vera: clinical implications for the role of JAK2 mutation analysis. Eur J Haematol 2006;77(1):57–60.

72. Briere JB. Essential thrombocythemia. Orphanet J Rare Dis 2007;2:3.

73. Akyildiz M, Karasu Z, Dheir H, et al. Fulminant Budd-Chiari syndrome associated with polycythemia rubra vera and factor V Leiden mutation. Eur J Intern Med 2006;17(1):66–7.

74. Colaizzo D, Amitrano L, Tiscia GL, et al. The JAK2 V617F mutation frequently occurs in patients with portal and mesenteric venous thrombosis. J Thromb Haemost 2007;5(1):55–61.

75. Ito H, Adachi Y, Arimura Y, et al. A 25-year clinical history of portopulmonary hypertension associated with latent myeloproliferative disorder. J Gastroenterol 2003;38(5):488–92.

76. Holcombe RF, Treseler PA, Rosenthal DS. Chronic myelomonocytic leukemia transformation in polycythemia vera. Leukemia 1991;5(7):606–10.

77. Assy N, Nasser G, Djibre A, et al. Characteristics of common solid liver lesions and recommendations for diagnostic workup. World J Gastroenterol 2009; 15(26):3217–27.

78. Dawood O, Mahadevan A, Goodman KA. Stereotactic body radiation therapy for liver metastases. Eur J Cancer 2009;45(17):2947–59.

79. Mylona S, Stroumpouli E, Pomoni M, et al. Radiofrequency ablation of liver metastases from cancer of unknown primary site. Diagn Interv Radiol 2009;15(4): 297–302.

80. Alexopoulou A, Koskinas J, Deutsch M, et al. Acute liver failure as the initial manifestation of hepatic infiltration by a solid tumor: report of 5 cases and review of the literature. Tumori 2006;92(4):354–7.

81. Jang HJ, Kim TK, Wilson SR. Imaging of malignant liver masses: characterization and detection. Ultrasound Q 2006;22(1):19–29.

82. Jang HJ, Yu H, Kim TK. Contrast-enhanced ultrasound in the detection and characterization of liver tumors. Cancer Imaging 2009;9:96–103.

83. Barugel ME, Vargas C, Krygier Waltier G. Metastatic colorectal cancer: recent advances in its clinical management. Expert Rev Anticancer Ther 2009;9(12): 1829–47.

84. Nguyen KT, Gamblin TC, Geller DA. World review of laparoscopic liver resection–2,804 patients. Ann Surg 2009;250(5):831–41.

85. Zhang L, Chen YJ, Shang CZ, et al. Total laparoscopic liver resection in 78 patients. World J Gastroenterol 2009;15(45):5727–31.

86. Lang H, Schlitt HJ, Schmidt H, et al. Total hepatectomy and liver transplantation for metastatic neuroendocrine tumors of the pancreas–a single center experience with ten patients. Langenbecks Arch Surg 1999;384(4):370–7.

87. Lang H, Oldhafer KJ, Weimann A, et al. Liver transplantation for metastatic neuroendocrine tumors. Ann Surg 1997;225(4):347–54.

88. Alberts SR. Updated options for liver-limited metastatic colorectal cancer. Clin Colorectal Canc 2008;7(Suppl 2):S58–62.

Hepatobiliary Manifestations of Gastrointestinal and Nutritional Disorders

Jason B. Samarasena, MD[a], Ke-Qin Hu, MD[b],*

KEYWORDS

- Hepatobiliary manifestations • Liver disease
- Primary sclerosing cholangitis • Celiac disease
- Whipple's disease • Parenteral nutrition

Hepatobiliary manifestations of gastrointestinal and nutritional disorders can occur as part of the clinical spectrum of the underlying disease or as a consequence of the treatment of the disease. These manifestations can be relatively common as is the association between primary sclerosing cholangitis (PSC) and ulcerative colitis, or very rare as in the hepatic manifestations in Whipple's disease. Their clinical significance can also vary from being inconsequential to a condition that could be severe. These conditions often represent a unique set of challenges for the practicing clinician. This article reviews aspects of the pathogenesis, diagnosis, and management of hepatobiliary manifestations associated with a selection of gastrointestinal and nutritional disorders.

HEPATOBILIARY MANIFESTATIONS OF INFLAMMATORY BOWEL DISEASE

Liver and biliary tract diseases commonly occur in patients with inflammatory bowel disease (IBD). In the case of PSC there is an unclear yet well-defined link between the intestinal disease and development of biliary tract abnormalities. In other cases, the agents used to treat IBD result in the development of liver disease such as with the use of thiopurines. The next section highlights these and other hepatobiliary manifestations related to IBD and its treatment.

PSC

PSC is a rare chronic cholestatic liver disease the cause of which is uncertain. It is characterized by segmental inflammation and fibrosing of the intrahepatic and/or

---

The authors have nothing to disclose.
[a] Division of Gastroenterology, University of California Irvine Medical Center, 101 The City Drive, City Tower, Suite 400, Zot 4092, Orange, CA 92868, USA
[b] Division of Gastroenterology and Hepatology, University of California, Irvine School of Medicine, 101 The City Drive, Orange, CA 92868, USA
* Corresponding author.
E-mail address: kqhu@uci.edu

Clin Liver Dis 15 (2011) 89–110
doi:10.1016/j.cld.2010.09.003
1089-3261/11/$ – see front matter © 2011 Elsevier Inc. All rights reserved.

extrahepatic bile ducts leading to the formation of multifocal bile duct strictures.[1] Approximately 60% to 80% of all patients with PSC have concomitant IBD[2] and PSC-IBD may represent a distinct phenotype of IBD.[3]

Epidemiology

The epidemiology of PSC in the general population has not been well defined but prevalence is estimated to be around 6.3 to 20 cases per 100,000 persons.[4–6] It is estimated that approximately 4% of patients with ulcerative colitis (UC) develop PSC and that UC is present in up to 70% to 80% of patients with PSC.[7] PSC is more prevalent in patients with UC pancolitis than those with distal colitis with 1 study showing a prevalence of approximately 5.5% and 0.5%, respectively.[8] Patients with UC and PSC more frequently have rectal sparing and backwash ileitis than patients with UC without PSC.[3] PSC also occurs in 1.4% to 3.4% of patients with Crohn's disease, which typically manifests as extensive colitis.[9] PSC is not believed to occur in association with Crohn's disease isolated to the small intestine.[9] Racial differences in the association between PSC and IBD likely exist, as concomitant IBD is seen in only 21% of Japanese patients with PSC.[10]

Causes and pathogenesis

The causes and pathogenesis of PSC remain poorly understood. Evidence supports that PSC represents an immunologic reaction in genetically susceptible persons who are exposed to environmental or toxic triggers. Proposed mechanisms include increased absorption of colonic toxins, portal bacteremia, viral infections, and ischemic injury.

Genetic factors First-degree relatives of patients with PSC are know to have an increased risk of PSC and UC, thus supporting a genetic predisposition.[11] The strongest association with susceptibility to PSC maps to HLA-B8 and HLA-DR3.[12] A relationship may exist between the non–major histocompatibility complex genes and PSC susceptibility, although this has yet to be confirmed.[13] No significant association between any of the IBD susceptibility genes and overall susceptibility to PSC has so far been observed.[14]

Immunologic factors Patients with PSC have increased levels of immunoglobulins, including autoantibodies. PSC is also associated with other autoimmune diseases; most commonly type 1 diabetes mellitus and Graves disease.[15] Antinuclear antibody (ANA) is present in 8% to 77% of patients with PSC, anti–smooth muscle antibody (SMA) is present in up to 83%. The prevalence of perinuclear antineutrophil cytoplasmic antibody (pANCA) ranges from 26% to 94% and a comparable prevalence of ANCA is reported in autoimmune hepatitis (AIH) and UC.[16] Antimitochondrial antibody (AMA) may represent one of the most useful autoantibodies in the diagnosis of cholestatic liver disease, because AMA is virtually absent in PSC patients compared with a 90% to 95% prevalence in primary biliary cirrhosis (PBC).[17] Other autoantibodies seen with PSC include anticardiolipin, antiendothelial cell, antithyroid peroxidase, antiglomerular basement membrane, antisulfite oxidase, and rheumatoid factor.[16] One study reported the presence of antibodies against isolated biliary epithelial cells (BEC) in 63% of patients with PSC. Anti-BEC antibody induced BEC to produce interleukin-6 (IL-6) and the adhesion molecule CD44, strongly suggesting pathogenetic importance.[18] A follow-up study showed that sera from patients with PSC with anti-BEC stimulated BEC to express toll-like receptors, leading to BEC cytokine production and recruitment of inflammatory cells,[19] further supporting that BECs may not only be targets of immune attack but may also be active participants and mediators of their own destruction potentially playing a significant role in PSC pathogenesis. However, the hypothesis that PSC is an autoimmune disease fails to explain some differences between PSC and autoimmunity, which include the absence of female predilection, the absence of disease specific autoantibodies, and a poor response to immunosuppressive medications.

Bacterial infection The strong association between PSC and colitis has led to the theory that increased permeability of the inflamed colon wall leads to penetration of infectious or toxic agents into the portal system leading to recurrent cholangitis, or chronic inflammation in the biliary tree.[20] However, the evidence to support this theory has been contradictory. Furthermore, the toxic injury hypothesis does not explain the observation that PSC is not associated with the severity of inflammation in patients with IBD and may develop years after total proctocolectomy.

Vascular injury The similar clinical, chemical, and cholangiographic appearance found after disruption of the biliary vascular supply after surgery has led to postulation that ischemia plays a role in the pathogenesis of PSC, but the data to support this theory are limited.[21]

Natural history and prognostic models
PSC is typically a progressive disease and may progress through 4 distinct clinical phases: asymptomatic phase, biochemical phase, symptomatic phase, and decompensated cirrhosis. According to one study the estimated time from diagnosis to death or orthotopic liver transplant (OLT) was 9.6 years with 39.6% of patients undergoing OLT.[4] Independent risk factors correlating with poor prognosis included age, hypoalbuminemia, persistently increased bilirubin for more than 3 months, splenomegaly, history of IBD, and histologic stage.[4,22,23] Small-duct PSC is characterized by histology consistent with PSC in the setting of normal cholangiography and its natural history is believed to be less aggressive than large-duct PSC. Multivariate prognostic models have been designed to predict survival in patients with PSC although recent guidelines recommend against their use as their ability to predict outcomes in an individual patient may be limited.[2]

Despite the strong association between PSC and UC, the 2 diseases often progress independently of each other. PSC may be diagnosed in a patient with UC years after proctocolectomy and conversely, newly diagnosed UC may occur after liver transplantation for end-stage liver disease as a result of PSC.[24] It is for this reason that a high index of suspicion for the development of IBD is warranted for patients with PSC. Full colonoscopy with random mucosal biopsies throughout the colon is recommended for all patients with a new diagnosis of PSC.[2] There is no conclusive evidence that the natural history of PSC varies between patients with and without IBD, however, it does seem that the bowel disease in patients with PSC tends to run a more quiescent course than in patients without PSC.[3]

Clinical features
The diagnosis of PSC is based on a combination of clinical symptoms, biochemical abnormalities, and most importantly cholangiographic and histologic findings. The most common symptoms at presentation are jaundice, fatigue, pruritus, and abdominal pain. Other associated symptoms include fevers, chills, night sweats, and weight loss. The most common clinical signs include hepatomegaly, jaundice, and splenomegaly. Disease onset is typically insidious and increasingly PSC is diagnosed at an asymptomatic stage likely because of the growing use of biochemical testing in patients with IBD and widespread availability of endoscopic retrograde

cholangiopancreatography (ERCP) and magnetic resonance cholangiopancreatography (MRCP) for evaluating increased serum alkaline phosphatase (ALP) levels.

Laboratory findings

Chronic increase in serum ALP levels, typically 3 to 5 times normal, is the biochemical hallmark of PSC, although normal ALP values may be found in up to 6% of patients with cholangiographically or biopsy proven PSC.[25] Serum aminotransferase levels are typically increased, although rarely to more than 4 to 5 times the upper limit of normal, except in the pediatric population.[26] Serum bilirubin levels can be increased and fluctuate with the disease course. Depending on the time of presentation, there may be coagulation abnormalities and reductions in serum albumin levels that may reflect hepatic synthetic dysfunction with advanced disease. As previously stated, levels of various immune markers can be abnormal in patients with PSC especially pANCA, although they rarely have a role in diagnosis.[2]

Imaging

Diagnosis of PSC is primarily established by demonstration of characteristic multifocal, short, annular strictures alternating with normal or slight dilation of intrahepatic and/or extrahepatic bile ducts (ie, the classic beaded appearance) on cholangiography by endoscopic retrograde cholangiography (ERC), magnetic resonance cholangiography (MRC), or percutaneous transhepatic cholangiography (PTC). ERC was regarded as the gold standard in diagnosing PSC, however given its invasive nature and potential complications, MRC has become the diagnostic modality of choice when PSC is suspected. However, ERC still has a useful role when MRC views may not be optimal.[2] Both intrahepatic and extrahepatic bile ducts are affected in 75% of cases of PSC, whereas intrahepatic duct involvement alone occurs in 15% to 20% of cases. Extrahepatic biliary tree abnormality alone is much less common. Major areas of focal, tight narrowing, known as dominant strictures, may be seen and often involve the common bile duct or the hepatic duct bifurcation.[27] Dominant strictures should raise suspicion for the presence of cholangiocarcinoma because this malignant complication occurs frequently as a stenotic lesion in the perihilar region (**Fig. 1**).[2]

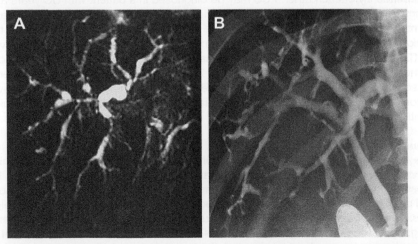

Fig. 1. Magnetic resonance cholangiogram (A) and endoscopic retrograde cholangiogram (B) in a patient with PSC. (*Courtesy of* Angela Levy, MD, Washington, DC.)

Pathology
Classic histologic features include bile duct proliferation, periductal fibrosis and inflammation, ductal obliteration, and loss of bile ducts. Histologic abnormalities typically are often nonspecific and distinction between other liver disorders, especially PBC, can often be difficult.[28] Fibrous obliterative cholangitis, a finding where interlobular and septal bile duct branches are obliterated entirely, is believed to be highly diagnostic for PSC although is present in only 5% to 10% of biopsy specimens.[29] As a result, in the presence of an abnormal cholangiogram, a liver biopsy is not required to establish a diagnosis of large-duct PSC. However, a liver biopsy is essential in the evaluation of patients with suspected small-duct PSC and with possible overlap syndromes.[2]

Complications
Complications common to chronic cholestasis develop in patients with PSC and include fatigue, pruritis, steatorrhea, fat-soluble vitamin deficiencies (A, D, E, K), and metabolic bone disease. Pruritis is one of the most common symptoms of PSC and can be debilitating and may severely affect quality of life. The pathogenesis of pruritis in chronic cholestasis is poorly understood. Nutritional deficiencies may occur because of poor absorption of fat-soluble vitamins A, D, E, and K as a result of reduced intestinal concentrations of conjugated bile acids. Metabolic bone disease, referred to as hepatic osteodystrophy, can result in osteoporosis in chronic cholestatic liver diseases. Bone mineral densitometry of the lumbar spine should be performed in patients with PSC at the time of diagnosis and thereafter at 2- to 3-year intervals to detect osteoporosis.[2] In patients with hepatic osteopenia, daily calcium and vitamin D should be supplemented. In patients with hepatic osteoporosis, in addition to calcium and vitamin D, bisphosphonate therapy should be used.[2] Cholelithiasis and choledocholithiasis are more common in patients with PSC than in the general population and may be present in 30% of patients,[30] often with pigmented calcium bilirubinate stones.[31] Patients with worsening jaundice or cholestasis should undergo ERCP or MRCP, which enables a search for choledocholithiasis and differentiation of biliary stone disease from a dominant stricture or cholangiocarcinoma.

Neoplasia PSC should be considered a premalignant condition as it increases the risk for cholangiocarcinoma (CCA), colorectal and gallbladder neoplasia. CCA is a feared complication of PSC and can arise from bile duct epithelium anywhere in the biliary tract. It unfortunately remains the leading cause of death in patients with PSC with a 10% to 15% lifetime risk and a 5-month median survival after diagnosis.[32] The pathogenesis of CCA is poorly understood although chronic inflammation is believed to predispose to epithelial dysplasia and malignant transformation. Risk factors for the development of CCA include UC with colonic dysplasia/carcinoma and the duration of IBD.[33] The diagnosis of cholangiocarcinoma is often challenging in patients with PSC as CCA tends to grow in sheets as opposed to a discrete mass and is often indistinguishable from the stricturing of progressive PSC. Several tumor markers for cholangiocarcinoma have been evaluated, with CA 19-9 being used most commonly. Sensitivity and specificity vary and are also dependent on the presence of cholangitis and biliary cholestasis.[34] One study showed sensitivity and specificity of 79% and 99%, respectively, for a patient with PSC with a serum CA 19-9 level greater than 129 U/mL, although the positive predictive value in this study was 59%.[35] Brush cytology performed at ERCP has a sensitivity of only as high as 40%, but in combination with tumor markers, diagnostic yield increases.[36] Recently, fluorescent in situ hybridization (FISH) has shown increased sensitivity for the diagnosis of CCA in patients with PSC than cytology alone.[37] Endoscopic ultrasound-guided fine-needle aspiration has also shown promise in the diagnosis of suspected cholangiocarcinoma.[38] Studies have not determined clear risk factors for cholangiocarcinoma and an optimal screening strategy has yet to be defined.[2]

Evidence suggests that patients with concomitant PSC and UC are at significantly higher risk for the development of colonic neoplasia than patients with UC alone with odds ratio (OR) of 4.79 (95% confidence interval [CI] 3.58–6.41).[39] The mechanism by which PSC confers added risk is unknown. Patients with PSC and UC should undergo surveillance colonoscopy at 1- to 2-year intervals from the time of diagnosis.[2]

PSC seems to confer an increased risk for gallbladder polyps and carcinoma.[40] As a result, patients with PSC should undergo an annual ultrasound examination to detect mass lesions, and cholecystectomy for patients with PSC in whom a mass lesion is detected regardless of the lesion size is recommended.[2]

Treatment
The management approach to PSC is multidisciplinary and includes medical and surgical therapies depending on stage of the disease.

Medical therapy No medical therapies to date have been shown to definitively alter the course of PSC. Ursodeoxycholic acid (UDCA) is a hydrophilic bile acid and is the most extensively studied of all medical treatments for PSC. UDCA is believed to work by protection of cholangiocytes against cytotoxic hydrophobic bile acids, stimulation of hepatobiliary secretion, and protection of hepatocytes against bile acid–induced apoptosis and induction of antioxidants.[41] At a dose of up to 15 mg/kg/d UDCA has shown efficacy in improving biochemical abnormalities, stabilizing liver inflammation, but has not resulted in a survival benefit or a delay in the need for liver transplantation.[42] Higher dose (20–30 mg/kg/d) UDCA may increase benefit, but it has been associated with higher rates of serious adverse events including a greater likelihood of reaching the primary end point of death, need for liver transplant, or development of varices.[43]

Liver transplantation Liver transplantation is the only specific therapy proved to improve the natural history of PSC and has also been shown to improve quality of life after transplantation.[44,45] Long-term outcomes for liver transplantation in PSC are good relative to transplantation for other indications and 5-year survival has been shown to be as high as 86%.[46] For patients with PSC there are special circumstances in which transplantation may be indicated despite a low priority Model for End-Stage Liver Disease score; these include recurrent or refractory cholangitis, intractable pruritus, and cholangiocarcinoma.[2]

IBD drug-induced hepatotoxicity
Thiopurines The thiopurine agents azathioprine and 6-mercaptopurine are commonly used for induction and maintenance of remission in patients with both UC and Crohn's disease. These medications can cause a spectrum of hepatic injury with the overall prevalence of thiopurine-induced liver disorders estimated to be 1% per patient per year of treatment.[47] A hypersensitivity syndrome can be seen usually within 2 to 3 weeks of medication onset and the laboratory picture is one of cholestatic injury with increased serum bilirubin and ALP levels with moderate increases in aminotransferases. Occasionally, a purely cholestatic pattern is seen and histologically this is accompanied by variable parenchymal necrosis. Nodular regenerative hyperplasia, venoocclusive disease, peliosis hepatis, fibrosis, and sinusoidal dilatation related to thiopurine toxicity are all believed to be dose-dependent and may occur between 3 months and 3 years after treatment.[47] The optimal liver test monitoring schedule

remains to be established, but some authorities state that a monthly liver test is the optimal frequency at the start of therapy.

Methotrexate Methotrexate is an immune modulating therapy used to treat Crohn's disease and UC and has been found to induce clinical remission more rapidly than azathioprine and 6-mercaptopurine. Methotrexate has been associated with macro-vesicular steatosis, hepatic fibrosis, and cirrhosis in a cumulative dose-response fashion. The incidence of increased alanine aminotransferase with methotrexate is estimated at 14%.[48] Patients using methotrexate should have liver function tests monitored at 4- to 12-week intervals based on duration of therapy. A pretreatment biopsy should be considered for patients with a history of excessive prior alcohol consumption, persistently abnormal baseline aspartate aminotransferase values, or chronic hepatitis B or C infection.[49]

HEPATOBILIARY MANIFESTATIONS OF CELIAC DISEASE

Celiac disease (CD), also known as gluten-sensitive enteropathy or celiac sprue, is defined as a permanent intolerance to ingested gluten, the storage protein components of wheat, barley, and rye. The disease results in immune-mediated damage to the mucosa of the small intestine characteristically inducing villous atrophy and crypt hyperplasia that resolves with the removal of gluten from the diet. Although the disease primarily affects the intestinal tract, CD is a typical example of a multi-system disorder with involvement of multiple other tissues and organs including the liver. Transglutaminase type 2 (TG2) has been identified as the main CD autoantigen and has a ubiquitous body distribution and therefore may play a large role in the systemic manifestations related to the disease. Systemic involvement may include skin, thyroid disease, pancreas, heart, joints, muscles, bones, reproductive system, central and peripheral nervous system, and the liver.[50] The following is a review of the hepatic manifestations of CD.

Prevalence of Liver Disease in CD

Celiac disease is often associated with a mild chronic increase in serum aminotransferase levels and this has been reported in about 40% of adults and 54% of children with a classic presentation of CD at the time of diagnosis.[51-53] In some cases of CD, hypertransaminasemia is the only clinical sign without any other gastrointestinal symptoms. CD may account for between 4% and 9% of abnormal liver function tests of unexplained cause.[50,54]

Pathogenesis

The mechanism underlying liver injury in CD is poorly understood. Aminotransferase levels seem to improve with removal of gluten from the diet suggesting a causal relationship between gluten intake, intestinal damage, and liver injury. Intestinal permeability is increased in CD and this may facilitate the entry of toxins, antigens, and inflammatory cytokines to the portal circulation. These mediators may have a role in the liver involvement seen in patients with CD.[53,55] Autoantibodies against tissue transglutaminase (tTG) are present in the liver raising the possibility of humoral-mediated liver injury.[56]

Clinical Manifestations

Most patients with liver injury associated with CD are asymptomatic but exhibit a mild chronic increase in serum aminotransferase levels with aspartate aminotransferase ranging from 29 to 80 IU/L and alanine aminotransferase ranging from 60 to 130 IU/L.[57]

CD rarely can also be associated with more severe forms of liver disease including cirrhosis, and CD has been found to be associated with an 8-fold increased risk of death from liver cirrhosis.[58] Hypoalbuminemia and prolonged prothrombin time may suggest cirrhosis, although can also be indirect markers of severe malabsorption.[59]

Histologic Findings

Histologic findings in patients with CD who undergo liver biopsy are generally mild and nonspecific and can include periportal inflammation, bile duct obstruction, increased number of Kupffer cells, mononuclear infiltration in the parenchyma, steatosis, and fibrosis.[60]

Response to a Gluten-free Diet

In patients with mild liver disease, a gluten-free diet (GFD) leads to normalization of serum transaminases in 75% to 90% of patients with CD usually within 6 to 12 months of good adherence.[51] Histologic changes of the liver also normalize after adherence to a GFD.[51,53,60] There has also been marked clinical improvement in patients with advanced liver disease and CD with improvement in bilirubin, internationalized normalized ratio, jaundice, and ascites reported. In one patient, liver transplantation was avoided.[61] Thus, CD needs to be excluded before a diagnosis of cryptogenic cirrhosis is established and CD should be suspected in those with risk factors including a positive family history of CD or dermatitis herpetiformis, those who have the HLA-DQ2 or HLA-DQ8 haplotypes, type 1 diabetes mellitus, premature osteoporosis, or osteomalacia.[62]

Autoimmune Liver Disorders Associated with Celiac Disease

Several autoimmune liver disorders including PBC, autoimmune hepatitis, and PSC have been associated with CD.

PBC

PBC is a progressive autoimmune disease of the liver. It is unique among autoimmune diseases in that 95% of those affected are female and rarely occurs in childhood or before the age of 30 years.[63] The incidence of PBC has been estimated to be 2.7 per 100,000 person years.[22] Fatigue and pruritis are the most common presenting symptoms.[64] Common findings in patients with PBC include hyperlipidemia, hypothyroidism, osteopenia, and coexisting autoimmune disease.[65] The diagnosis of PBC is based on the presence of detectable antimitochondrial antibodies in serum, increased liver enzymes (most commonly alkaline phosphatase) for more than 6 months, and histologic findings that are compatible with the disease.

The association of CD and PBC was originally reported by Logan and colleagues[66] in 1978. More recently, 2 large population-based studies have strongly supported an association between CD and PBC,[67,68] which has prompted screening for CD in patients with PBC with the reported prevalence ranging between 0% and 11%.[69] Loss of weight, malabsorption, osteopenic bone disease, steatorrhea, and increased alkaline phosphatase are common features of both diseases, so that early in their coexistence, CD or PBC may not be easily appreciated.

Several pathophysiologic processes are shared in CD and PBC. Increased intestinal permeability is an abnormality in CD that has also been shown in PBC and can lead to increased exposure to the liver of intestine-derived antigens via the portal circulation.[70,71] An immunologic mechanism in both the pathogenesis of PBC and CD is supported by the observation that PBC and CD are frequently associated with other autoimmune disorders such as scleroderma, autoimmune thyroid disease, and kera-toconjunctivitis sicca.[65]

Studies evaluating the effect of a GFD on patients with both CD and PBC have failed to show improvement in liver blood tests and clinical symptoms of PBC. One study showed that liver blood tests did not improve in patients with silent CD and PBC after 12 to 24 months on a GFD despite the disappearance of antiendomysial antibody in the serum.[70,71] Despite this, the early recognition and treatment of CD is recommen-ded, as GFD improves symptoms attributable to CD and can reduce the risk of compli-cations including malabsorption, osteoporosis, and malignant neoplasms.[69,72]

Autoimmune hepatitis

The prevalence of CD in patients with AIH was found to be 4% and 6.4% in two studies and was found in type 1 and type 2 AIH.[73,74] In one study after 6 months of GFD, there was overall clinical improvement with regrowth of small intestinal mucosa and improved absorption of nutrients but autoimmune liver disease was largely unaffected by the GFD.[50,73] At this time, the data on concurrent AIH and CD is limited and the clin-ical effect of GFD on the liver disease of patients with IH remains to be elucidated. Nevertheless, the benefits of early detection and treatment of CD in patients with AIH includes normal absorption of medication and calcium with maintenance of skel-etal integrity and prevention of osteoporosis in patients with AIH treated with corticosteroids.[50]

PSC

PSC was initially found to be associated with celiac disease in 1988 in 3 patients with diarrhea and steatorrhea.[75] Since then, the relationship between CD and PSC has been substantiated in multiple reports[50] with the prevalence of CD in patients with PSC estimated at 1.6%.[76] CD and PSC are both believed to be immune-mediated diseases and there seems to be a shared immunogenetic basis that may partially explain the association between the two diseases. The HLA-DR3/DQ2 heterozygous genotype was found to be associated with a rapidly progressive course of PSC[77] and this same genotype is considered one of the major genetic risk factors for the development of CD.[78] It is unclear if the clinical course of PSC is affected by GFD.[75,79,80]

Viral Hepatitis and Celiac Disease

There is no clear association between CD and viral hepatitis C and the prevalence of CD in hepatitis C virus (HCV)-related chronic hepatitis is not different from that of CD in the general population. Nevertheless, because these diseases are relatively common, CD should be considered in patients who develop unexplained diarrhea during treatment.

Patients with CD may have a significant genetic predisposition to not responding to the standard hepatitis B vaccine with 2 studies showing failure rates of 54% in children and 68% in adults with CD. The defective vaccine response seems to be linked to the HLA genotype DQ2.[81]

Diagnosis of Celiac Disease in Patients with Chronic Liver Disorders

Antitissue transglutaminase antibody (tTGA) is used largely as a screening tool for CD, however false-positive results are more likely to occur in patients with chronic liver disease.[82] In the first generation of tTGA tests, tTG derived from guinea pig liver was used and false-positives may have been caused by antigens present in the crude extract of pig liver. Specificity improved when tTG derived from human red cells or generated recombinantly from human tTG sequences was used. However, false-positives could still occur.[83] As a result, a proposed algorithm for evaluating for CD in a patient with chronic liver disease includes following up a positive tTG with the endomysial antibody test and then, if this is positive, confirming with an intestinal biopsy.[69]

HEPATOBILIARY MANIFESTATIONS OF WHIPPLE'S DISEASE

Whipple's disease is an extremely rare chronic systemic disease that can affect almost any organ in the body and is caused by a gram-positive bacillus related to Actinomycetes named *Tropheryma whipplei* (formerly called *Tropheryma whippelii*).[84] The disorder has a striking predilection for white males of European descent.[85] The pathogenesis of the disease remains unclear. Invasion or uptake of the bacillus is widespread throughout the body including the intestinal epithelium, macrophages, capillary and lymphatic endothelium, colon, liver, brain, heart, lungs, synovium, kidney, bone marrow, and skin with all of these sites showing a remarkable lack of inflammatory response to the bacillus. The diagnosis is established by small bowel biopsy, which shows inclusions in macrophages of the lamina propria positive with periodic acid-Schiff (PAS) stain. Polymerase chain reaction testing of various tissues and fluid can also be used to make the diagnosis.[86] The 4 cardinal clinical manifestations of the disease include arthralgias, weight loss, diarrhea, and abdominal pain. Patients usually present with migratory arthralgias of the large joints, which may precede other symptoms by many years. Later in the disease, diarrhea and weight loss often progress. Depending on organ involvement, symptoms related to cardiac disease, pleuropulmonary disease, or neurologic disease can ensue. While untreated the disease is chronic, progressive, and fatal but many patients treated with antibiotics achieve rapid clinical remission.[87]

Liver involvement of Whipple's disease is uncommon and is described in only a few case reports. Patients may present with right upper quadrant pain, abnormal liver function tests, hepatomegaly, and rarely jaundice. One case report describes a patient who presented with painless hepatomegaly and fever who was found to have diagnostic small bowel biopsies and granulomas on liver biopsy.[88] Another report describes a case of Whipple's disease complicated by fatal hepatitis.[89] Misra and colleagues[90] describe a case of Whipple's disease with diagnostic bacillary bodies on liver and appendiceal biopsies.

The treatment of Whipple's disease is antibiotic therapy, and the antibiotic regimen is often tailored for specific organ involvement. For patients who are severely ill, recommended antibiotics included parenteral ceftriaxone (2 g, once daily) or penicillin (2 MU, every 4 hours) for 2 weeks followed by trimethoprim and sulfamethoxazole (TMP-SMX) (1 double strength tablet twice daily) for at least 1 year to prevent relapse. Other antibiotics used successfully for treatment include doxycycline and streptomycin.[87]

HEPATOBILIARY MANIFESTATIONS OF TOTAL PARENTERAL NUTRITION

Total parenteral nutrition (TPN) has become established as a life-saving treatment of patients with acute and chronic intestinal failure. Both children and adults receiving TPN are at risk for developing a range of hepatic complications related to this treatment. TPN-induced hepatobiliary complications range from mild increases in liver transaminase levels to severe hepatic dysfunction including cirrhosis. The range of hepatobiliary complications related to TPN, the risk factors for development of parenteral nutrition–associated liver disease (PNALD), and management strategies is reviewed in the following sections.

Prevalence of TPN-related Hepatobiliary Complications

The reported prevalence rates of PNALD vary greatly among studies and the issue is complicated further because most studies have relied on liver enzyme and bilirubin concentrations to define hepatic dysfunction rather than liver biopsy. Hepatobiliary complications are common in both infants and adults receiving TPN. In the pediatric age group, the prevalence has been reported in the range of 20% to 90% with cholestasis being the most common abnormality. In adults, a wide range of hepatobiliary derangements have been reported in 15% to 85% of patients undergoing TPN.[91] One of the few prospective studies that evaluated the prevalence of PNALD in adults showed that 65% of patients developed chronic cholestasis and 41.5% developed severe TPN-related liver disease characterized by extensive fibrosis or cirrhosis.[92]

Clinical Spectrum of TPN-related Hepatobiliary Disorders

The main types of hepatobiliary disorders associated with TPN include steatosis, cholestasis, and gallbladder stones and sludge.[93] Steatosis, or hepatic fat accumulation, is predominant in adults and is generally benign. It typically presents as mild to moderate increases in serum aminotransferase levels and less pronounced increases in serum ALP and bilirubin concentration than cholestasis. Increases generally occur within 2 weeks of TPN therapy and may return to normal even with TPN continued. Steatosis is generally believed to be a nonprogressive lesion, although cases of hepatic steatosis progressing to fibrosis or cirrhosis have been reported.[92]

Cholestasis is a condition of impaired secretion of bile and is the most common type of PNALD occurring in both children and adult patients. TPN-induced cholestasis has been defined as an increase in serum conjugated bilirubin of 2 mg/dL or more, which may be accompanied by increases in γ-glutamyl transpeptidase, ALP, and serum transaminases.[94] TPN-associated cholestasis is a serious complication because it may progress to cirrhosis and liver failure. If TPN is stopped before irreversible hepatic damage occurs, complete liver recovery is expected and serum conjugated bilirubin concentrations typically return to normal within 2 months.[95]

TPN therapy often leads to gallbladder stasis and the resultant development of gallstones and gallbladder sludge, with subsequent cholecystitis. It can occur in both adult and pediatric patients and is likely related to the lack of enteral stimulation and decreased cholecystokinin (CCK) release and therefore impaired bile flow and gallbladder contractility. The development of biliary sludge and gallstones seems to correlate with the duration of TPN therapy.[96]

Histopathologic Findings

TPN-induced hepatic steatosis is characterized by centrilobular and midzonal microvesicular and macrovesicular fatty change with fat cysts. Steatohepatitis is characterized by the presence of mixed inflammatory infiltrates and focal necrosis that can be associated with fibrosis or cirrhosis.[97] Intrahepatic cholestasis is commonly characterized by biliary plugging, extramedullary hematopoiesis, bile duct hyperplasia, pigmented Kupffer cells, pseudoacinar formation, pericellular and portal fibrosis, and occasionally cirrhosis.[98]

Risk Factors for TPN-associated Liver Disease

Several conditions have been well associated with the pathogenesis of TPN-associated liver disease and these should be assessed when managing PNALD.

Prematurity and low birth weight
There is an association between development of cholestasis in infants who are premature and of low birth weight. This is attributed to the relative immaturity of the biliary secretory system, a decreased bile acid pool, and impaired hepatic mitochondrial function.[99]

Sepsis
The presence of sepsis is an important precipitant of cholestasis in neonates and of abnormal liver function tests in adults receiving TPN. Patients on long-term TPN are predisposed to blood stream infections, particularly from bacterial migration along the indwelling central venous catheters. The exact mechanism of sepsis-induced cholestasis is unknown. Bacterial overgrowth of the small intestine is relatively common in both children and adults with intestinal failure because of intestinal stasis. It can be identified by hallmark symptoms including bloating, gas, cramps, foul-smelling stool or ostomy output, and diarrhea. Bacterial overgrowth is believed to cause liver dysfunction by translocation of bacteria and endotoxins causing release of cytokines with resulting hepatic inflammation, altered bile canaliculi membrane function, and reduced bile flow.[100]

Intestinal anatomy
Massive intestinal resection has been identified as a risk factor for PNALD and small bowel length less than 50 cm is an independent risk factor for cholestasis. Some investigators have proposed that short-bowel syndrome predisposes to liver dysfunction through interruption of the enterohepatic bile circulation, resulting in abnormal bile acid metabolism.[92]

Lack of enteral nutrition
Lack of enteral nutrition has been shown to reduce the secretion of several gastrointestinal hormones including gastrin, motilin, pancreatic polypeptide, insulinotropic polypeptide, and glucagon.[101] This reduction in secretion can lead to intestinal stasis, enterocyte hypoplasia with decreased gastrointestinal lymphoid tissue function with reduced IgA secretion and impaired gut immunity, which may favor bacterial overgrowth and endotoxin-mediated liver injury. Lack of enteral nutrition leads to decreased CCK release and consequent decreased emptying of the gallbladder resulting in bile stasis and depletion of the enterohepatic bile circulation.[94]

Nutrient deficiency
Deficiencies of several methionine metabolites, such as carnitine, choline, and taurine may also play a role in PNALD. Carnitine, choline, and taurine are not routinely administered as part of the parenteral formulations and there is evidence that levels are low in individuals receiving parenteral nutrition.[102,103] Carnitine is involved in the transport of long-chain fatty acids across the mitochondrial membrane so that they can undergo beta-oxidation. In deficiency states when carnitine is less than 10% of normal levels, hepatic steatosis can develop. However, intervention studies have failed to show any benefit of parenteral carnitine supplementation in patients receiving long-term parenteral nutrition with regard to hepatic abnormalities.[104]

Studies have shown that choline levels are low in more than 90% of patients receiving TPN.[102] Choline deficiency in patients receiving TPN has been shown to correlate with increased transaminase levels and steatosis.[105] Small studies have shown that both parenteral choline supplementation and high-dose oral supplementation can reverse these abnormalities.[105,106]

Taurine solubilizes bile salts and is therefore necessary for adequate biliary secretion and ileal reabsorption.[107] Taurine deficiency in neonates is associated with cholestatic liver disease and studies have shown that supplementation may improve this condition.[103] One study has shown that supplementing TPN solutions with taurine in adult patients with chronic cholestasis also improved liver function tests.[108]

It has been proposed that individuals receiving TPN may be deficient in antioxidants such as glutathione, β-carotene, and vitamin E and increased oxidative stress may lead to hepatic dysfunction.[109] From animal models it seems that mitochondria-associated apoptosis triggered by oxidative damage may play an important role in this process.[110]

Nutrient toxicity

Early TPN formulations provided an excess of calories, particularly in the form of carbohydrate. US guidelines suggest a carbohydrate administration via TPN greater than 20 to 25 kcal/kg/d exceeds the mean oxidation rate of glucose, and leads to hyperinsulinemia and fatty liver infiltration.[111] The replacement of a proportion of glucose energy with parenteral lipid has been shown to reduce the incidence of steatosis.[11] However, excess lipid has also been shown to result in hepatic dysfunction and in one study a parenteral lipid intake of 1 g/kg of body weight per day or more of a soybean-based lipid emulsion was an independent risk factor for liver disease, with a relative risk of cholestasis of 2.3 and a relative risk of advanced liver disease of 5.5.[92] The exact mechanism of hepatic dysfunction remains largely unknown but soybean-based lipid emulsions comprise primarily long-chain fatty acids or linoleic acid and these have been associated with increased insulin resistance and hepatic lipogenesis. Recent studies have shown that lipid emulsions with a lower soybean oil component such as with replacement with medium-chain triglycerides, olive oil, or fish oil either alone or in combination may be associated with less hepatic dysfunction.[112-114]

Management

When a patient receiving TPN develops liver complications, all aspects of the patient's care must be reviewed to identify and treat reversible factors that may be contributing to liver injury. This includes a detailed review of the medications and herbal supplements that may be causing hepatotoxicity. Other strategies include maximizing enteral nutrition, treatment of sepsis and bacterial overgrowth, optimizing TPN composition, and in refractory cases transplantation (**Box 1**).

Maximize oral and enteral nutrition

Oral and enteral nutrition are known to reverse intestinal mucosal hypoplasia and preserve the immunologic integrity of the gut. In addition, enteral nutrition stimulates motility, thus reducing intestinal stasis, bacterial translocation, and cytokine and endotoxin production. Enteral nutrition also stimulates CCK secretion and gallbladder stimulation, which will reduce the risk of biliary sludge and stone formation.[115]

Treatment of sepsis

Sepsis has been recognized as a major cause of PNALD. Infection should be aggressively treated with antimicrobial agents and measures should be taken to minimize recurrence. Strict catheter care procedures should be followed in both the hospital and home setting, including minimizing catheter manipulation, using proper hand hygiene and aseptic technique when accessing the catheter, and using proper site care.[116]

Box 1
Management strategies for TPN-associated liver complications

1. Rule out other causes of liver injury

    Previous history of a pathologic liver condition before TPN was initiated

    Hepatotoxic medications and herbal supplements

    Biliary obstruction

    Sepsis

2. Modifications to the TPN formulation and administration

    Limit TPN calories to less than 25 kcal/kg/d

    Decrease dextrose

    Decrease intravenous fat emulsion to 1 g/kg/d

    Consider the use of intravenous fat emulsions containing medium-chained fatty acids, fish oil, or olive oil

    Cyclic infusion

    Consider supplementation of deficient methionine metabolites (taurine, choline)

3. Maximize enteral nutrition

    Encourage oral diet

    Start low-rate tube feeding

4. Medical therapy

    Treat bacterial overgrowth

    Enteral antibiotics (metronidazole, augmentin, neomycin, rifaximin)

    Consider promotility agents in patients with chronic intestinal pseudoobstruction

    Treat sepsis with appropriate antimicrobials

    Consider starting ursodeoxycholic acid (10–30 mg/kg/d)

5. Surgical therapy

    Intestinal transplantation

    Combined intestine and liver transplantation

Optimizing TPN composition and timing

Adjustments in TPN composition and infusion parameters can often improve PNALD. Overfeeding patients can lead to deleterious effects related to excess glucose and lipid as mentioned earlier. With the growing evidence that lipid emulsions containing a mixture of long-chain and medium-chain triglycerides may be less hepatotoxic than soybean-based emulsions, a switch to this type of lipid emulsion may be favorable.

Cyclic infusion of TPN refers to the infusion of a daily supply of TPN components within a 24-hour period (generally 8–12 hours), allowing a period in the day free of TPN. Cyclic infusion of TPN has been shown to result in a reduction of serum liver enzyme and bilirubin levels in adult and pediatric patients compared with continuous infusion.[95,117]

Treating bacterial overgrowth

Treatment of bacterial overgrowth seems to play an important role in preventing and managing PNALD. Treatment with enteral administration of antibiotics seems to be more effective than the intravenous route because the intestine is the target site for activity. For small intestinal bacterial overgrowth (SIBO) resulting as a complication of intestinal failure, the condition may prove to be more refractory to antibiotic therapy than SIBO unrelated to intestinal failure. As a result, treatment may require more repeated courses of antibiotics or continuous antibiotic therapy. For continuous antibiotic therapy, rotating antibiotic regimens are recommended to prevent the development of resistance.[93] The choice of antibiotic is generally empiric and may include metronidazole 250 mg 3 times daily, amoxicillin-clavulanic acid 500 mg 3 times daily, neomycin 500 mg 4 times daily, or rifaximin 400 mg 3 times daily.[93]

Pharmacotherapy

Ursodiol (ursodeoxycholic acid [UDCA]), a secondary bile acid that reduces cholesterol crystallization by reducing the concentrations of promoting factors, has been used widely in the treatment of cholestatic liver disorders.[94] The use of ursodiol to improve parenteral nutrition-associated cholestasis (PNAC) has been studied more extensively in children than adults. In 1 small study evaluating UDCA 30 mg/kg/d on PNAC in children with intestinal failure, full remission or partial improvement occurred in more than 90% of the patients.[118] Similar studies in neonates have also shown benefit with UDCA with doses in the range of 10 to 30 mg/kg/d. In adults, UDCA 10–15 mg/kg/d has shown some improvement in markers of cholestasis.[118]

Small intestine and liver transplantation

Impending or overt liver failure associated with PNALD is recognized as an indication for small intestinal transplantation and PNALD is one of the most common reasons for performing intestinal transplantation.[119] Significant hepatic fibrosis and liver dysfunction may regress after intestinal transplantation.[120] There has also been a case of reversal of liver cirrhosis after isolated small intestinal transplantation.[121] This is encouraging as the outcomes for patients who require combined liver and intestinal transplantation are poor, and mortality of patients waiting for combined liver-intestinal transplantation on transplant waiting lists is high.[122]

SUMMARY

The gastrointestinal tract and the liver are closely related anatomically, physiologically, and pathologically. Our understanding of the hepatobiliary manifestations of gastrointestinal and nutritional disorders is evolving. A close link between UC and PSC has been recognized for a long time, but it is now known that the IBD phenotype of a patient with PSC differs from that of a patient with IBD without PSC. The hepatic manifestations of CD are relatively common and usually mild, although in rare instances CD can be associated with severe liver disease. As a result, CD should be ruled out before a diagnosis of cryptogenic cirrhosis is made because the improvement in liver dysfunction with a GFD can be significant. Whipple's disease, although a rare disorder, should still be considered in a patient with multisystem signs and symptoms including liver disease. TPN-associated liver disease remains a very common issue with few effective therapies for severe disease except intestinal transplantation. Liver disease related to TPN, such as hepatobiliary complications of many gastrointestinal and nutritional disorders, is the subject of much debate and research. Despite our growing understanding, management of many of these diseases and complications still remain challenging.

ACKNOWLEDGMENTS

The authors thank Dr Angela Levy from the Department of Radiology, Georgetown University, Washington, DC, for the MRC and ERC images of PSC.

REFERENCES

1. Vierling JM, Amankonah TD. Primary sclerosing cholangitis. In: Afdhal NH, editor. Gallbladder and biliary tract diseases. New York: Marcel Dekker; 2000. p. 659–703.
2. Chapman R, Fevery J, Kalloo A, et al. Diagnosis and management of primary sclerosing cholangitis. Hepatology 2010;51(2):660–78.
3. Loftus EV Jr, Harewood GC, Loftus CG, et al. PSC-IBD: a unique form of inflammatory bowel disease associated with primary sclerosing cholangitis. Gut 2005; 54:91–6.
4. Tischendorf JJ, Hecker H, Kruger M, et al. Characterization, outcome, and prognosis in 273 patients with primary sclerosing cholangitis: a single center study. Am J Gastroenterol 2007;102:107–14.
5. Kaplan GG, Laupland KB, Butzner D, et al. The burden of large and small duct primary sclerosing cholangitis in adults and children: a population-based analysis. Am J Gastroenterol 2007;102:1042.
6. Bambha K, Kim WR, Talwalkar J, et al. Incidence, clinical spectrum, and outcomes of primary sclerosing cholangitis in a united states community. Gastroenterology 2003;125:1364.
7. Loftus EV, Sandborn WJ, Lindor KD, et al. Interactions between chronic liver disease and inflammatory bowel disease. Inflamm Bowel Dis 1997;3: 288–302.
8. Olsson R, Danielsson A, Jarnerot G, et al. Prevalence of primary sclerosing cholangitis in patients with ulcerative colitis. Gastroenterology 1991;100:1319.
9. Fausa O, Schrumpf E, Elgjo K. Relationship of inflammatory bowel disease and primary sclerosing cholangitis. Semin Liver Dis 1991;11:31–9.
10. Takikawa H, Manabe T. Primary sclerosing cholangitis in Japan–analysis of 192 cases. J Gastroenterol 1997;32:134.
11. Bergquist A, Montgomery SM, Bahmanyar S, et al. Increased risk of primary sclerosing cholangitis and ulcerative colitis in first-degree relatives of patients with primary sclerosing cholangitis. Clin Gastroenterol Hepatol 2008;6:939.
12. Karlsen TH, Schrumpf E, Boberg KM. Genetic epidemiology of primary sclerosing cholangitis. World J Gastroenterol 2007;13:5421–31.
13. Wiencke K, Louka AS, Spurkland A, et al. Association of matrix metalloproteinase-1 and -3 promoter polymorphisms with clinical subsets of Norwegian primary sclerosing cholangitis patients. J Hepatol 2004;41:209.
14. Karlsen TH, Hampe J, Wiencke K, et al. Genetic polymorphisms associated with inflammatory bowel disease do not confer risk for primary sclerosing cholangitis. Am J Gastroenterol 2007;102:115–21.
15. Saarinen S, Olerup O, Broome U. Increased frequency of autoimmune diseases in patients with primary sclerosing cholangitis. Am J Gastroenterol 2000;95: 3195.
16. Hov JR, Boberg KM, Karlsen TH. Autoantibodies in primary sclerosing cholangitis. World J Gastroenterol 2008;14:3781–91.
17. Invernizzi P, Lleo A, Podda M. Interpreting serological tests in diagnosing autoimmune liver diseases. Semin Liver Dis 2007;27:161–72.

18. Xu B, Broome U, Ericzon BG, et al. High frequency of autoantibodies in patients with primary sclerosing cholangitis that bind biliary epithelial cells and induce expression of CD44 and production of interleukin 6. Gut 2002; 51:120–7.
19. Karrar A, Broome U, Sodergren T, et al. Biliary epithelial cell antibodies link adaptive and innate immune responses in primary sclerosing cholangitis. Gastroenterology 2007;132:1504–14.
20. Sasatomi K, Noguchi K, Sakisaka S, et al. Abnormal accumulation of endotoxin in biliary epithelial cells in primary biliary cirrhosis and primary sclerosing cholangitis. J Hepatol 1998;29:409.
21. Terblanche J, Allison HF, Northover JM. An ischemic basis for biliary strictures. Surgery 1983;94:52.
22. Kim WR, Lindor KD, Locke GR III, et al. Epidemiology and natural history of primary biliary cirrhosis in a U.S. community. Gastroenterology 2000;119: 1631.
23. Talwalkar JA, Lindor KD. Natural history and prognostic models in primary sclerosing cholangitis. Best Pract Res Clin Gastroenterol 2001;15(4):563–75.
24. Papatheodoridis GV, Hamilton M, Mistry PK, et al. Ulcerative colitis has an aggressive course after orthotopic liver transplantation for primary sclerosing cholangitis. Gut 1998;43:639.
25. Balasubramaniam K, Wiesner RH, LaRusso NF. Primary sclerosing cholangitis with normal serum alkaline phosphatase activity. Gastroenterology 1988;95: 1395.
26. El-Shabrawi M, Wilkinson ML, Portmann B, et al. Primary sclerosing cholangitis in childhood. Gastroenterology 1987;92:1226.
27. Cameron JL, Gayler BW, Sanfey H, et al. Sclerosing cholangitis: anatomical distribution of obstructive lesions. Ann Surg 1984;200:54.
28. Lefkowitch J. Primary sclerosing cholangitis. Arch Intern Med 1982;142:1157.
29. Ludwig J, Czaja AJ, Dickson ER, et al. Manifestations of nonsuppurative cholangitis in chronic hepatobiliary diseases: morphologic spectrum, clinical correlations and terminology. Liver 1984;4:105.
30. Brandt DJ, MacCarty RL, Charboneau JW, et al. Gallbladder disease in patients with primary sclerosing cholangitis. Am J Roentgenol 1988;150:571.
31. Kaw M, Silverman WB, Rabinovitz M, et al. Biliary tract calculi in primary sclerosing cholangitis. Am J Gastroenterol 1995;90:72.
32. Rosen CB, Nagorney DM, Wiesner RH, et al. Cholangiocarcinoma complicating primary sclerosing cholangitis. Ann Surg 1991;213:21.
33. Broome U, Lofberg R, Veress B, et al. Primary sclerosing cholangitis and ulcerative colitis: evidence for increased neoplastic potential. Hepatology 1995;22: 1404–8.
34. Kim HJ, Kim MH, Myung SJ, et al. A new strategy for the application of CA19-9 in the differentiation of pancreaticobiliary cancer: analysis using a receiver operating characteristic curve. Am J Gastroenterol 1999;94:1941.
35. Levy C, Lymp J, Angulo P, et al. The value of serum CA 19-9 in predicting cholangiocarcinoma in patients with primary sclerosing cholangitis. Dig Dis Sci 2005;50:1734.
36. Siqueira E, Schoen RE, Silverman W, et al. Detecting cholangiocarcinoma in patients with primary sclerosing cholangitis. Gastrointest Endosc 2002;56:40.
37. Moreno Luna LE, Kipp B, Halling KC, et al. Advanced cytologic techniques for the detection of malignant pancreatobiliary strictures. Gastroenterology 2006; 131:1064–72.

38. Fritscher-Ravens A, Broering DC, Knoefel WT, et al. EUS-guided fine-needle aspiration of suspected hilar cholangiocarcinoma in potentially operable patients with negative brush cytology. Am J Gastroenterol 2004;99:45.
39. Soetikno RM, Lin OS, Heidenreich PA, et al. Increased risk of colorectal neoplasia in patients with primary sclerosing cholangitis and ulcerative colitis: a meta-analysis. Gastrointest Endosc 2002;56:48–54.
40. Said K, Glaumann H, Bergquist A. Gallbladder disease in patients with primary sclerosing cholangitis. J Hepatol 2008;48:598–605.
41. Paumgartner G, Beuers U. Ursodeoxycholic acid in cholestatic liver disease: mechanisms of action and therapeutic use revisited. Hepatology 2002;36:525.
42. O'Brien CB, Senior JR, Arora-Mirchandani R, et al. Ursodeoxycholic acid for the treatment of primary sclerosing cholangitis: a 30-month pilot study. Hepatology 1991;14:838–47.
43. Lindor KD, Kowdley KV, Luketic VA, et al. High-dose ursodeoxycholic acid for the treatment of primary sclerosing cholangitis. Hepatology 2009;50(3): 808–14.
44. Gross CR, Malinchoc M, Kim WR, et al. Quality of life before and after liver transplantation for cholestatic liver disease. Hepatology 1999;29:356.
45. Saldeen K, Friman S, Olausson M, et al. Follow-up after liver transplantation for primary sclerosing cholangitis: effects on survival, quality of life, and colitis. Scand J Gastroenterol 1999;34:535.
46. Graziadei IW, Wiesner RH, Marotta PJ, et al. Long-term results of patients undergoing liver transplantation for primary sclerosing cholangitis. Hepatology 1999; 30:1121.
47. Gisbert JP, González-Lama Y, Maté J. Thiopurine-induced liver injury in patients with inflammatory bowel disease: a systematic review. Am J Gastroenterol 2007; 102(7):1518–27.
48. Berkowitz RS, Goldstein DP, Bernstein MR. Ten year's experience with methotrexate and folinic acid as primary therapy for gestational trophoblastic disease. Gynecol Oncol 1986;23:111.
49. Saag KG, Teng GG, Patkar NM, et al. American College of Rheumatology 2008 recommendations for the use of nonbiologic and biologic disease-modifying antirheumatic drugs in rheumatoid arthritis. Arthritis Rheum 2008;59:762.
50. Volta U. Pathogenesis and clinical significance of liver injury in celiac disease. Clin Rev Allergy Immunol 2009;36(1):62–70.
51. Bardella MT, Franquelli M, Quatrini M, et al. Prevalence of hypertransaminasemia in adult celiac patients and effect of gluten-free diet. Hepatology 1995;22: 833–6.
52. Bonamico M, Pitzalis G, Culasso F, et al. Hepatic damage during celiac disease in childhood. Minerva Pediatr 1986;38:959–63.
53. Hagander B, Brandt L, Sjolund K, et al. Hepatic injury in adult celiac disease. Lancet 1977;2:270–2.
54. Lo Iacono O, Petta S, Venezia G, et al. Anti-tissue transglutaminase antibodies in patients with abnormal liver tests: is it always coeliac disease? Am J Gastroenterol 2005;100:2472.
55. Volta U, De Franceschi L, Lari F, et al. Celiac disease hidden by cryptogenic hypertransaminasemia. Lancet 1998;352:26–9.
56. Korponay-Szabo IR, Halttunen T, Szalai Z, et al. In vivo targeting of intestinal and extraintestinal transglutaminase 2 by celiac autoantibodies. Gut 2004;53:641–8.
57. Bardella MT, Vecchi M, Conte D, et al. Chronic unexplained hypertransaminasemia may be caused by occult celiac disease. Hepatology 1999;29:654.

58. Peters U, Askling J, Gridley G, et al. Causes of death in patients with celiac disease in a population-based Swedish cohort. Arch Intern Med 2003;163: 1566–72.
59. Rostom A, Murray JA, Kagnoff MF. American Gastroenterological Association (AGA) Institute technical review on the diagnosis and management of celiac disease. Gastroenterology 2006;131:1981–2002.
60. Jacobsen MB, Fausa O, Elgjo K, et al. Hepatic lesions in adult celiac disease. Scand J Gastroenterol 1990;25:656–62.
61. Kaukinen K, Halme L, Collin P, et al. Celiac disease in patients with severe liver disease: gluten-free diet may reverse hepatic failure. Gastroenterology 2002; 122:881.
62. Farrell RJ, Kelly CP. Celiac sprue - current concepts. N Engl J Med 2002;346: 180–8.
63. Kaplan MM. Primary biliary cirrhosis. N Engl J Med 2005;353:1261.
64. Bergasa NV. Pruritus and fatigue in primary biliary cirrhosis. Clin Liver Dis 2003; 7:879–900.
65. Watt FE, James OF, Jones DE. Patterns of autoimmunity in primary biliary cirrhosis patients and their families: a population-based cohort study. QJM 2004;97:397–406.
66. Logan RF, Fergusson A, Finlayson ND, et al. Primary biliary cirrhosis and celiac disease: an association? Lancet 1978;1:230–3.
67. Sorensen HT, Thulstrup AM, Blomqvist P, et al. Risk of primary biliary liver cirrhosis in patients with celiac disease: Danish and Swedish cohort study. Gut 1999;44:736–8.
68. Lawson A, West J, Aithal GP, et al. Autoimmune cholestatic liver disease in people with celiac disease: a population-based study of their association. Aliment Pharmacol Ther 2005;21:401–5.
69. Rubio-Tapia A, Murray J. The liver in celiac disease. Hepatology 2007;46: 1650–959.
70. Dickey W, McMillan SA, Callender ME. High prevalence of celiac sprue among patients with primary biliary cirrhosis. J Clin Gastroenterol 1997;25(1):328–9.
71. Feld JJ, Meddings J, Heathcote EJ. Abnormal intestinal permeability in primary biliary cirrhosis. Dig Dis Sci 2006;51:1607–13.
72. Murray JA, Watson T, Clearman B, et al. Effect of a gluten-free diet on gastrointestinal symptoms in celiac disease. Am J Clin Nutr 2004;79:669–73.
73. Volta U, DeFranceschi L, Molinaro N, et al. Frequency and significance of anti-gliadin and anti-endomysial antibodiesin autoimmune hepatitis. Dig Dis Sci 1998;43:2190–5.
74. Villalta D, Girolami D, Bidoli E, et al. High prevalence of celiac disease in auto-immune hepatitis detected by anti-tissue transglutaminase autoantibodies. J Clin Lab Anal 2005;19:6–10.
75. Hay JE, Wiesner RH, Shorter RG, et al. Primary sclerosing cholangitis and celiac disease. A novel association. Ann Intern Med 1988;109:713–7.
76. Volta U, Rodrigo L, Granito A, et al. Celiac disease in autoimmune cholestatic liver disorders. Am J Gastroenterol 2002;97:2609–13.
77. Boberg KM, Spurkland A, Rocca G, et al. The HLA-DR3, DQ2 heterozygous genotype is associated with an accelerated progression of primary sclerosing cholangitis. Scand J Gastroenterol 2001;8:886–90.
78. Tollefsen S, Arentz-Hansen H, Fleckenstein B, et al. HLA-DQ2 and -DQ8 signatures of gluten T cell epitopes in celiac disease. J Clin Invest 2006; 116:2226–36.

79. Fracassetti O, Delvecchio G, Tambini R, et al. Primary sclerosing cholangitis with celiac sprue: two cases. J Clin Gastroenterol 1996;22:71–2.

80. Venturini I, Cosenza R, Miglioli L. Adult celiac disease and primary sclerosing cholangitis: two case reports. Hepatogastroenterology 1998;45:2344–7.

81. Noh KW, Poland GA, Murray JA. Hepatitis B vaccine nonresponse and celiac disease. Am J Gastroenterol 2003;98:2289–92.

82. Carroccio A, Giannitrapani L, Soresi M, et al. Guinea pig transglutaminase immunolinked assay does not predict celiac disease in patients with chronic liver disease. Gut 2001;49:506–11.

83. Vecchi M, Folli C, Donato MF, et al. High rate of positive anti-tissue transglutaminase antibodies in chronic liver disease. Role of liver decompensation and of the antigen source. Scand J Gastroenterol 2003;38:50–4.

84. Relman DA, Schmidt TM, MacDermott RP, et al. Identification of the uncultured bacillus of Whipple's disease. N Engl J Med 1992;327:293.

85. Puéchal X. Whipple disease and arthritis. Curr Opin Rheumatol 2001;13:74–9.

86. Fenollar F, Laouira S, Lepidi H, et al. Value of Tropheryma whipplei quantitative polymerase chain reaction assay for the diagnosis of Whipple disease: usefulness of saliva and stool specimens for first-line screening. Clin Infect Dis 2008;47:659.

87. Marth T. New insights into Whipple's disease – a rare intestinal inflammatory disorder. Dig Dis 2009;27:494–501.

88. Saint-Marc Girardin MF, Zafrani ES, Chaumetter MT, et al. Hepatic granulomas in Whipple's disease. Gastroenterology 1984;86:753–6.

89. Minkari T, Pars B, Erbengi T, et al. A case of Whipple's disease complicated by fatal hepatitis. Hepatogastroenterology 1980;27(4):322–6.

90. Misra PS, Lebwohl P, Laufer H. Hepatic and appendiceal Whipple's disease with negative jejunal biopsies. Am J Gastroenterol 1981;75(4):302–6.

91. Luman W, Shaffer JL. Prevalence, outcome and associated factors of deranged liver function tests in patients on home parenteral nutrition. Clin Nutr 2002;21(4): 337–43.

92. Cavicchi M, Beau P, Crenn P, et al. Prevalence of liver disease and contributing factors in patients receiving home parenteral nutrition for permanent intestinal failure. Ann Intern Med 2000;132:525–32.

93. Quigley EM, Quera R. Small intestinal bacterial overgrowth: roles of antibiotics, prebiotics, and probiotics. Gastroenterology 2006;130(2 Suppl 1):S78–90.

94. Guglielmi FW, Regano N, Mazzuoli S, et al. Cholestasis induced by total parenteral nutrition. Clin Liver Dis 2008;12(1):97–110, viii.

95. Btaiche IF, Khalidi N. Parenteral nutrition-associated liver complications in children. Pharmacotherapy 2002;22:188–211.

96. Messing B, Bories C, Kunstlinger F, et al. Does total parenteral nutrition induce gallbladder sludge formation and lithiasis? Gastroenterology 1983;84:1012–9.

97. Briones ER, Iber FL. Liver and biliary tract changes and injury associated with total parenteral nutrition pathogenesis and prevention. J Am Coll Nutr 1995; 14:219–28.

98. Payne-James JJ, Silk DB. Hepatobiliary dysfunction associated with total parenteral nutrition. Dig Dis 1991;9:106–24.

99. Hofmann AF. Defective biliary secretion during total parenteral nutrition: probable mechanisms and possible solutions. J Pediatr Gastroenterol Nutr 1995;20:376–90.

100. Gonnella PA, Helton WS, Robinson M, et al. O-side chain of Escherichia coli endotoxin 0111:B4 is transported across the intestinal epithelium in the rat: evidence for

increased transport during total parenteral nutrition. Eur J Cell Biol 1992;59(1): 224–7.

101. Greenberg GR, Wolman SL, Christofides ND, et al. Effect of total parenteral nutrition on gut hormone release in humans. Gastroenterology 1981;80(5 pt 1):988–93.

102. Buchman AL, Moukarzel A, Jenden DJ, et al. Low plasma free choline is prevalent in patients receiving long term parenteral nutrition and is associated with hepatic aminotransferase abnormalities. Clin Nutr 1993;12:33–7.

103. Spencer AU, Yu S, Tracy TF, et al. Parenteral nutrition-associated cholestasis in neonates: multivariate analysis of the potential protective effect of taurine. JPEN J Parenter Enteral Nutr 2005;29:337–43.

104. Bowyer BA, Miles JM, Haymond MW, et al. L-Carnitine therapy in home parenteral nutrition patients with abnormal liver tests and low plasma carnitine concentrations. Gastroenterology 1988;94:434–8.

105. Buchman A, Ament M, Sohel M, et al. Choline deficiency causes reversible hepatic abnormalities in patients receiving parenteral nutrition: proof of a human choline requirement: a placebo-controlled trial. JPEN J Parenter Enteral Nutr 2001;25:260–8.

106. Buchman AL, Dubin M, Jenden D, et al. Lecithin increases plasma free choline and decreases hepatic steatosis in long-term total parenteral nutrition patients. Gastroenterology 1992;102(4 Pt 1):1363–70.

107. Howard D, Thompson DF. Taurine: an essential amino acid to prevent cholestasis in neonates? Ann Pharmacother 1992;26(11):1390–2.

108. Schneider SM, Joly F, Gehrardt MF, et al. Taurine status and response to intravenous taurine supplementation in adults with short-bowel syndrome undergoing long-term parenteral nutrition: a pilot study. Br J Nutr 2006;96(2):365–70.

109. Cai W, Wu J, Hong L, et al. Oxidative injury and hepatocyte apoptosis in total parenteral nutrition-associated liver dysfunction. J Pediatr Surg 2006;41(10): 1663–8.

110. Hong L, Wang X, Wu J, et al. Mitochondria-initiated apoptosis triggered by oxidative injury play a role in total parenteral nutrition-associated liver dysfunction in infant rabbit model. J Pediatr Surg 2009;44(9):1712–8.

111. Mirtallo J, Canada T, Johnson D, et al. Safe practices for parenteral nutrition. JPEN J Parenter Enteral Nutr 2004;28:S39–69.

112. Calder PC. Hot topics in parenteral nutrition. Rationale for using new lipid emulsions in parenteral nutrition and a review of the trials performed in adults. Proc Nutr Soc 2009;68(3):252–60.

113. Piper SN, Schade I, Beschmann RB, et al. Hepatocellular integrity after parenteral nutrition: comparison of a fish-oil-containing lipid emulsion with an olive-soybean oil-based lipid emulsion. Eur J Anaesthesiol 2009;26(12):1076–82.

114. Meguid MM, Akahoshi MP, Jeffers S, et al. Amelioration of metabolic complications of conventional total parenteral nutrition. A prospective randomized study. Arch Surg 1984;119:1294–8.

115. Jawaheer G, Pierro A, Lloyd DA, et al. Gall bladder contractility in neonates: effects of parenteral and enteral feeding. Arch Dis Child Fetal Neonatal Ed 1995;72(3):F200–202.

116. Mermel LA, Farr BM, Sherertz RJ, et al. Centers for disease control and prevention. Guidelines for the prevention of intravascular catheter-related infections. MMWR Morb Mortal Wkly Rep 2002;51:1–29, 53.

117. Hwang TL, Lue MC, Chen LL. Early use of cyclic TPN prevents further deterioration of liver functions for the TPN patients with impaired liver function. Hepatogastroenterology 2000;47:1347–50.

118. De Marco G, Sordino D, Bruzzese E, et al. Early treatment with ursodeoxycholic acid for cholestasis in children on parenteral nutrition because of primary intestinal failure. Aliment Pharmacol Ther 2006;24(2):387–94.

119. Grant D, Abu-Elmagd K, Reyes J, et al. 2003 report of the intestine transplant registry: a new era has dawned. Ann Surg 2005;241:607–13.

120. Fiel MI, Sauter B, Wu HS, et al. Regression of hepatic fibrosis after intestinal transplantation in total parenteral nutrition liver disease. Clin Gastroenterol Hepatol 2008;6(8):926–33.

121. Fiel MI, Wu HS, Iyer K, et al. Rapid reversal of parenteral-nutrition-associated cirrhosis following isolated intestinal transplantation. J Gastrointest Surg 2009; 13(9):1717–23.

122. Fryer J, Pellar S, Ormond D, et al. Mortality in candidates waiting for combined liver-intestine transplants exceeds that for other candidates waiting for live transplants. Liver Transpl 2003;9:748–53.

Infectious Diseases and the Liver

Rohit Talwani, MD[a], Bruce L. Gilliam, MD[b], Charles Howell, MD[c],*

KEYWORDS

- Hepatitis • Bacterial • Virus • Protozoa

The liver contains approximately one-third of the reticuloendothelial system mass in humans. As the recipient of both the portal and systemic circulation, the liver plays an important role in host defense against invasive microorganisms. The effect of microbial pathogens on the liver can vary greatly, presenting with a wide variety of manifestations from asymptomatic increases in aminotransaminases, acute liver failure, hepatic fibrosis, and cirrhosis. This article reviews the involvement of the liver during systemic infections with organisms that are not considered to be primarily hepatotropic (**Table 1**).

VIRUSES

Epstein-Barr Virus

Epstein-Barr virus (EBV) is a member of the herpes virus group, and up to 95% of the adult population is seropositive for EBV. The virus typically causes an infectious mononucleosis syndrome (fever, sore throat, and lymphadenopathy) in adolescents and young adults who have not had prior exposure. A minority of patients (2%–15%) will have gastrointestinal complaints such as nausea and abdominal pain, and less than 5% will have jaundice. On examination, up to 14% of patients have hepatomegaly and one-half have splenomegaly.[1] Severe, fulminant hepatitis occurs rarely and usually in immunosuppressed patients. Despite the infrequency of liver-related complaints and findings observed clinically, most patients with EBV-associated mononucleosis have abnormal liver function tests. In excess of 90% of patients will have mild increases of aminotransferases (2–3 times the upper limit of

[a] Division of Infectious Diseases, Department of Medicine, Institute of Human Virology, University of Maryland School of Medicine, 725 West Lombard Street Room N150, Baltimore, MD 21201, USA
[b] Division of Infectious Diseases, Department of Medicine, Institute of Human Virology, University of Maryland School of Medicine, 725 West Lombard Street Room N545, Baltimore, MD 21201, USA
[c] Division of Gastroenterology and Hepatology, Department of Medicine, University of Maryland School of Medicine, 22 South Greene Street, Room M3W50, Baltimore, MD 21201, USA
* Corresponding author. Division of Gastroenterology, University of Maryland School of Medicine, 22 South Green Street Room N3W50, Baltimore, MD 21201.
E-mail address: chowell@medicine.umaryland.edu

Clin Liver Dis 15 (2011) 111–130
doi:10.1016/j.cld.2010.09.002
1089-3261/11/$ – see front matter © 2011 Elsevier Inc. All rights reserved.

Table 1
Summary of pathogens reviewed

Viruses	Bacteria and Mycobacteria	Parasites	Fungi
Epstein-Barr virus	*Salmonella enterica* serotype typhi	*Schistosoma* species (schistosomiasis)	*Candida* species
Cytomegalovirus	*Mycobacterium tuberculosis*	*Plasmodium* species (malaria)	*Histoplasma capsulatum*
Herpes simplex virus and other herpes viruses	*Brucella* species		
Yellow fever virus	*Coxiella bunerii* (Q fever)		
Dengue virus	*Leptospira* and other spirochetes		

normal), which typically manifest in the second week of the illness and resolve by week 6. Mild increases in alkaline phosphatase (60% of patients) and bilirubin (45%) are also observed, with cholestasis occurring in less than 5% of cases.[1–3] EBV replicates primarily in nasopharyngeal epithelial cells and B lymphocytes. However, infection of hepatocytes by EBV has been shown in patients with posttransplant lymphoproliferative disease.[4] The mechanism of liver damage has not been well defined, but likely involves the host immune responses to EBV antigens.[5,6]

The diagnosis of EBV infection usually relies on serology or a positive heterophile antibody. Typically, patients with EBV infections will have a positive immunoglobulin M (IgM) antibody. Liver biopsy findings vary, but typically include a sinusoidal infiltrate of mononuclear cells in a single file, the so-called Indian bead or Indian file pattern, mixed portal tract inflammatory infiltrate, and mild hepatocyte ballooning and vacuolization. Epithelioid granuloma formation and steatosis have also been described.[7] More specific adjunctive molecular testing, including in situ hybridization and polymerase chain reaction (PCR) testing, have been successfully used in both transplant and native liver specimens. Conflicting results have been reported on the usefulness of immunohistochemical staining of EBV antigens in liver biopsy specimens.[7–9]

The treatment of EBV-associated hepatitis is generally supportive; however, there are case reports of successful treatment with severe EBV hepatitis in both patients who are immunocompetent[5] and after liver transplant.[10]

Cytomegalovirus

Like EBV, cytomegalovirus (CMV) is a member of the herpes virus family with high (60%–100%) seroprevalence rates in adults.[11] CMV also causes an infectious mononucleosis syndrome with concomitant hepatitis. The mononucleosis syndrome caused by CMV in immunocompetent hosts is similar to EBV-associated illness except that splenomegaly is less frequent. Aminotransferase increases are also common with abnormal aspartate aminotransferase (AST) levels in up to 91% of immunocompetent patients; only 2.8% had a total bilirubin level greater than 2.0.[12] The characteristics of liver biopsies among immunocompetent patients are a sinusoidal and portal lymphocytic infiltrate and granulomas.[12–14] Owl's eye nuclear inclusion bodies may also be found in hepatocytes and bile duct epithelium.[12,13]

Diagnosis of an acute CMV syndrome is confirmed by the presence of IgM antibodies. However, the disease course and diagnostics workup are different among immunocompromised hosts, including liver transplant recipients. Clinical features, prevalence, diagnosis, and management of systemic CMV infection, and possible association with rejection after liver transplant are well described elsewhere.[15] The incidence of CMV hepatitis following liver transplantation varies from 2% to 34%.[16,17] Factors including immunosuppressive regimen, use of antiviral prophylaxis, and donor and recipient serostatus likely contribute to this variability in incidence. A large retrospective study of more than 1146 liver transplant recipients between 1988 and 2000 found CMV hepatitis in 24 (2%) patients.[17] Of those cases, 18 occurred in seronegative patients, 5 in seropositive patients, and 1 had an unknown serostatus. Most cases occurred between weeks 4 and 8 after transplant and only 3 cases were noted after 1996 (after which roughly half of the patients positive for the CMV matrix protein pp65, a protein that can be detected before symptoms of disease, received oral ganciclovir preemptively). Twenty-two of the 24 patients had isolated hepatitis, with 2 having disseminated disease; all of these patients had lower graft survival rates comparable with those without CMV hepatitis. A multivariate analysis indicated that the significant risk factors for the development of CMV hepatitis included donor positive/recipient negative serostatus, OKT3 treatment, and human leukocyte antigen-D–related matches. Diagnosis is aided by molecular techniques including quantitative CMV DNA PCR from blood, and special staining for viral antigens. The histopathologic findings of CMV hepatitis after liver transplant may include viral inclusion bodies. However, this is not consistent,[18] and microabscesses have also been found to be more prevalent in the transplant setting. Treatment of immunocompetent patients is generally supportive, whereas ganciclovir and valganciclovir are generally used in immunocompromised patients, including transplant recipients.[15]

Herpes Simplex Virus and Other Herpes Viruses

Herpes simplex virus (HSV)-1 typically causes orolabial infections and has an estimated seroprevalence of 62%. HSV-2 causes genital disease and has an estimated seroprevalence in the United States of 17% among adolescents and young adults.[19] Hepatic involvement during infections with HSV-1 and HSV-2 is rare, and most cases in the medical literature have had acute liver failure. Thus, the full spectrum of liver involvement during disseminated HSV is not well characterized and may be biased toward the more severe hepatitis cases. Of the approximately 100 cases described in the literature, fewer than 10 were described in immunocompetent patients. The remainder of cases had varying degrees of impaired immunity, including neonates, malnourished children, pregnant women, and patients receiving immunosuppressive medications.[20] Clinical presentation[21] includes fever (82%), severe abdominal pain (33%), concomitant lesions suggestive of HSV (57%), and hepatomegaly (45%). Jaundice was uncommon. Laboratory findings typically include abnormal liver tests (71%), white blood cell count of less than 5000/mm^3 (43%), and thrombocytopenia (45%). Other reviews describe large increases of transaminases (up to 100 times the upper limit of normal)[22] with only minor increases in bilirubin.[20] Liver biopsy typically reveals extensive necrosis with hemorrhage, minimal inflammatory cells, and hepatocytes with intranuclear inclusions. The diagnosis of HSV-associated hepatitis is often difficult, with only 12 of the 52 cases having a correct diagnosis established before death in one case series.[21] The finding of acute liver failure with fever, leucopenia, and thrombocytopenia without jaundice, even in the absence of suspicious mucocutaneous lesions, should arouse suspicion for HSV hepatitis. Adjunctive immunohistochemical staining for HSV may help in establishing the diagnosis. Hepatitis associated with other herpes viruses, including HHV-6 and HHV-7 in immunocompromised patients and disseminated varicella-zoster infections, have also been reported.

The pathogenesis of HSV hepatitis remains speculative and proposed mechanisms include a large inoculum of HSV, an impaired immune response including possible hypersensitivity reactions, enhanced virulence of certain HSV strains, and directly viral cytopathy.[21]

Early treatment with acyclovir seems to be associated with improved survival, reinforcing the need to establish the diagnosis promptly.[21,23] In one review of treated cases, 13 of 21 patients survived.[24] Given the severity of this syndrome, some investigators recommend treatment with acyclovir at a dose of 10 mg/kg intravenously every 8 hours.

Yellow Fever

Yellow fever is an arthropod-borne viral hemorrhagic fever syndrome caused by the yellow fever virus. A member of the Flavivirus genus, yellow fever virus is unique among the viral hemorrhagic fevers in its capacity to cause hepatitis and jaundice. Ninety percent of the estimated 200,000 annual cases occur in Africa, and the other 10% occur in South America.[25] The incidence of infection seems to fluctuate, in many instances occurring in epidemics (with infection incidences that may be as high as 20%) that are either seasonal, or caused by war and other events that interrupt health care delivery. More cases are reported in regions with low yellow fever vaccine coverage. The scope of infection is unknown, especially in more remote areas of Africa and South America, because of lack of disease reporting, limited health care resources for diagnosis, and presence of asymptomatic or mild cases. Between 1970 and 2002, there were 9 reported cases (8 fatal) of yellow fever among unvaccinated travelers from the United States and Europe.[25]

The virus is spread by the Aedes species mosquitoes in Africa and the Haemoagogus species in South America. Person-to-person transmission does not occur. The clinical spectrum of yellow fever ranges from asymptomatic infection (5%–50%) to a febrile multisystem hemorrhagic illness.[26] The incubation period is 3 to 6 days after acquisition of infection via bite by an infected mosquito, after which time peak viral levels are maintained, usually between 10^5 and 10^6 viral particles per milliliter of blood. Most of the understanding of the clinical course of disease is descriptive, given its occurrence in areas with limited resources. The disease is described in 3 phases. The first phase, or period of infection, occurs when virus levels peak, and is characterized by an acute onset of fevers, chills, myalgias, nausea, and vomiting. Patients appear acutely ill and may have conjunctival injection, and temperature-pulse dissociation (Faget sign). This phase lasts 3 to 6 days. Other findings during this phase include modest increase of transaminases, leukopenia, and lack of jaundice. The second phase is a brief (<24 hours) recovery phase (period of remission), at which time symptoms and fever abate. Patients may recover from this phase and develop lifelong immunity. Fifteen to twenty-five percent progress to the third phase, the period of intoxication, which lasts from 3 to 8 days. During this phase, patients may have fever, emesis, abdominal pain, jaundice, coagulopathy with bleeding diathesis, and renal failure. Transaminase levels peak and are directly proportional to the severity of disease. In one study, average AST and alanine transaminase (ALT) levels among fatal cases were 2766 IU/L and 660 IU/L, and were 929 IU/L and 351 IU/L among survivors with jaundice. AST levels are higher than ALT levels because of myocardial and skeletal muscle injury. Liver pathology typically reveals midzonal hepatocyte necrosis and injury often with sparing of the central vein and portal tracts, minimal inflammatory cell infiltrates, and preserved reticulin framework. Infected hepatocytes undergo apoptosis with characteristic eosinophilic condensed nuclear chromatin called Councilman bodies.[27] Among patients who develop jaundice, mortality is estimated at 20% to 50%, usually 7 to 10 days afterward. The pathogenesis of severe disease is not fully understood. Proposed mechanisms include undetermined host genetic factors that confer susceptibility to infection, direct viral cytopathic effect, and host cytokine dysregulation. Direct viral infection of hepatocytes and ischemia contribute to the liver injury observed in yellow fever.

Diagnosis is usually established on clinical grounds in persons with an appropriate travel history. Other febrile illnesses that cause jaundice include bacterial sepsis, acute HSV hepatitis, leptospirosis, severe malaria, relapsing fever from *Borrelia recurrentis* infection, dengue hemorrhagic fever, and acute hepatitis A, B, or E infection (although fever is less likely with these hepatotropic viruses). Commercially available tests include immunoglobulin G (IgG) and IgM enzyme-linked immunosorbent assays (ELISAs), which may cross-react with other flaviviruses, whereas PCR testing is available in research laboratories. There are no specific antiviral therapies available for yellow fever. A 17D live-attenuated vaccine is available for travelers to endemic regions, but is contraindicated in pregnancy, and immunosuppressed persons. Reports of serious infection with the attenuated vaccine strain have been reported but are exceedingly rare; fewer than 1 per million vaccinations.

Dengue and Dengue Hemorrhagic Fever

Dengue is an acute, usually self-limited febrile zoonotic illness commonly referred to as breakbone fever. Dengue virus is a flavivirus with 4 antigenically similar types (1–4); however, human infection with one type does not consistently or completely confer immunity to the other types. The World Health Organization estimates that dengue virus infects 50 million people annually.[28] The virus is spread by a mosquito, *Aedes aegypti*, and the disease distribution generally occurs within the vector's distribution (largely tropical and subtropical regions of Africa, the Caribbean, the Americas, Asia, and Australia). The incubation period ranges from several days to 1 to 2 weeks. The symptoms and severity of disease vary with age. Infections are often asymptomatic in children. Classic dengue presents with fever, severe myalgias, arthralgias, headache, retro-orbital pain, gastrointestinal symptoms, and rash. Minor bleeding from mucosal surfaces, hemoptysis, and gastrointestinal hemorrhage can occur.[29] In contrast, dengue hemorrhagic fever (DHF) and dengue shock syndrome (DSS) are characterized by increased vascular permeability, spontaneous hemorrhage, and hypotension.

Serum aminotransaminases are increased in most cases (60%–80%) and can be accompanied by symptoms of acute hepatitis including right upper quadrant pain, hepatomegaly, and jaundice. The enzyme increases peak on day 9 and return to normal levels within 2 to 3 weeks.[30,31] Although the presence of hepatic dysfunction generally does not confer a worse prognosis, liver involvement has been reported to be more severe in DHF and DSS, and fulminant hepatic failure can occur.[31–34] Dengue virus has been isolated and antigen detected in hepatocytes, suggesting that hepatocytes may support viral replication.[34,35] Recently, one group has reported that liver injury in dengue is caused by direct infection of Kupffer cells and hepatocytes.[33] Pathologic evaluation of the liver reveals findings similar to those seen in yellow fever and can include centrilobular necrosis, fatty alterations, hyperplasia of the Kupffer cells, Councilman bodies, and monocyte alteration of the portal tracts.[31,36]

The differential diagnosis of dengue is similar to that of yellow fever. There is no effective antiviral treatment at this time and treatment is supportive. Although there are vaccine candidates in development, there are currently no approved vaccines for dengue.

BACTERIA

Systemic bacterial infections can affect many organ systems, including the liver. The indirect effect of these infections, which is seen with syndromes such as sepsis, are discussed elsewhere in this issue. Formation of abscesses in the liver is a complication of many bacterial infections. Although not a focus of this review, **Table 2** describes the pathogens that have been reported to cause liver abscesses. This topic has also been reviewed in depth elsewhere.[37,38] This article focuses on bacteria with specific liver manifestations.

Typhoid Fever

Salmonella enterica serotype typhi is the causative agent of typhoid fever, which is an enteric fever syndrome characterized by acute onset of fever and abdominal pain. There are approximately 16 million cases of typhoid fever and 600,000 deaths annually.[39] Most of the cases reported in the United States occur either among travelers in endemic areas such as Asia and Central America or during point source outbreaks.[40] Infection usually occurs 1 to 2 weeks after ingestion of the organism. In addition to fever and abdominal pain, other clinical features of typhoid fever are variable and nonspecific, and include headache, relative bradycardia, leukopenia, hepatomegaly, and splenomegaly. Constipation may occur as frequently as diarrhea in otherwise healthy adults, whereas diarrhea occurs more frequently in children and patients infected with human immunodeficiency virus.[41] One of the classically described features, rose spots, which are 2- to 4-mm erythematous papules typically observed on the abdomen and chest, are seen in 5% to 30% of cases.[41] Most cases go untreated or are managed in an outpatient setting. Intestinal perforation occurs in 1% to 3% of those admitted for typhoid fever.[42] Hepatic involvement with *Salmonella* occurs via both hematogenous seeding of the liver during bacteremic periods and from infection of cells of the reticuloendothelial system. Hepatic manifestations of typhoid fever include incidental findings of hepatomegaly and abnormal liver function tests, which occur in 50% of cases. A severe form of disease with jaundice can occur in 0.4% to 26% of cases. The increases in serum transaminases are usually 3 to 5 times the upper limit of normal, with AST usually being higher than the ALT. Twenty-three percent of cases have increases in serum bilirubin, and alkaline phosphatase levels are normal to slightly increased.[43] The diagnosis of typhoid fever is established by positive blood cultures, which are positive in 60% to 80% of cases. Bone marrow cultures have a higher yield and may remain positive even after initiation of antibiotics.[41] Treatment generally entails a 7- to 10-day course of a fluoroquinolone.[41] Live oral and parenteral polysaccharide vaccines are available for travelers to endemic areas and have a protective efficacy that ranges from 50% to 96%.[41]

Mycobacterium Tuberculosis

There are a variety of clinical manifestations of hepatic tuberculosis, prompting some investigators[44] to further classify the various forms as miliary, granulomatous, and localized hepatic tuberculosis. Miliary or disseminated tuberculosis accounts for 50% to 80% of cases.[45] Granulomatous disease refers to cases of caseating granulomatous hepatitis and fever that respond to empiric antitubercular therapy. Localized hepatic tuberculosis may occur either with or without biliary involvement. This last form includes hepatic tuberculous abscesses and tuberculomas, but occurs in less than 1% of tuberculosis in various case series.[46,47] However, localized hepatic tuberculosis accounts for most case series and reports of hepatic tuberculosis cited in the literature and, thus, are the focus of this review. Clinical features of hepatic tuberculosis noted in a review of 4 case series (more than 400 total patients) included fever in 60% to 90% of cases, weight loss in 55% to 75%, hepatomegaly in 80% to 95%, splenomegaly in 25% to 57%, and jaundice in 11% to 35%. Another review of 14 cases noted a median time from the onset of symptoms to presentation for

Table 2
Infectious pathogens isolated from cystic or mass lesions of the liver

	Bacteria					Parasites	Fungi
	Aerobes		Anaerobes				
Gram-negative	Gram-positive	Gram-negative	Gram-positive	Other			
Escherichia coli	Streptococcus species	Bacteroides species	Streptococcus species	Mycobacterium species	Entamoeba histolytica	Candida species	
Klebsiella pneumoniae and other Klebsiella species	Viridans streptococcus (facultatively anaerobic)	Fusobacterium species	Peptococcus species	Chlamydia species	Echinococcus	Cryptococcus	
Pseudomonas aeruginosa	Streptococcus pyogenes	Prevotella	Peptostreptococcus species				
Enterobacter species	Streptococcus pneumoniae	Eikenella	Clostridium species				
Proteus species	Staphylococcus species	Brucella species	Lactobacillus species				
Citrobacter species	Staphylococcus aureus	Veillonella species	Eubacterium				
Morganella species	Staphylococcus epidermidis	Yersinia species	Actinomyces				
Providencia species	Enterococcus species		Propionibacterium acnes				
Salmonella species	Diphtheroid species						
Hemophilus species	Listeria monocytogenes						
Serratia species	Bacillus cereus						
Legionella pneumophila							
Yersinia species							
Burkholderia							
Capnocytophaga canimorsus (facultatively anaerobic)							
Pasteurella species							
Acaligenes xylosoxidans							

medical evaluations of more than 40 days.[47] Diagnostic tests showed modest increases of transaminases (35%–70%), abnormal chest radiographs (65%–78%), and hepatic calcifications of plain abdominal films (50%). On computed tomography (CT), both solitary and multiple lesions were found, and were often difficult to distinguish from malignancy and amebic or pyogenic abscesses. Caseating granulomas were observed in 51% to 83% of cases. In some instances, the tuberculous lesions were described as having a hard, gritty sensation during liver biopsy.[44] Chalky hepatic and bile duct calcifications have also been described.[48] Caseating granulomas may be observed in other infections such as coccidiomycosis,[49] brucellosis,[50] and Hodgkin disease.[51] Noncaseating granulomas have also been observed. The yield of acid-fast bacillus smear and culture are low, ranging from 0% to 45% and 10% to 60% respectively.[52,53] Tissue PCR for *Mycobacterium tuberculosis* may have a higher sensitivity and specificity and allow for more rapid diagnosis.[52,54–56] Treatment entails standard 4-drug antitubercular therapy for at least 1 year. The role of adjunctive drainage is debated, and instances of biliary involvement may necessitate endoscopic retrograde cholangiopancreatography and stent placement.

Brucellosis

Brucellosis is a systemic febrile illness caused by zoonotic infection with *Brucella* species, which are small, intracellular gram-negative diplococci. The 4 species responsible for disease in humans and their main domestic animal hosts include *Brucella melitensis* (sheep, goat), *Brucella abortus* (cows), *Brucella canis* (dogs), and *Brucella suis* (pigs, boar). Most human infections are caused by *B melitensis*. Exposure to domestic animals is the usual mode of transmission. Infection can occur through direct contact with infected animal hides and carcasses, inhalation of aerosols, and ingestion of contaminated milk or milk products. The incubation period is variable and may be up to several months. Apart from fevers, chills, and constitutional symptoms, clinical manifestations of brucellosis can vary widely because multiple organ systems may be involved. One of the most common findings is hepatomegaly, which occurs in 20% to 40% of patients.[57] A review of 530 cases of *B melitensis* infection found hepatomegaly as the most common physical finding, occurring in 38% of cases.[58] The next most common physical finding from the same review was osteoarticular involvement, which was seen in 23% of cases. Increases in aminotransferase levels occur in 25% of cases (range 5%–40%). Jaundice is a rare finding and in a large study 5/432 had jaundice. In one series of 14 brucellosis patients with known hepatic involvement, the average ALT was 152 IU/mL (51–460 IU/mL) and AST was 106 IU/mL (46–240 IU/mL).[57] The extent of liver involvement in brucellosis varies, and may even be species dependent. Hepatitis associated with *Brucella* seems to be mild, with no reports of acute liver failure. In its more severe form, *Brucella* can cause hepatic abscesses, traditionally associated with *B suis*. A correlation with cirrhosis has been observed but is not definitive. Histopathology also varies, with the most common finding being hepatic granulomas, inflammatory cell infiltrates, and mild, localized parenchymal necrosis.[57]

Diagnosing brucellosis is challenging. Serologic assays are the most common diagnostic test used to make the diagnosis. The most commonly available assay is the serum agglutination assay; a titer greater than 1:160 in the presence of a compatible illness is considered diagnostic. Titers generally remain high for prolonged periods. However, this test does not detect *B suis* infections and is not specific, because other organisms may cross-react with the test. ELISA may offer improved sensitivity and specificity, and PCR from blood and tissue specimens is promising but not yet widely available. Blood cultures have a sensitivity of 15% to 70%. Modern blood culture systems seem to have a higher yield. Bone marrow cultures have a higher yield of organisms. In both cases, laboratory personnel should be alerted to the suspicion of brucellosis.

The World Health Organization (WHO) recommends treatment with doxycycline 200 mg daily for 6 weeks combined with either rifampin 600 to 900 mg daily for 6 weeks or intramuscular streptomycin 1 gm daily for 2 weeks.[59]

Q Fever

Q fever is a worldwide zoonotic infection caused by *Coxiella burnetii*, an intracellular gram-negative coccobacillus formerly classified as a rickettsiae. Many animals are reservoirs of infection, with cattle, goats, and sheep being the most frequent sources of human infection. The organism is shed in animals' urine, feces, and milk and is found in high concentrations in placental tissue. Infection typically arises after inhalation of aerosolized infectious particles, usually from parturient livestock or carcasses, although animal contact is notably absent in some cases.[60] Consumption of unpasteurized milk may also lead to infection.

The clinical spectrum of illness caused by this pathogen varies from asymptomatic infection to acute and chronic Q fever. Acute Q fever may manifest as a flulike illness, hepatitis, and pneumonia. Illness is characterized by the acute onset of high fever, headache, and myalgias. When present, pneumonia is usually mild, without characteristic chest radiograph findings. Hepatitis typically manifests as fever and mild asymptomatic increases (2–3 times the upper limit of normal) of transaminases.[61] Other gastrointestinal symptoms, including nausea, vomiting, and abdominal pain, are uncommon. Chronic Q fever may also present as endocarditis, osteomyelitis, arteritis with aneurysm formation, and hepatitis.[62] Q fever hepatitis is seen in younger patients[63] and may even vary geographically because it seems to be more common among cases reported in Spain. In a retrospective review of more than 1000 cases of Q fever in France, 40% presented with hepatitis, and only 8 patients were suspected of having chronic hepatitis.[63] One patient had acute jaundice and liver failure necessitating transplant. Jaundice is reportedly rarely in other case series, usually in less than 1% of cases. It may be difficult to distinguish Q fever hepatitis from other cases of acute hepatitis except for the presence of severe headache and fever. As with other self-limited illnesses with abnormal liver function, biopsy may not be performed, but it can prove useful. Liver pathology reveals minimal hepatic necrosis,[64] a granulomatous hepatitis, and the presence of a characteristic fibrin ring or doughnutlike granulomas, which are fibrin rings surrounding a lipid vacuole. Fibrin ring granulomas have also been observed with CMV, EBV, mycobacterial infections, typhoid fever, and lymphomas.[65] The pathogenesis of liver disease is believed to arise from Kupffer cells, not direct hepatocyte infection, with ensuing granulomatous inflammatory response.[66]

The diagnosis of Q fever is usually established by positive serology, usually indirect immunofluorescent assays.[62] Treatment of symptomatic acute fever is doxycycline for 14 days, whereas much longer (18–36 months) courses with the addition of hydroxychloroquine are required for chronic Q fever, especially endocarditis.

Leptospirosis

Leptospirosis, caused by spirochetes of the genus *Leptospira*, is one of the most widespread zoonotic infections in the world. Human infection is usually acquired through contact with urine from infected animals, most commonly rodents and other small mammals. Infections usually peak during late summer/early fall in temperate regions and the rainy season in the tropics. The clinical presentation of the disease is variable. Subclinical infection occurs in most cases, which, in general, do not seek medical attention. Symptomatic disease generally consists of biphasic illness that can occur in 2 forms: anicteric and icteric (Weil disease). Anicteric disease, generally a self-limited illness, occurs in approximately 90% of infections and presents with an abrupt onset of high fever, chills, rigors, headache, and malaise. Conjunctival suffusion occurs in 30% to 99% of cases, and is an important diagnostic sign. The acute phase can last 5 to 7 days and then is followed a brief period of improvement. A second (or immune) phase is characterized by recurrence of the symptoms and signs seen in the acute phase and may last from 4 to 30 days. Notably, the headache may be severe and throbbing. Other symptoms and signs include nausea, vomiting, abdominal pain, and diarrhea. Aseptic meningitis has been reported in up to 80% of cases and rash may occur in 2% to 30%.[67,68] Increased transaminases and bilirubin are uncommon in this phase, but hepatomegaly can occur.

Icteric disease(Weil disease) is a severe form of the disease that develops in 5% to 10% of cases. In this form, jaundice may occur in the acute phase and last for weeks. The immune phase follows without the period of brief improvement. This phase presents with high fever, hepatic failure, and renal failure. Hemorrhagic complications, likely a result of immune complex–mediated capillary injury, are common and thrombocytopenia may occur in the absence of disseminated intravascular coagulation.[69] Although conjugated bilirubin levels may increase to 80 mg/dL, transaminase increases are usually mild to moderate(<200 U/L). Hepatic histology is usually nonspecific but may reveal intrahepatic cholestasis, hypertrophy of Kupffer cells, and, in severe cases, erythrophagocytosis.[70] Hepatocyte necrosis is usually not seen.

The disease is diagnosed by blood or urine cultures and serologies are used for confirmation of the diagnosis. Doxycycline is effective in mild disease or when used as disease prophylaxis. Penicillin or ceftriaxone are generally used in more severe disease.[71]

Other Spirochetes (Syphilis, Borrelia)

Hepatic involvement during the various stages of syphilis is a rare event in the postantibiotic era. Mild increases in serum aminotransferase levels occur in about 10% of cases of secondary syphilis,[72] whereas, in a large series of more than 30,000 patients, the incidence of acute syphilitic hepatitis was 0.24%.[73] Liver damage is variable and may include evidence of gummas, caseating and noncaseating granulomas, and focal necrosis around the central vein. Hepatic architecture remains intact with cirrhosis occurring rarely.[74,75]

Lyme disease, caused by *Borrelia burgdorferi*, may also be accompanied by hepatitis, usually manifesting as incidental, asymptomatic increases in aminotransferases. This condition has been reported in 20% to 50% of patients with erythema migrans, the initial stage of Lyme disease.[76] Patients presenting with hepatitis as the primary manifestation of Lyme disease are exceedingly rare and, in these instances, diagnosis requires a high index of suspicion. There are 2 cases reported in the literature of granulomatous hepatitis presumably caused by Lyme disease.[77,78]

PARASITES

Evaluation of parasitic infections requires a careful clinical history including travel and exposures to direct further workup. Many parasitic infections may cause liver disease, as outlined in **Table 3**. Schistosoma and malaria are 2 of the most common parasitic infections globally.

Table 3
Parasitic infections of the liver

Parasitic Disease/Agent	Liver Disorder Associated with Infection
Ascariasis	Biliary hyperplasia
Babesiosis	Kupffer cell hyperplasia or infection
Capillariasis	Granulomatous hepatitis
Clonorchiasis	Cholangitis, biliary hyperplasia and obstruction, cholangiocarcinoma
Cryptosporidiosis	Biliary strictures, cholangitis
Echinococcosis	Cystic lesions
Entamoeba histolytica	Hepatic abscess
Fascioliasis	Hepatic fibrosis and necrosis, cholangitis, biliary obstruction, biliary cirrhosis
Opisthorchiasis	Cholangitis, biliary hyperplasia and obstruction, cholangiocarcinoma
Plasmodium species (malaria)	Kupffer cell hyperplasia, rarely hepatic necrosis
Schistosomiasis	Portal fibrosis, portal hypertension
Strongyloidiasis	Periportal inflammation, granulomatous hepatitis
Toxocariasis	Granulomatous hepatitis
Toxoplasmosis	Hepatitis, hepatocyte necrosis
Trypanosoma cruzi	Kupffer cell infection, fatty degeneration, fibrosis
Visceral leishmaniasis	Kupffer cell infection, rare noncaseating granulomas

Schistosomiasis

Schistosomiasis is a parasitic infection caused by trematode blood flukes referred to as schistosomes. The 4 main species capable of producing hepatic complications during human infection include *Schistosoma mansoni*, *Schistosoma japonicum*, *Schistosoma mekongi*, and *Schistosoma intercalatum*. The fifth major species, *Schistosoma haematobium* is classically associated with genitourinary complications and only rarely affects the liver.[79] There are more than 200 million people worldwide with schistosomiasis, about 60% with symptomatic disease. Approximately 20 million suffer from more severe disease that causes an estimated 100,000 deaths annually.[80,81] The geographic distribution of schistosomiasis varies by species and endemic locales are present across tropical and subtropical regions of Africa, Asia, South America, and the Caribbean. Schistosomes have a complicated life cycle, with snails as an intermediate host and humans as the definitive host. Infected humans excrete eggs of the parasite in feces and urine, which can contaminate fresh, warm water, especially in areas with poor sanitation. The eggs hatch, releasing miracidia that infect susceptible snails, reproduce asexually, and emerge as cercariae. The cercariae then penetrate the human skin and transform into schistosomula. The schistosomula traverse through blood and lymph, making their way to the left side of the heart and eventually into mesenteric and portal vessels where the maturing worms take up residence about 3 to 6 weeks after initial infection. The subsequent sexual reproduction with egg deposition in various organs elicits an immune response responsible for tissue damage and disease.[80,82,83]

Clinical syndromes from schistosomiasis include asymptomatic infection, a self-limited cercarial dermatitis (swimmer's itch), acute schistosomiasis, and chronic schistosomiasis. Most infections occur in inhabitants of endemic regions, and the severity of infection is generally proportional to the organism burden. Infections in travelers to endemic regions with brief freshwater exposures have been reported. Most patients with the chronic form will have eosinophilia. Acute schistosomiasis may manifest as Katayama fever, an illness similar to serum sickness and characterized by acute onset of fever, chills, headache, arthralgias, myalgias, diarrhea, and abdominal pain, sometimes accompanied by hepatomegaly. Chronic schistosomiasis can present as intestinal or hepatosplenic disease. Hepatic disease is usually caused by S mansoni, S japonicum, or S mekongi. The spectrum and severity of liver disease seen in schistosomiasis varies according to duration of infection and organism load. Early in the disease, egg deposition in portal vein tributaries elicits an immune response with granuloma formation, hepatomegaly, and splenomegaly. This inflammatory hepatic form of schistosomiasis is usually seen in children. Between 5% and 10% percent of infected young and middle-aged adults who have been infected for several years develop periportal or Symmer pipestem fibrosis as a consequence of the chronic inflammation. Hepatic parenchymal perfusion is usually preserved, thus hepatocyte dysfunction is generally not observed, and lobular architecture remains intact.[82,83] Liver chemistries may be normal. Nonetheless, the fibrosis can progress leading to clinical sequelae of portal hypertension including splenomegaly, bleeding esophageal varices, and, with decompensated disease, encephalopathy and ascites. Stigmata of chronic liver disease are noticeably absent.[83] Patients with concomitant liver disease such as alcoholic hepatitis B or C may have an accelerated disease course.[82]

Diagnosis is based on clinical findings in patients with appropriate exposure history and microscopic examination of feces or urine for eggs. Eosinophilia is present in 33% to 66% of cases.[84,85] Serologic assays, including ELISAs for the various schistosome species, have variable sensitivities, and cannot distinguish acute from chronic infection.[83] Praziquantel 40 to 60 mg/kg divided into 1 to 3 doses for 1 day is the treatment of choice.[82,86]

Malaria

Malaria is caused by 1 of 4 species of the protozoan parasite, Plasmodium: Plasmodium falciparum, Plasmodium vivax, Plasmodium malariae, and Plasmodium ovale. The WHO estimates that there were 246 million cases of malaria in 2006, which led to close to 1 million deaths.[87] It is transmitted through the bite of an infected anopheline mosquito and commonly occurs in areas where this mosquito flourishes, primarily underdeveloped tropical countries. The life cycle of all of the Plasmodium species has 2 phases. The bite of the anopheline mosquito introduces sporozoites into the bloodstream, which, after circulating for a short period of time, invade hepatocytes in the liver. The sporozoites then mature into tissue schizonts, a hepatocyte infected by a sporozoite, which can each produce thousands of merozoites. When the hepatocyte ruptures to release the merozoites, each merozoite can invade a human erythrocyte and produce an additional 20 to 30 merozoites through asexual replication. Infected erythrocytes then rupture to release the merozoites, which are able to repeat this cycle, termed erythrocytic schizogony. In P vivax and P ovale, which can cause relapsing malaria, sporozoites also can become dormant hypnozoites when they invade hepatocytes. These hypnozoites may remain dormant for months after an initial infection, without any symptoms of disease, before they mature to tissue schizonts and produce symptomatic infection.

The classic presentation of malaria is cyclic fever occurring every 48 to 72 hours. Shaking chills usually precede the high fever. Fever coincides with schizont rupture and can be accompanied by cough, headache, nausea, vomiting, abdominal pain, diarrhea, backache, and tachycardia. After several hours, the febrile phase is followed by severe diaphoresis and fatigue. Severe cases of *P falciparum* infection can also present with hypotension, altered consciousness and central nervous system complications, hypoglycemia, renal failure, pulmonary edema, and, occasionally, hepatic failure. Although the exact pathogenesis of all of these complications is not clear, obstruction of the microvasculature related to cytoadherence of *P falciparum* to vessel endothelia, binding of infected erythrocytes to noninfected erythrocytes, reduced erythrocyte deformability, and platelet-mediated clumping of infected erythrocytes of parasitized erythrocytes are believed to be the central process.[88]

Approximately 60 percent of patients with *P falciparum* or *P vivax* may have hepatomegaly and/or splenomegaly.[89] The reports of jaundice seen with malaria vary greatly, from 2.58% to 5.3% of patients with falciparum malaria; however, jaundice has been reported in 11% to 62% of patients during epidemics.[90–92] Jaundice has been reported more commonly in falciparum compared with vivax malaria.[92] Both unconjugated and conjugated hyperbilirubinemia have been reported.[91] Causes of jaundice in malaria include hepatocellular dysfunction; intravascular hemolysis of parasitized red blood cell, septicemic hepatitis, microangiopathic hemolysis associated with disseminated intravascular coagulation, G6PD-related hemolysis, antimalarial drug–induced, coexisting acute viral hepatitis, and underlying chronic hepatitis.[92] Moderate increases of serum aminotransferase levels are commonly seen in malaria. However, severe falciparum malaria may mimic hepatic failure with marked transaminase increases usually accompanied by multiorgan dysfunction.[92] Liver biopsy demonstrates Kupffer cell hyperplasia with pigment deposition caused by phagocytosis of erythrocytes (parasitized and unparasitized). Hepatocyte necrosis, portal inflammation, steatosis, and cholestasis may also be observed, especially in fatal cases.[93]

Peripheral blood smears(thick and thin) can be diagnostic for malaria; however, in many cases, the number of organisms may be low, especially in mild cases. Evaluation by an experienced examiner is recommended in these situations. Clinical history and physical examination are also important in making the diagnosis of malaria. Treatment of malaria depends on the species and the prevalence of antimalarial drug resistance in the region where the malaria was acquired. For chloroquine-sensitive malaria, the treatment is usually chloroquine 600 mg base initially followed by 300 mg base at 6, 24, and 48 hours. Other agents used in the treatment of uncomplicated malaria include mefloquine, quinine plus doxycycline, atovaquone-proguanil, and artemether plus lumefantrine. For patients infected with *P vivax* or *P ovale*, chloroquine treatment is followed by 14 days of primaquine to eradicate hypnozoites. Primaquine is contraindicated in patients with G6PD deficiency.

FUNGI
Candida

Liver infection with *Candida* species usually manifests as hepatosplenic candidiasis, a complication of disseminated candida infection that is usually seen among patients with hematologic malignancies who are recovering from a prolonged severe neutropenia. Before the more widespread use of antifungal chemoprophylaxis among patients at high risk with hematologic malignancies, the incidence of disseminated hepatosplenic candidiasis in various case series varied from 3% to 7%.[94,95] The incidence seems to be decreasing with the more widespread use of antifungal prophylaxis among patients at high risk.[96,97] The pathogenesis of disease is believed to arise from seeding of fungal organisms into liver and spleen after chemotherapy-induced damage to intestinal mucosa. Clinically, the classic symptom of hepatosplenic candidiasis is prolonged fever despite broad spectrum antibiotics in a patient with recovering neutropenia. The patients may also have abdominal pain, and 50% will have hepatomegaly or splenomegaly, or both. Laboratory abnormalities are notable for a substantially increased serum alkaline phosphatase level (3–5 times the upper limit of normal) in 86%[98] and either normal or modest increases in serum aminotransferases. Imaging is the mainstay of diagnosis, with multiple, small, round lesions noted on either CT or magnetic resonance imaging in almost 90% of patients. The characteristic bull's eye appearance, or target lesions, is well described in hepatosplenic candidiasis. Diagnosis is usually made on clinical grounds, precluding the need for more invasive measures. When performed, liver biopsy may reveal granulomatous inflammation with character-istic fungal elements shown with special staining techniques. The treatment of hepatos-plenic candidiasis is usually an induction course of liposomal amphotericin B, because the deoxycholate preparation does not penetrate well into liver tissue[96] and has been associated with treatment failure and relapse.[99] After induction, therapy usually consists of a prolonged course of oral fluconazole in doses of 400 to 800 mg and serial monitoring of imaging (usually CT).[96,100] Optimal duration is unknown but is at least several months, and most patients respond by 6 months.[99]

Other Fungi

Other fungi may involve the liver and do so in a similar manner to Candida (ie, during disseminated infection in immunocompromised hosts). There do not seem to be fungi with a peculiar proclivity for liver tissue, perhaps accounting for the rarity of hepatic fungal infections in the absence of disseminated disease. Candida species normally inhabit the gastrointestinal tract, explaining the frequency with which hepatosplenic candidiasis is seen. Other fungal infections, such as those with endemic mycoses such as Histoplasma capsulatum, are acquired exogenously and typically disseminate in immunocompromised hosts, most commonly those with acquired immune defi-ciency syndrome. Disseminated histoplasmosis is a rare event after acute infection, occurring in about 1 in 2000 cases.[101,102] However, the liver is involved in up to 90% of cases of disseminated histoplasmosis.[103] The pattern of liver involvement is not well characterized and, in one review of 36 cases with hepatic infection, liver involvement was characterized by hepatomegaly and a more diffuse infiltrative infec-tion; focal lesions were only seen in 17% of cases. When present, the focal lesions were small nodules ranging from 0.2 to 1.0 cm. In this series, the yield of visualizing organisms through special fungal stains, such as methenamine silver staining, was high. Presumably, this occurs through liver seeding during dissemination of infection because of the organisms' affinity for the reticuloendothelial system. Liver biopsy find-ings are variable and include sinusoidal Kupffer cell hyperplasia and granulomatous changes in 19% of cases.[104] Diagnosis[105] and treatment of disseminated histoplas-mosis[106] are reviewed elsewhere. Because hepatic involvement by fungi occurs almost exclusively in the context of disseminated infection in immunocompromised hosts, the diagnosis of hepatic fungal infections (with the exception of hepatosplenic candidiasis) is usually established by positive cultures or antigen tests in blood or other extrahepatic sites. Liver biopsy with fungal stains may be a useful diagnostic adjunct in difficult or atypical cases.

SUMMARY

Because of its role as a filter, the liver is exposed to many systemic infectious patho-gens. These pathogens may directly or indirectly affect the liver depending on the characteristics of the pathogen. Liver disease in this setting may frequently be multi-factorial, with the pathogen, other pathogens, and disease states and drug treatments all contributing. In evaluating the liver manifestations of a potential infectious pathogen, diagnosis of some of the less common infectious pathogens is dependent on a high level of suspicion and recognition of some of the key diagnostic clues. Successful diagnosis can only be accomplished through a careful history, including travel and exposures, physical examination, and appropriate microbiologic studies.

REFERENCES

1. Crum NF. Epstein Barr virus hepatitis: case series and review. South Med J 2006;99(5):544–7.
2. Finkel M, Parker GW, Fanselau HA. The hepatitis of infectious mononucleosis: experience with 235 cases. Mil Med 1964;129:533–8.
3. Hinedi TB, Koff RS. Cholestatic hepatitis induced by Epstein-Barr virus infection in an adult. Dig Dis Sci 2003;48:539–41.
4. Randhawa PS, Jaffe R, Demetries AJ, et al. Expression of Epstein-Barr virus-encoded small RNA (by the EBER-1gene) in liver specimens from transplant recipients with post-transplantation lymphoproliferative disease. N Engl J Med 1992; 327:1710–4.
5. Adams LA, Bastiaan B, Jeffrey G, et al. Ganciclovir and the treatment of Epstein-Barr virus hepatitis. J Gastroenterol Hepatol 2006;21:1758–60.
6. Kimura H, Nagasaka T, Hoshino Y, et al. Severe hepatitis caused by Epstein-Barr virus without infection of hepatocytes. Hum Pathol 2001;32:757–62.
7. Suh N, Liapis H, Misdraji J, et al. Epstein-Barr virus hepatitis: diagnostic value of in situ hybridization, polymerase chain reaction, and immunohistochemistry on liver biopsy from immunocompetent patients. Am J Surg Pathol 2007;31(9): 1403–9.
8. Barkholt L, Reinholt FP, Teramoto N, et al. Polymerase chain reaction and in situ hybridization of Epstein-Barr virus in liver biopsy specimens facilitate the diagnosis of EBV hepatitis after liver transplantation. Transpl Int 1998;11:336–44.
9. Lones MA, Shintaku IP, Weiss LM, et al. Posttransplant lymphoproliferative disorder in liver allograft biopsies: a comparison of three methods for the demonstration of Epstein-Barr virus. Hum Pathol 1997;28:533–9.
10. Fereanchak A, Tyson RW, Narkewicz MR, et al. Fulminant Epstein-Barr viral hepatitis: orthotopic liver transplantation and review of the literature. Liver Transpl Surg 1998;4:469–76.
11. de Jong MD, Galasso GJ, Gazzard B, et al. Summary of the 11 International Symposium on Cytomegalovirus. Antiviral Res 1998;39:141–62.
12. Horwitz CA, Henle W, Henle G, et al. Clinical and laboratory evaluation of cytomegalovirus-induced mononucleosis in previously healthy individuals. Report of 82 cases. Medicine 1986;65(3):124–34.
13. Ten Napel CHH, Houthoff HJ, The TH. Cytomegalovirus hepatitis in normal and immune compromised hosts. Liver 1984;4:184–94.
14. Kanno A, Abe M, Yamada M, et al. Clinical features of cytomegalovirus hepatitis in previously healthy adults. Liver 1997;17:129–32.
15. Razonable RR. Cytomegalovirus infection after liver transplantation: current concepts and challenges. World J Gastroenterol 2008;14(31):4849–60.
16. Colina F, Juca NT, Moren E, et al. Histological diagnosis of cytomegalovirus hepatitis in liver allografts. J Clin Pathol 1995;48:351–7.

17. Seehofer D, Rayes N, Tullius SG, et al. CMV hepatitis after liver transplantation: incidence, clinical course and follow up. Liver Transpl 2002;8:1138–46.

18. Lautenschlager I, Halme L, Hockerstedt K, et al. Cytomegalovirus infection of the liver transplant: virological, histological, immunological, and clinical observations. Transpl Infect Dis 2006;8:21–30.

19. Xu F, Sternberg MR, Kottiri BJ, et al. Trends in herpes simplex virus type 1 and type 2 seroprevalence in the United States. JAMA 2006;296:964–73.

20. Fahy RJ, Crouser E, Pacht ER. Herpes simplex type 2 causing fulminant hepatic failure. South Med J 2000;93(12):1212–6.

21. Kaufman B, Gandhi SA, Louie E, et al. Herpes simplex virus hepatitis: case report and review. Clin Infect Dis 1997;24(3):334–8.

22. Aboguddah A, Stein H, Phillips P, et al. Herpes simplex hepatitis in a patient taking prednisone and methotrexate. Report and review of the literature. J Rheumatol 1991;18:1406–12.

23. Sevilla J, Fernandez-Plaza S, Gonzalez-Vincent M, et al. Fatal hepatic failure secondary to acute herpes simplex virus infection. J Pediatr Hematol Oncol 2004;26(10):686–8.

24. Klein NA, Mabie WC, Shaver DC, et al. Herpes simplex virus in pregnancy. Two patients successfully treated with acyclovir. Gastroenterology 1991;100(1):239–44.

25. Barnett ED. Yellow fever: epidemiology and prevention. Clin Infect Dis 2007;44:850–6.

26. Vaughan DW, Barrett A, Solomon T. Flaviviruses. In: Mandell GL, Bennett JE, Dolin R, editors. Mandell, Douglas, and Bennett's principles and practice of infectious diseases. 7th edition. Philadelphia: Churchill Livingstone; 2010. p. 2133–50.

27. Monath TP. Yellow fever: an update. Lancet Infect Dis 2001;1:11–20.

28. WHO. Dengue and dengue haemorrhagic fever. Factsheet No 117, revised. Geneva (Switzerland): World Health Organization; 2009. Available at: http://www.who.int/mediacentre/factsheets/fs117/en/. Accessed October 11, 2010.

29. Tsai CJ, Kuo CH, Chen PC, et al. Upper gastrointestinal bleeding in dengue fever. Am J Gastroenterol 1991;86:33–5.

30. de Souza LJ, Gonçalves Carneiro H, et al. Hepatitis in dengue shock syndrome. Braz J Infect Dis 2002;6(6):322–7.

31. Gulati S, Maheshwari A. Atypical manifestations of dengue. Trop Med Int Health 2007;12(9):1087–95.

32. Mohan B, Patwari AK, Anand VK, et al. Hepatic dysfunction in childhood dengue infection. J Trop Pediatr 2000;46:40–3.

33. Ling LM, Wilder-Smith A, Leo YS. Fulminant hepatitis in dengue haemorrhagic fever. J Clin Virol 2007;38(3):265–8.

34. Miagostovich MP, Santos FB, De Simone TS, et al. Genetic characterization of dengue virus type 3 isolates in the State of Rio de Janeiro, 2001. Braz J Med Biol Res 2002;35:1–4.

35. Nogueira RMR, Miagostovich MP, Schatzmayr HG, et al. Virological study of a dengue type 1 epidemic in Rio de Janeiro. Mem Inst Oswaldo Cruz 1988; 83:219–25.

36. Burke T. Dengue haemorrhagic fever: a pathological study. Trans R Soc Trop Med Hyg 1968;62(5):682–92.

37. Lederman ER, Crum NF. Pyogenic liver abscess with a focus on Klebsiella pneumoniae as a primary pathogen: an emerging disease with unique clinical characteristics. Am J Gastroenterol 2005;100(2):322–31.

38. Johannsen EC, Sifri CD, Madoff LC. Pyogenic liver abscesses. Infect Dis Clin North Am 2000;14(3):547–63.

39. Ivanoff B. Typhoid fever: global situation and WHO recommendations. Southeast Asian J Trop Med Public Health 1995;26(Suppl 2):1–6.
40. Ackers ML, Puhr ND, Tauxe RV, et al. Laboratory-based surveillance of *Salmonella* serotype typhi infections in the United States: antimicrobial resistance on the rise. JAMA 2000;283:2668–73.
41. Parry CM, Tinh Hien T, Dougan G, et al. Typhoid fever. N Engl J Med 2002; 347(22):1770–82.
42. Bitar RE, Tarpley J. Intestinal perforation in typhoid fever: a historical and state-of-the-art review. Rev Infect Dis 1985;7:257–71.
43. Pramoolsinap C, Viranuvatti V. Salmonella hepatitis. J Gastroenterol Hepatol 1998;13:745–50.
44. Alvarez SZ. Hepatobiliary tuberculosis. J Gastroenterol Hepatol 1998;13:833–9.
45. Morrie E. Tuberculosis of the liver. Am Rev Tuberc 1930;22:585–92.
46. Kok KY, Yapp SK. Isolated hepatic tuberculosis: report of five cases and review of the literature. J Hepatobiliary Pancreat Surg 1999;6:195–8.
47. Chong VH. Hepatobiliary tuberculosis: a review of presentations and outcomes. South Med J 2008;101(4):356–61.
48. Maglinte DT, Alvarez SZ, Ng AC, et al. Patterns of calcifications and cholangiographic findings in hepatobiliary tuberculosis. Gastrointest Radiol 1998;3: 331–5.
49. Paggagianis D. Coccidioidiomycosis. In: Samter M, editor. Immunological diseases. Boston: Little Brown; 1971. p. 652–61.
50. Spink WW. Brucellosis immunological mechanisms relating to pathogenesis, diagnosis, and treatment. In: Samter M, editor. Immunological diseases. Boston: Little Brown; 1971. p. 662–7.
51. Johnson LN, Iseri D, Knodell RG. Caseating hepatic granulomas in Hodgkin's lymphoma. Gastroenterology 1990;99:1837–40.
52. Huang WT, Wang CC, Chen W, et al. The nodular form of hepatic tuberculosis: a review with five additional new cases. J Clin Pathol 2003;56:835–9.
53. Chen HC, Chao YC, Shyu RY, et al. Isolated tuberculous liver abscesses with multiple hyperechoic masses on ultrasound: a case report and review of the literature. Liver Int 2003;23:346–50.
54. Diaz ML, Herrera T, Vidal YL, et al. Polymerase chain reaction for the detection of *mycobacterium tuberculosis* DNA in tissue and assessment in of its utility in the diagnosis of hepatic granulomas. J Lab Clin Med 1996;127:359–63.
55. Popper H, Winter E, Hofler G. DNA of *Mycobacterium tuberculosis* in formalin-fixed paraffin-embedded tissues by polymerase chain reaction. Am J Clin Pathol 1994;101:738–41.
56. Ghossein RA, Ross DG, Salomon RN, et al. Rapid detection and species identification of mycobacteria in paraffin-embedded tissues by polymerase chain reaction. Diagn Mol Pathol 1992;1:185–9.
57. Akritidis N, Tzivras M, Delladetsima I, et al. The liver in brucellosis. Clin Gastroenterol Hepatol 2007;5:1109–12.
58. Colmenero JD, Reguera JM, Martos F, et al. Complications associated with *Brucella melitensis* infection: a study of 530 cases. Medicine 1996;75(4): 195–211.
59. Pappas G, Akritidis N, Bosilkovski M, et al. Brucellosis. N Engl J Med 2005; 352(22):2325–36.
60. Tissot-Dupont H, Torres S, Nezri M, et al. Hyperendemic focus of Q fever related to sheep and wind. Am J Epidemiol 1999;150:67–74.
61. Marrie TJ. Liver involvement in acute Q fever. Chest 1988;94:896–8.

62. Tissot-Dupont H, Raoult H. Q fever. Infect Dis Clin North Am 2008;22:505–14.
63. Raoult D, Tissot-Dupont H, Drancourt M, et al. Q fever 1985–1998: clinical and epidemiologic features of 1938 infections. Medicine (Baltimore) 2000;79(2): 109–23.
64. Lai C-H, Chin C, Chung H-C, et al. Acute Q fever hepatitis in patients with and without underlying hepatitis B or C infection. Clin Infect Dis 2007;45:e52–9.
65. Bonilla M-F, Kaul DR, Saint S, et al. Ring around the diagnosis. N Engl J Med 2006;354:1937–42.
66. Maurin M, Raoult D. Q fever. Clin Microbiol Rev 1999;12:518–53.
67. Bharti AR, Nally JE, Ricaldi JN, et al. Leptospirosis: a zoonotic disease of global importance. Lancet Infect Dis 2003;3(12):757–71.
68. Feigin RD, Anderson DC. Human leptospirosis. Crit Rev Clin Lab Sci 1975;5: 413–65.
69. Edwards CN, Nicholson GD, Hassell TA, et al. Thrombocytopenia in leptospirosis: the absence of evidence for disseminated intravascular coagulation. Am J Trop Med Hyg 1986;35(2):352–4.
70. Levett PN. Leptospirosis. Clin Microbiol Rev 2001;14:296–326.
71. Griffith ME, Hospenthal DR, Murray CK. Antimicrobial therapy of leptospirosis. Curr Opin Infect Dis 2006;19:533–7.
72. Jorsa L, Timmer M, Somogyi T, et al. Hepatitis syphilitica. A clinico-pathological study of 25 cases. Acta Hepatogastroenterol 1977;24:344–7.
73. Harn RD. Syphilis of the liver. Am J Syph Gonorrhea Vener Dis 1943;27:529–62.
74. Veeravahu M. Diagnosis of liver involvement in early syphilis. A critical review. Arch Intern Med 1985;145:132–4.
75. Maincent G, Labadie H, Fabre M, et al. Tertiary hepatic syphilis a treatable cause of multinodular liver. Dig Dis Sci 1997;42(2):447–50.
76. Horowitz HW, Dworkin B, Forester G, et al. Liver function in early Lyme disease. Hepatology 1996;23(6):1412–7.
77. Zanchi AC, Gringold AR, Theise ND, et al. Necrotizing granulomatous hepatitis as an unusual manifestation of Lyme disease. Dig Dis Sci 2007;52:2629–32.
78. Chavet P, Pillon D, et al. Granulomatous hepatitis associated with Lyme disease. Lancet 1987;330:623–4.
79. Abdel-Wahab MF, Esmat G, Ramzy I, et al. *Schistosoma haematobium* infection in Egyptian schoolchildren: demonstration of both hepatic and urinary tract morbidity by ultrasonography. Trans R Soc Trop Med Hyg 1992;86:406–9.
80. Maguire J. Trematodes (schistosomes and other flukes). In: Mandell GL, Bennett JE, Dolin R, editors. Mandell, Douglas, and Bennett's principles and practice of infectious diseases. 7th edition. Philadelphia: Churchill Livingstone; 2010. p. 3595–605.
81. Chitsulo L, Loverde P, Engels D. Schistosomiasis. Nat Rev Microbiol 2004;2: 12–3.
82. Gyssels B, Polman K, Clerinx J, et al. Human schistosomiasis. Lancet 2006;368: 1106–18.
83. Bica I, Hamer DH, Stadecker JS. Hepatic schistosomiasis. Infect Dis Clin North Am 2000;14(3):583–604.
84. Gundersen SG, Ravin J, Haagensen I. Early detection of circulating anodic antigen (CAA) in a case of acute *Schistosomiasis mansoni* with Katayama fever. Scand J Infect Dis 1992;24:549–52.
85. Mahmoud AA. The ecology of eosinophils in schistosomiasis. J Infect Dis 1982; 145:613–22.

86. World Health Organization. The control of schistosomiasis. World Health Organ Tech Rep Ser 1985;728:1–113.
87. WHO. Malaria. Factsheet No 94. Geneva (Switzerland): World Health Organization; 2009. Available at: http://www.who.int/mediacentre/factsheets/fs094/en/. Accessed October 11, 2010.
88. Fairhurst RM, Wellems TE. *Plasmodium* species (malaria). In: Mandell GL, Bennett JE, Dolin R, editors. Mandell, Douglas, and Bennett's principles and practice of infectious diseases. 7th edition. Philadelphia: Churchill Livingstone; 2010. p. 3438.
89. Ramachandran S, Perea MV. Jaundice and hepatomegaly in primary malaria. J Trop Med Hyg 1976;79:207–10.
90. Mehta SR, Naidu G, Chandar V, et al. Falciparum malaria: present day problems: an experience with 425 cases. J Assoc Physicians India 1989;37:264–7.
91. Anand AC, Ramji C, Narula AS, et al. Malarial hepatitis: a heterogeneous syndrome? Natl Med J India 1992;5:59–62.
92. Anand AC, Pankaj P. Jaundice in malaria. J Gastroenterol Hepatol 2005;20:1322–32.
93. Rupani AB, Amarapurkar AD. Hepatic changes in fatal malaria: an emerging problem. Ann Trop Med Parasitol 2009;103(2):119–27.
94. Anttila VJ, Elonen E, Nordling S, et al. Hepatosplenic candidiasis in patients with acute leukemia: incidence and prognostic implications. Clin Infect Dis 1997;24:375–80.
95. Blade J, Lopez-Guillermo A, Roman C, et al. Chronic systemic candidiasis in acute leukemia. Ann Hematol 1992;64:240–4.
96. Kontoyiannis DP, Luna MA, Samuela BI, et al. Hepatosplenic candidiasis. A manifestation of chronic disseminated candidiasis. Infect Dis Clin North Am 2000;14(3):721–39.
97. Van Burik JH, Leisenring W, Myerson D, et al. The effect of prophylactic fluconazole on the clinical spectrum of fungal diseases in bone marrow transplant recipients with special attention to hepatic candidiasis. An autopsy study of 355 patients. Medicine (Baltimore) 1998;77:246–54.
98. Pagano L, Mele L, Fianchi L, et al. Chronic disseminated candidiasis in patients with hematologic malignancies. Clinical features and outcome of 29 episodes. Haematologica 2002;87:535–41.
99. Anaissie E, Bodey GP, Kantarijan H, et al. Fluconazole therapy for chronic disseminated candidiasis in patients with leukemia and prior amphotericin B therapy. Am J Med 1991;91:142–50.
100. Pappas PG, Kauffman CA, Andes D, et al. Clinical practice guidelines for the management of candidiasis: 2009 update by the Infectious Diseases Society of America. Clin Infect Dis 2009;48:503–35.
101. Sathapatayavongs B, Batteiger BE, Wheat LJ, et al. Clinical and laboratory features of disseminated histoplasmosis during two large urban outbreaks. Medicine (Baltimore) 1983;62:263–70.
102. Wheat LJ, Connoly-Stringfield PA, Baker RL, et al. Disseminated histoplasmosis in the acquired immune deficiency syndrome: clinical findings, diagnosis and treatment, and review of the literature. Medicine (Baltimore) 1990;69:361–74.
103. Goodwin RA, Shapiro JL, Thurman GH, et al. Disseminated histoplasmosis: clinical and pathologic correlations. Medicine (Baltimore) 1980;59:1–33.

104. Lamps LW, Molina CP, West AB, et al. The pathologic spectrum of gastrointestinal and hepatic histoplasmosis. Am J Clin Pathol 2000;113:64–72.

105. Wheat LJ. Improvements in the diagnosis of histoplasmosis. Expert Opin Biol Ther 2006;6:1207–21.

106. Wheat LJ, Freifield AG, Kleiman MB, et al. Clinical practice guidelines for the management of patients with histoplasmosis: 2007 update by the Infectious Diseases Society of America. Clin Infect Dis 2007;45:807–25.

HIV Infection and the Liver: The Importance of HCV-HIV Coinfection and Drug-Induced Liver Injury

Shehzad N. Merwat, MD[a,b,c], John M. Vierling, MD[a,b,c],*

KEYWORDS

- Human immunodeficiency virus • HAART • Hepatitis C virus
- HCV-HIV coinfection • Pegylated interferon • Ribavirin
- Hepatotoxicity

Coinfection with hepatitis C virus (HCV) and human immunodeficiency virus (HIV) is common, as both viruses share similar routes of transmission (**Box 1**). The prevalence of chronic hepatitis C infection in patients with HIV has been reported in the range of 25% to 30%.[1] The prevalence, however, is substantially higher in HIV-infected injection drug users, and may be more than 85%.[2,3] With the advent of highly active antiretroviral therapy (HAART) for the treatment of HIV, premature deaths due to complications of acquired immune deficiency syndrome (AIDS) have decreased substantially. As life expectancies have increased in patients treated for HIV infection, however, the morbidity and mortality due to advanced liver disease caused by HCV has worsened in coinfected patients. It is now clear that deleterious hepatic outcomes in HCV-HIV coinfected patients are significantly more common among coinfected patients than those in patients infected with HCV alone.[4,5] However, it is important to note that only a minority (approximately 33%) of HCV-HIV coinfected patients currently receives treatment for HCV.[6,7] Because a sustained viral response (SVR,

[a] Hepatology and Liver Transplantation Program, Baylor College of Medicine, and St Luke's Episcopal Hospital, Houston, TX, USA
[b] Department of Medicine, Baylor College of Medicine, 1709 Dryden Street, Suite 1500, Houston, TX 77030, USA
[c] Department of Surgery, Baylor College of Medicine, 1709 Dryden Street, Suite 1500, Houston, TX 77030, USA
* Corresponding author. Department of Medicine, Baylor College of Medicine, 1709 Dryden Street, Suite 1500, Houston, TX 77030.
E-mail address: vierling@bcm.tmc.edu

Clin Liver Dis 15 (2011) 131–152
doi:10.1016/j.cld.2010.09.012
1089-3261/11/$ – see front matter © 2011 Elsevier Inc. All rights reserved.

Box 1
Shared modes of parenteral transmission for both HCV and HIV

Injection drug use

Multiple sexual partners

Men who have sex with men

Blood product transfusion or organ transplant recipient prior to 1992

Vertical transmission from mother to newborn child

Occupational exposure (eg, needle stick)

---

defined as undetectable HCV RNA 24 weeks or more after completion of antiviral therapy) predicts a durable long-term response[8] and a decreased risk of progression to advanced liver disease,[9] identification and appropriate treatment of both HCV and HIV infections represents an unmet need.

The goals of this review are threefold. The first is to review the epidemiology, significance, and consequences of HCV-HIV coinfection. The second is to identify and advocate for the removal of barriers HCV-HIV coinfected patients face in obtaining antiviral therapy for chronic hepatitis C. The final goal is to champion the urgent need for studies of drug-drug interactions between new Specifically Targeted Antiviral Therapy for HCV (STAT-C) agents and HAART regimens, so that combination therapy with STAT-C agents with pegylated interferon and ribavirin can be offered to coinfected patients as soon as possible.

EPIDEMIOLOGY

Approximately 250,000 to 300,000 people in the United States have HCV-HIV coinfection,[7,10] which comprises nearly 25% of all persons infected with HIV and 8% of all persons infected with HCV.[2] The prevalence of HCV-HIV coinfection appear to be similar in Europe, and in one large cohort of 5957 patients with HIV, 33% were HCV seropositive.[11] In another HIV-infected cohort of 1017 European patients, 8% were coinfected with HCV. In accord with United States data, the prevalence of HCV-HIV coinfection was highest among injection drug users.[12]

HCV, HIV, and hepatitis B virus (HBV) share similar routes of parenteral transmission, which include exposures to infected blood or blood products, sexual transmission among heterosexuals and men who have sex with men, and vertical transmission from an infected mother to her neonate during childbirth. However, the efficiency of transmitting HCV and HIV infections varies substantially among these routes of transmission. The greatest risk of HCV and HIV transmission is associated with exposure to contaminated blood during injection drug use. In injection drug users the prevalence of HCV-HIV coinfection approaches 85%, whereas coinfection among persons with only risk factors for sexual transmission is less than 10%.[13] Even though the overall risk of HCV being vertically transmitted is low compared with that with injection drug use, the risk of transmitting HCV to an infant is nearly doubled when the mother is coinfected with HCV and HIV (odds ratio [OR] 1.9; 95% confidence interval [CI] 1.36–2.67) compared with that of mothers infected with HCV alone.[14] In either case, the risk of vertical transmission of HCV is directly proportional to the maternal serum levels of HCV RNA, with increased levels conferring a higher risk of transmission.[15]

While the majority of HCV-HIV coinfected individuals are injection drug users, the incidence of each infection varies in this high-risk population. Specifically, the incidence of HCV is 8 to 10 times higher than that of HIV; thus, it is likely that the majority of coinfected individuals acquire HIV after having been already infected with HCV.[7] However, it is important to note that a person infected with HIV who later becomes infected with HCV is much less likely to clear the acute HCV infection spontaneously.[16,17] The mode of HCV transmission also plays a role in the rate of chronicity in such persons. The ability to clear an acute HCV infection is less likely when a person infected with HIV acquires HCV through injection drug use as compared with acquiring HCV through sexual transmission.[18]

SIGNIFICANCE OF HIV AND HCV COINFECTION
The Impact of HCV on the Natural History of HIV Infection

Most early studies focused on the effects of HIV infection and how it affects liver disease in patients coinfected with HCV and HIV.[19–22] Recently, greater emphasis has been placed on understanding the impact of HCV on the natural history of HIV infection. An initial report from Switzerland after the introduction of HAART for HIV noted that HCV-HIV coinfected patients had greater risks of death or development of an AIDS-related illness.[23] Prospective data on the clinical progression in 1157 patients with HCV-HIV coinfection from a cohort of 3111 patients with HIV infection were analyzed. Multivariate Cox regression analyses showed that the probability of progression to death or a new AIDS-defining clinical event was independently associated with HCV seropositivity (hazard ratio [HR] 1.7; 95% CI 1.26–2.30).[23] However, these findings remain controversial, since a large multicenter longitudinal study of medical records in the United States from 1998 to 2004 concluded that that HCV infection did not increase the risk of death or AIDS-related opportunistic infections after controlling for common confounders. The study population of 10,481 HIV-infected patients included 1991 (19%) with HCV-HIV coinfection.[24] Greub and colleagues[23] conducted a meta-analysis to address the question of whether coinfection with HCV impaired CD4 cell recovery in HIV-infected persons. The study, which included 8 trials involving 6216 patients, found that the mean CD4 T-cell count in patients with HCV-HIV coinfection was 33 cells/mm^3 (95% CI 24–43 cells/mm^3) less than that of patients with HIV infection alone.[25] However, this difference has not been observed in patients on HAART with maximal viral suppression (viral load <50 copies/mL).[26] The clinical significance of these findings remains unclear. Overall, there is no validated evidence that HCV coinfection significantly alters the natural history of HIV infection.[27]

The Impact of HIV on the Natural History of HCV Infection

In contrast to the paucity of data indicating that HCV coinfection alters the natural history of HIV infection, it is now clear that HIV infection has a detrimental impact on the natural history of HCV infection. Prior to the use of HAART, patients infected with HIV succumbed to AIDS-related complications rather rapidly. With the advent of HAART, however, HIV infections became controllable, and the morbidity and mortality caused by AIDS-related complications significantly decreased. As HIV-infected patients lived longer, mortality related to the progression of HCV-related advanced liver disease and its complications of liver failure, variceal hemorrhage, and hepatocellular carcinoma became major causes of mortality in HCV-HIV coinfected patients.[28,29] In the large, prospective Data Collection on Adverse Events of Anti-HIV Drugs (D.A.D.) trial, advanced liver disease HCV-HIV coinfected patients was second only to AIDS as the cause of death (14.5% of all deaths).[30] An increasing rate of liver-related mortality in HCV-HIV coinfected patients was also observed in the French GERMIVIC study, which used serial surveys to assess HIV-related mortality in hospitalized patients from 1995 to 2005. In the 1995 and 1997 surveys, relative mortality rates from liver disease ranged from 1.5% to 6.6%.[31] By the time of the 2005 survey, mortality due to liver disease had increased to 16.7%, whereas AIDS-related mortality had decreased.[32]

The Impact of CD4 Cell Count on Progression of HCV-Related Liver Disease in Patients with HCV-HIV Coinfection

Reports of the impact of CD4 cell counts on the progression of HCV-related liver disease in HCV-HIV coinfection have provided inconsistent results. In a study of 204 patients with HCV infection, 84 (41%) of whom were coinfected with HIV, a CD4 count of less than 500 cells/mm^3 at the time of liver biopsy was significantly associated with advanced fibrosis in those with HCV-HIV coinfection.[33] In another study of 122 coinfected patients, a CD4 cell count of less than 200 cells/mm^3 was significantly associated with a greater rate of fibrosis progression.[34] Finally, a multivariate analysis conducted by Mohsen and colleagues[35] found that a CD4 count of less than 250 cells/mm^3 was the only independent risk factor significantly associated with advanced fibrosis. Although these results indicate an inverse relationship between the CD4 count and hepatic fibrosis in patients with HCV-HIV coinfections, significant fibrotic progression also can occur in coinfected patients with relatively high CD4 cell counts.[36] By contrast, a prospective study of 184 HCV-HIV coinfected patients with at least 2 liver biopsies for comparison (median interval 2.9 years), showed no association between the CD4 count and progression of fibrosis, including amongst those patients with CD4 cell counts of less than 200/mm^3.[37] While a low CD4 cell count may or may not predispose to fibrosis in HCV-HIV coinfection, it is clear that a normal CD4 cell count does not protect against fibrosis progression in either coinfected patients or those infected only with HCV.

The Impact of HCV-HIV Coinfection on Progression of Hepatic Fibrosis in Coinfected Patients

Whereas 14% to 45% of patients with acute HCV monoinfections immunologically clear HCV within 6 months, only about 5% of patients with HIV infection spontaneously clear an acute HCV infection, and those with lower CD4 cell counts do so even less frequently.[17,19,20,38] In addition, liver disease appears to progress more quickly to advanced fibrosis and cirrhosis in patients with HCV-HIV coinfection who do not develop AIDS-related illnesses. In HCV monoinfected patients, progression to cirrhosis occurs in less than 10% after up to 25 years.[17,39] In contrast, several natural history studies in patients with HCV-HIV coinfection showed that the presence of HIV accelerated the rate of fibrosis progression to cirrhosis.[34,35,40] Two meta-analyses have been performed to assess this clinically important issue. First, Graham and colleagues[41] selected 8 studies that included 601 patients with HCV-HIV coinfection out of 1871 patients with HCV infection. These investigators demonstrated that HCV-HIV coinfection significantly increased the risk of cirrhosis on liver biopsy (relative risk [RR] 2.07; 95% CI 1.40–3.07) and the risk of developing decompensation (RR 6.14; 95% CI 2.86–13.20) compared with patients infected with HCV alone. The second, more recent, meta-analysis included 27 studies with a total of 3567 patients with HCV-HIV coinfection. The prevalence of cirrhosis after 20 years and 30 years was 21% and 49%, respectively, which was significantly higher than the prevalence in patients infected with HCV alone (RR 2.1; 95% CI 1.5–3.0).[42] A retrospective study of the rates of progression of hepatic fibrosis included 4852 patients with diverse causes of liver disease, including monoinfection with HCV, HCV-HIV coinfection, monoinfection with HBV, HBV-hepatitis D virus coinfection, alcoholic liver disease, primary biliary cirrhosis, hereditary hemochromatosis, and autoimmune hepatitis found that the most rapid rates of fibrosis progression occurred in patients with HCV-HIV coinfection.[43]

The Impact of HCV-HIV Coinfection in Patients with Decompensated Cirrhosis

The survival of HCV-HIV coinfected patients with decompensated cirrhosis appears to be inferior to that of patients with HCV monoinfection. In a prospective Spanish study of 153 HCV-HIV coinfected consecutive patients followed from the time of their initial presentation with hepatic decompensation, Merchante and colleagues[4] found the median survival was only 13 months. The cumulative probability of survival at 1, 3, and 5 years was 50%, 30%, and 26%, respectively. Multivariate analysis identified the following independent risk factors for mortality: higher Child-Turcotte-Pugh (CTP) score, the presence of hepatic encephalopathy at the time of initial decompensation, and CD4 cell counts lower than 100 cells/mm^3 at the time of first hepatic decompensation. A multicenter, case-control study of 1037 Spanish patients with HCV monoinfection and 180 with HCV-HIV coinfection patients also showed worse outcomes for HCV-HIV coinfected cirrhotics after onset of decompensation than cirrhotics with HCV monoinfection. Specifically, the 1-year and 5-year survival rates were 74% for the HCV monoinfected cirrhotics and 44% for the HCV-HIV coinfected cirrhotics. Median survival for patients with HCV monoinfection was significantly greater than that of HCV-HIV coinfected patients (median survival 48 vs 16 months; RR 2.26, 95% CI 1.51–3.38). Multivariate analysis identified HCV-HIV coinfection as an independent predictor of mortality ($P<.001$).[5] High mortality rates in HCV-HIV coinfected patients and in patients with HIV monoinfections undergoing orthotopic liver transplantation (OLT) evaluation also have been reported. A prospective study conducted in the United States found that only 26% of HIV-infected transplant candidates (76% of whom were coinfected with HCV) underwent OLT, compared with 63% of candidates without HIV infection. This disparity in rates of OLT in part reflected the fact that 36% of the HIV-infected candidates died on the waiting list compared with only 15.5% of HIV-negative candidates ($P<.001$).[44]

Occurrence of spontaneous bacterial peritonitis (SBP) in cirrhotic patients with HIV infection indicated a poor prognosis. A report of 35 cirrhotic patients with HIV infection who had developed SBP during a 12-year period of observation documented HIV infection as an independent risk factor for mortality after the first episode of SBP (HR 9.81; 95% CI 4.03–23.84). In addition, SBP in HIV-infected patients was more often due to infection with *Streptococcus pneumoniae* than observed in patients without HIV infection (22% vs 8%, $P = .02$).[45]

The Significance of HCV-HIV Coinfection and Hepatocellular Carcinoma

At present, the incidence of hepatocellular carcinoma (HCC) in patients with cirrhosis caused by chronic HCV infection varies between 2% and 8% per year.[46] The fact that HCC does not develop in HCV-infected patients before development of cirrhosis means that most immunocompetent patients have had a chronic HCV infection for 20 to 30 years before progressing to cirrhosis. The incidence of HCC in HCV-HIV coinfection appears to be higher than observed in HCV infection. Examination of the incidence of HCC in a large retrospective study of 14,018 HIV-infected male United States veterans showed a significantly increased incident risk ratio (IRR) for HCC in HIV positive veterans than in HIV-negative veterans (IRR 1.68; 95% CI 1.02–2.77). After adjusting for HCV infection and alcohol abuse/dependence, HIV infection was no longer independently associated with a risk for HCC (IRR 0.96; 95% CI 0.56–1.63). Thus, the increased risk of HCC was primarily in veterans who had HCV-HIV coinfection or HIV and alcoholic liver disease.[47] In another large retrospective study of *hospitalized* United

States veterans, including 11,678 with HIV monoinfection and 4761 with HCV-HIV coinfection, Giordano and colleagues[48] also found the incidence of HCC to be greater in coinfected patients (adjusted HR for HCC 5.35 in coinfected compared with HIV monoinfected, 95% CI 2.34–12.20; P<.001). Among veterans diagnosed after the introduction of HAART for HIV infection, the HR for HCC was 5.07 (95% CI 1.72–14.99; P = .003). Of note, the prevalence of HCC in HCV-HIV coinfection may be lower than that in HCV monoinfected patients. In one retrospective study from 8 centers in Spain, a cohort of 180 decompensated, cirrhotic patients with HCV-HIV coinfection were compared with 1037 patients with HCV infection alone.[49] HCC was diagnosed in 234 (23%) patients with HCV monoinfection compared with only 4 (2%) HCV-HIV coinfected subjects (P<.001). One explanation for this disparity in cumulative prevalence is that an increased mortality in HCV-HIV coinfected cirrhotics occurred before HCC could develop.[49] With widespread use of HAART to prevent AIDS-related complications, it is possible that the prevalence of HCC in cirrhotic patients with HCV-HIV coinfection may begin to approximate that of cirrhotic patients with HCV infection alone.

TREATMENT
Evolution of Antiviral Therapy for HCV Infection

Evidence of increased morbidity and mortality caused by progression of chronic hepatitis C in HCV-HIV coinfected patients in the HAART era underscores the urgent need for safe, well tolerated, and effective therapies for both HCV and HIV. Attempts to treat the HCV infection in patients coinfected with HIV has paralleled the evolution of antiviral therapy for chronic HCV, beginning with monotherapy with interferon alone, advancing to combination treatment with interferon and ribavirin, and culminating in the current standard-of-care combination of pegylated interferon and ribavirin. The application of these evolving therapies for HCV to HCV-HIV coinfected patients also paralleled the development of multiple new agents for HAART and an increasing need to tailor HAART based on each individual's pattern of HIV resistance mutations. To optimize the therapeutic impact of combinations of agents in HAART, careful studies were required to determine the impacts of each agent on the bioavailability, pharmacodynamics, and pharmacokinetics of all agents to be used in combination. Because antiviral therapy for HCV has not involved, to date, introduction of agents beyond pegylated interferon and ribavirin, there has not been a need for similar studies of their impacts on agents used in HAART.

Goals of Therapy for HCV Infection

The goals of HCV antiviral treatment are to prevent: (1) progression of liver disease and development of complications of portal hypertension and hepatocellular carcinoma; and (2) liver-related mortality and need for OLT. The surrogate marker for these goals is the SVR, which is defined as the absence of detectable serum HCV RNA using a sensitive polymerase chain reaction (PCR) test at the end of treatment and again 24 weeks or more after cessation of treatment. Long-term follow up studies have demonstrated that an SVR is extremely durable, and for 99% of patients represents a permanent elimination of HCV infection.[8,50]

Antiviral Therapy for HCV in Patients Coinfected with HCV and HIV

The safety, efficacy, and tolerability of pegylated interferon and ribavirin for the treatment of HCV in HCV-HIV coinfected patients was assessed in 4 pivotal studies (Table 1) reported in 2004.[51–54] Overall, the rates of SVR were lower than those observed in patients with HCV infection alone, which was in part due to excessive rates of

Table 1
Comparison of 4 large randomized controlled therapeutic trials in patients with HCV-HIV coinfection

	APRICOT[52]	ACTG[51]	Barcelona Trial[54]	RIBAVIC[53]
Location	Multinational	USA	Spain	France
n=	868	133	95	412
PEG-IFNα	α 2a	α 2a	α 2b	α 2b
Ribavirin dosing	800 mg	600–1000 mg	800–1200 mg (weight based)	800 mg
Treatment duration	48 wk	48 wk	24 wk in genotype 2, 3 & HCV VL <800,000 IU/mL 48 wk in all others	48 wk
CD4 count status	>200/mm³ or 100–200/mm³ and HIV RNA <5000 c/mL	>100/mm³ and HIV RNA <10,000 c/mL	>250/mm³ and HIV RNA <10,000 c/mL	>200/mm³
SVR genotypes 1, 4	29%	14%	38%	17%
SVR genotypes 2, 3	62%	73%	53%	44%
Discontinuation rate (all causes)	25%	12%	15%	39%

Abbreviations: c, copies; IU, international units; PEG-IFN, pegylated interferon; SVR, sustained virological response.

discontinuation because of adverse events and poor tolerability. The results of these 4 studies were combined with 2 other randomized controlled trials[55,56] in a meta-analysis.[57] In accord with results in patients with HCV infection alone, patients with HCV-HIV coinfection treated with pegylated interferon and ribavirin were more likely to achieve an SVR than those treated with standard interferon and ribavirin (OR 2.94, 95% CI 1.70–5.08; $P = .0001$). Neither safety nor compliance was significantly different between patients treated with pegylated interferon and ribavirin and those treated with standard interferon and ribavirin. The likelihood of achieving SVR with pegylated interferon and ribavirin compared with that using standard interferon and ribavirin was greater with genotypes 1 and 4 (OR 4.38, 95% CI 2.85–6.75; $P<.00001$) than with genotypes 2 and 3 (OR 2.33, 95 CI 0.80–6.77; $P = .12$). The likelihood of achieving SVR with pegylated interferon and ribavirin was also greater than that observed using pegylated interferon without ribavirin (OR 2.65, 95% CI 1.87–3.76; $P<.0001$).

Ribavirin, SVR, and Anemia

Adequate doses of ribavirin are required for an optimal treatment response to antiviral therapy in HCV monoinfected patients, and weight-based dosing has become the standard of care.[58] This also was found to be the case in HCV-HIV coinfected patients in the recent PRESCO trial. Most prior trials used a ribavirin dose of 800 mg/d,[52,53,59] which would be considered too low a dose for patients weighing more than 59 kg. In the PRESCO trial, patients received standard weight-based dosing of ribavirin: 1000 mg/d for weight 74 kg or less and 1200 mg/d for weight 75 kg or more. Overall, the SVR rate of 50% exceeded the rates of SVR in the previous trials.[60]

Recent data indicate that SVR in patients treated with pegylated interferon and weight-based ribavirin is correlated with the development of anemia caused by ribavirin-induced hemolysis.[61–63] The correlation between anemia and SVR has suggested that anemia is a surrogate marker for the adequacy of effective ribavirin concentrations in the liver. Although definitive evidence is lacking, many experts advocate using erythropoietin-stimulating agents when hemoglobin levels decrease to less than 10 g/dL to maintain adequate dosing of ribavirin instead of addressing the anemia by reducing the ribavirin dose.

Selection of HCV-HIV Coinfected Patients for HCV Treatment

Antiviral therapy for HCV should be considered for every HCV-HIV coinfected patient because achieving SVR can prevent or retard liver-related complications and premature mortality. However, in the absence of an antiviral therapy for HCV that is completely safe, highly effective, and well tolerated in all stages of disease progression, multiple factors should be considered in the selection of candidates for HCV therapy. To fulfill the obligation of *primum non nocere*, it is essential to avoid antiviral therapy with pegylated interferon and ribavirin in patients with decompensated cirrhosis, advanced cirrhosis with a high risk of decompensation, significant cytopenias, active infections, immune-mediated diseases (eg, rheumatoid arthritis, psoriasis, ulcerative colitis, and Crohn disease), and autoimmune diseases (eg, systemic lupus erythematosus, Graves disease, myasthenia gravis, autoimmune hepatitis, primary biliary cirrhosis, primary sclerosing cholangitis) to reduce the risk of liver failure, significant toxicities, and exacerbations of preexisting immunologic diseases (**Table 2**). Patients with decompensated cirrhosis, defined as the presence of ascites, gastroesophageal varices, hepatic encephalopathy, and severe hypersplenism, have an unacceptably high risk of complications when treated with conventional doses of interferon and ribavirin.[50] A CTP score of 7 or more or model for end-stage liver disease (MELD) score of 15 or more also portend an unacceptable rate of complications. It is notable that a minority of patients with decompensated cirrhosis due to HCV infection awaiting OLT have been successfully treated using a low-dose accelerating regimen (LDAR), in which dose escalation is pursued only in patients who tolerate the interferon and ribavirin.[64] However, access to OLT for patients who clinically deteriorate during therapy is a key safety provision of this protocol. Thus, an escalating dose approach should not be considered for patients with decompensated cirrhosis unless actively listed for OLT. The levels of pretreatment cytopenias also influence selection of candidates for antiviral therapy for HCV infection. Because weight-based ribavirin predictably causes hemolytic anemia, baseline hemoglobin must be greater than 12 g/dL in men and more than 11 g/dL in women. At baseline, the absolute neutrophil count should be more than 1500/cm^3, and the platelet count greater than 75,000/cm^3.[10]

Alanine aminotransferase in selection for antiviral therapy

Approximately 25% of HCV monoinfected patients have persistently normal alanine aminotransferase (ALT) levels, based on conventional laboratory ranges.[65–67] Normal values of ALT are more commonly observed in women[68] and in patients infected with genotype 4.[69–71] HCV-HIV coinfected patients, however, most often have elevated ALT levels, even in the absence of significant fibrosis on liver biopsy. Two reports identified normal ALT levels in only 7% to 9% of HCV-HIV coinfected patients. Despite the absence of ALT elevations, 25% to 40% of these patients had significant fibrosis on biopsy.[71,72] This prevalence of aminotransferase elevation is higher than the 10% to 30% of monoinfected patients who have ALT elevation.[68,73] Thus, normal ALT levels in HCV-HIV coinfected patients should not be regarded as evidence that antiviral therapy for HCV is unwarranted. On the contrary, such patients should be treated to prevent the possibility of progression to advanced liver fibrosis.[74]

Table 2
Important considerations regarding antiviral therapy for HCV infection in patients with HCV-HIV coinfection

Factors	Comments
Cirrhotics: –CTP or MELD score –Hyperbilirubinemia –Coagulopathy –Renal impairment	Decompensated cirrhosis is a contraindication for HCV antiviral therapy Must assess potential to decompensate during HCV antiviral therapy in all cirrhotics
Genotype	Probability of SVR Related to Genotype: Genotypes 2 > 3 >> 4 >> 1
Liver biopsy	Not required but may be considered if the risks versus benefits of treatment are unclear. Noninvasive tests may have some role in assessing degree of underlying fibrosis
ALT	Patients with persistently normal ALT should be considered candidates for treatment
CBC	Preexisting cytopenias are relative contraindications for therapy
Illicit substance abuse	Active abuse may not be an absolute contraindication if with appropriate monitoring and patient compliance
Alcohol abuse	Alcohol abuse promotes hepatic fibrogenesis and hepatic alcohol metabolism may interfere with response to HCV therapy. Abstinence recommended
Mental illness	Significant history of mental illness may be a contraindication for therapy. Psychiatric clearance for HCV therapy required for patients with significant depression or bipolar disorder
Seizure disorder	Uncontrolled seizure disorder is absolute contraindication for HCV therapy Neurologic clearance for HCV therapy required for patients using antiseizure medications
Smoking	Should be discouraged because of associated risk for upper and lower respiratory infection but not a contraindication for therapy

Abbreviations: ALT, alanine aminotransferase; CBC, complete blood count; CTP, Child-Turcotte-Pugh; MELD, model for end-stage liver disease; SVR, sustained viral response.

Liver biopsy in selection for antiviral therapy

A liver biopsy provides important diagnostic and prognostic information about primary and comorbid liver diseases. In HCV infection, both the grade of inflammation and stage of fibrosis can be quantified, and both features have prognostic significance.[75] Recently revised Practice Guidelines from the American Association for the Study of Liver Diseases recommended that liver biopsy be considered in HCV monoinfected patients when the patient and physician need to use the grade of inflammation and stage of fibrosis to determine the patient's prognosis without therapy.[50] In addition, a biopsy showing cirrhosis (stage 4 fibrosis) would also indicate the need to initiate surveillance imaging and α-fetoprotein testing every 6 months. Because the risk of progressive fibrosis is increased in HCV-HIV coinfected patients, antiviral therapy should not be withheld, even with a biopsy showing stage 0 or 1 fibrosis. Noninvasive markers of fibrosis are increasingly available as alternatives to liver biopsy.[10,74] A recent meta-analysis of noninvasive fibrosis tests included 5 studies of appropriate design containing a total of 574 HCV-HIV coinfected patients.[76] Four fibrosis tests based on the measurement of various serum markers yielded favorable results. The different serum marker panels reviewed included the FibroTest (a composite of 5 markers to include α2-microglobulin, apolipoprotein A1, haptoglobin, γ-glutamyl-transpeptidase [GGT], and bilirubin), APRI (aspartate aminotransferase-platelet ratio index) (n = 4 studies), Forns index (age, GGT, cholesterol, and platelets) (n = 2 studies), and SHASTA (hyaluronic acid, aspartate aminotransferase, and albumin). In a retrospective cross-sectional study of 398 HCV-HIV coinfected patients, the accuracy of the Forns index and APRI serum tests for detection of hepatic fibrosis were found to have less diagnostic accuracy when compared with results obtained from previous studies of these indices in HCV monoinfected patients.[77] By contrast, another study did not detect any differences in the reliability of noninvasive tests for the detection of fibrosis in HCV-HIV coinfected patients (n = 97).[78] Given that advanced HIV infection predisposes to opportunistic infection and subsequent inflammation with resultant biochemical abnormalities, in addition to the biochemical abnormalities that may be caused by prescription drug therapy for HIV infection, such as bilirubin elevations with atazanavir, γ-glutamate transaminase elevations with nonnucleoside reverse transcriptase inhibitors, and hypercholesterolemia observed with some protease inhibitors, interpretation of serum markers of fibrosis is less reliable.[74] Recently, magnetic resonance imaging elastometry has shown promise by achieving excellent correlations with the biopsy stage of fibrosis.[79,80] Based on current recommendations, it is clear that there is little need for staging hepatic fibrosis to aid in decisions about treatment of HCV-HIV coinfected patients with pegylated interferon and ribavirin. Thus, neither liver biopsy nor noninvasive tests for fibrosis are mandatory before initiating therapy.

Effects of HIV Treatment on the Progression of HCV-Related Liver Disease

Hepatologists are increasingly consulted to evaluate the status of liver disease and develop plans for treatment and management of HCV-HIV coinfected patients receiving HAART. The results from several recent studies have indicated that liver-related outcome in confected patients receiving HAART are superior to those in coinfected patients not receiving HAART. In a Spanish prospective study of 153 HCV-HIV coinfected patients, the cumulative probability of survival in patients receiving HAART was 60% at 1 year and 40% at 3 years, compared with 38% at 1 year and 18% at 3 years in patients not receiving HAART (P<.0001).[4] Benhamou and colleagues[81] assessed liver biopsies from 182 consecutive patients with HCV-HIV coinfection, and found that fibrosis stage was lower in patients receiving protease inhibitors (PIs) for HIV than observed in patients who had never received PIs (P = .03). Comparing the cumulative prevalence of cirrhosis at 5, 15, and 25 years showed that antiretroviral treatment with PIs reduced the rate (2%, 5%, and 9% with PIs vs 5%, 18%, and 27% in patients never treated with a PI; P = .0006). Among 210 HCV-HIV coinfected patients followed at an HIV clinic, 64% had received HAART within 2 years of liver disease assessment, and HAART was associated with the absence of significant fibrosis.[82] Shorter cumulative exposure to HAART was associated with greater necroinflammatory activity (adjusted OR per year of exposure, 0.8; 95% CI 0.70–0.96). Moreover, hepatic inflammation was minimal in those in whom HAART had suppressed HIV RNA to undetectable levels (P<.01). The relationship between HAART-related aminotransferase elevation and degree of liver fibrosis was studied. Amongst 12% of individuals (n = 26) who had previous HAART-associated liver enzyme elevations (biochemical grades 3–4), those in whom the liver enzymes normalized did not have more severe liver fibrosis than individuals who did not have liver enzyme elevations. On the other hand, liver fibrosis was more severe in persons in whom liver enzyme elevations remained persistent (biochemical grades 1–4).[82] Similarly, Verma and colleagues[83] and Brau and colleagues[84] found that HCV-HIV coinfected patients with undetectable HIV viral load had liver histologic findings similar to HCV monoinfected patients. In the larger of these 2 studies,[84] 274 HCV-HIV coinfected patients were recruited from two centers, one in Puerto Rico and the other in New York. Fibrosis progression rates (FPR) were assessed after patients were stratified according to CD4 counts and HIV viral load at the time of biopsy. The investigators observed that HCV-HIV coinfected patients with HIV viral loads less than 400 copies/mL had similar FPR to those of HCV monoinfected patients (0.122 Ishak fibrosis units/year vs 0.128 units/year, $P = .52$). In contrast, HCV-HIV coinfected patients with HIV viral loads greater than 400 copies/mL had higher FPR compared with HCV monoinfected patients (0.151 units/year vs 0.128 units/year, $P = .015$) and with coinfected subjects with HIV viral load less than 400 copies/mL (0.151 units/year vs 0.122 units/year, $P = .013$). HIV viral load, but not CD4 count, was an independent predictor of the rate of progression of hepatic fibrosis. There is well described hepato-toxicity associated with HAART; however, taking the above current evidence into account, HAART therapy appears to be of benefit from both the HIV and liver disease point of view, and should be considered in all coinfected patients.[85]

Treatment of Acute HCV Infection in Patients Infected with HIV

Patients with HIV infection are much less likely to clear an acute HCV infection than are persons without HIV.[17,19,20,38] Higher rates of HCV transmission occur in HIV-infected patients who are injection drug users or men who have sex with men. An analysis of acute HCV infections in men who have sex with men conducted in HIV and genitouri-nary clinics in the London and Brighton areas showed that the incidence of new HCV infections had increased from 6.86 per 1000 in 2002 to 11.58 per 1000 in the period January to June 2006.[86] Because acute HCV infection is most often asymptomatic, diagnosis is always difficult. In addition, the diagnostic utility of testing for anti-HCV antibodies to detect acute HCV infection is compromised by a delayed time serocon-version in patients with HIV.[38] Thus, it is more reasonable and accurate to use HCV RNA PCR to test for acute HCV infection in HIV-infected patients. Because HIV infec-tion reduces the probability of spontaneous clearance of an acute HCV infection, early antiviral therapy to prevent chronic HCV infection is especially appropriate. Because spontaneous clearance of HCV primarily occurs within the first 12 weeks of infection, antiviral therapy for HCV infection can be postponed until after this period without compromising efficacy.[87] In one study, 10 out of 11 HIV-infected patients with acute HCV infection permanently cleared HCV with interferon or interferon and ribavirin.[88] In another study, 19 HIV-infected patients were treated for acute HCV infection with pegylated interferon α-2a (180 μg/wk) and ribavirin (800 mg/d) for 24 weeks. Fourteen finished 24 weeks of antiviral therapy, and 10 (53% based on intention to treat anal-ysis) achieved an SVR.[89] While it remains unclear whether the addition of ribavirin to pegylated interferon increases the probability of a HIV-infected patient eliminating HCV during an acute infection, lower rates of spontaneous clearance of HCV by an HIV-infected patient argue for treatment with both pegylated interferon and ribavirin for 24 weeks.[16,74] **Fig. 1** shows a proposed scheme for the diagnosis and therapy of HCV-HIV coninfected patients using standard-of-care antiviral therapy.

BARRIERS TO TREATMENT

Barriers to treatment clearly exist for HCV-HIV coinfected patients (**Box 2**). One barrier involves physicians' recommendations against initiation of antiviral therapy for HCV in coinfected patients. In the observational study of HCV-HIV coinfected patients by Cacoub and colleagues,[90] physicians recommended against antiviral therapy in 84% of cases. Their reasons included concern about excessive alcohol consumption

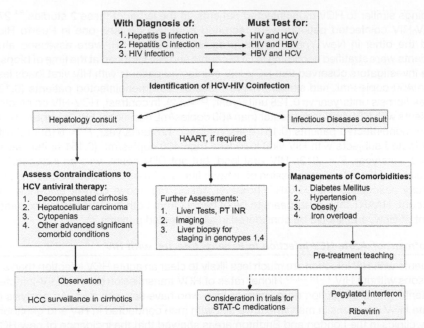

Fig. 1. Proposed scheme for the diagnosis and management of patients with HCV-HIV coinfection. INR, international normalized ratio; PT, prothrombin time.

and/or active drug use, concern about poor patient compliance, and identification of relative contraindications for combination therapy with interferon and ribavirin. In another study of 149 HCV-HIV coinfected patients, 70% were deemed ineligible for treatment because of failure to keep medical appointments (23%), use of drugs or alcohol in the preceding 6 months (23%), active psychiatric diseases (21%) and decompensated liver disease (13%).[6] These studies highlight the challenges of using antiviral therapy for chronic HCV infection in HCV-HIV coinfected patients but do not diminish the urgent need to provide antiviral therapy to all eligible patients. Based on the success of Sylvestre[91] in providing successful antiviral therapy for HCV infection in patients with active substance and alcohol abuse, the emerging model for improved care is a multidisciplinary team approach involving hepatologists, substance and alcohol abuse counselors, psychiatrists, and psychologists.[90,92]

HEPATOTOXICITY OF MEDICATIONS
Interactions Between HAART and Antiviral Medications for the Treatment of HCV Infection

Because treatments for both HIV and HCV involve multidrug regimens, there is legitimate concern about possible deleterious drug-drug interactions that could compromise the effectiveness of HAART as well as the clinical impact of drug toxicities (**Table 3**). The deleterious interaction between ribavirin and didanosine, resulting in increased incidence of pancreatitis, lactic acidosis, and decompensation of cirrhosis, serves as a historical reminder of the issue.[93,94] Ribavirin appears increase the intracellular inosine monophosphate pool, which acts as phosphate donor for the conversion of didanosine into dideoxy-IMP (inosine monophosphate) that is then metabolized into dideoxy-ATP, inhibiting both HIV reverse transcriptase and mitochondrial DNA polymerase γ, hence increasing mitochondrial DNA depletion.[95–97] The risk of additive

Box 2
Barriers to HCV antiviral therapy in patients with HCV-HIV coinfection

Physician -Related:	**Patient Related:**
Refusal of recommended liver biopsy	Limited access to HCV antiviral therapy
US evidence of hepatic lesions (hemangiomas?)	Refusal of HCV antiviral therapy
Physician convinced of poor compliance among patients with HCV-HIV coinfection	Significant substance abuse
HIV considered only priority for treatment	History of non-noncompliance
HCV therapy deemed unnecessary because of minimal liver disease	Failure to return for appointments
Unaware of potential for successful HCV therapy in patients with active substance abuse	Financial concerns about medications, laboratory tests, and required appointments
Concern for female patients of childbearing age to practice 2 modes of contraception	
Medical Conditions:	
Advanced fibrosis or cirrhosis	
Cytopenias	
Significant psychiatric disease	
Immune-mediated or autoimmune diseases	
Significant cardiovascular or respiratory diseases	
Retinopathy	
Uncontrolled diabetes mellitus	
Uncontrolled hypertension	
Autoimmune disorders	

toxicities also exists, as illustrated by the increased magnitude of cytopenias observed in patients treated with zidovudine and ribavirin.[98] Another concern is that combinations of drugs may reduce efficacy in the absence of toxicity. For example, the use of abacavir with ribavirin appears to reduce the virological response to HCV treatment.[99]

Hepatotoxicity of HAART

Hepatotoxicity as a complication of various regimens of HAART has been well described (**Table 4**). The severity of the hepatotoxicities ranges from asymptomatic elevations of aminotransferase levels to fatal acute liver failure.[100,101] HCV infection, HBV infection, and alcohol abuse have been identified as risk factors for hepatotoxicity caused by HAART, and are especially associated with severe grade 3 and 4

Table 3	
Adverse interactions between ribavirin and components of HAART	
Drug Combination	**Interaction**
Didanosine and ribavirin	Potentially fatal mitochondrial toxicity with lactic acidosis Combination absolutely contraindicated
Zidovudine and ribavirin	Substantially greater anemia or neutropenia than observed with either agent alone Combination to be avoided
Abacavir and ribavirin	Potential for decreased efficacy of HCV antiviral therapy with this regimen Combination to be avoided

Table 4
Hepatotoxicity associated with components of HAART

Type of Hepatotoxicity	Drugs
Early onset (1–4 wk) Non–dose related Immune-mediated hypersensitivity	Nevirapine, abacavir
Late onset (4–8 mo) Dose related Mediated by direct toxicity	Didanosine, stavudine, nevirapine, ritinovir, tipranavir

events.[102–105] Two groups have reported that HCV genotype 3 was associated with a higher incidence of hepatotoxicity due to HAART.[70,104] The underlying mechanisms for HAART hepatotoxicity are poorly understood and difficult to analyze, because HAART regimens are not uniform and often require individualization because of HIV drug-resistant mutants. The most important theoretical mechanisms of hepatotoxicity of HAART include: (1) direct toxicity from individual component drugs; (2) mitochondrial toxicity of nucleoside agents; (3) idiosyncratic hypersensitivity reactions; (4) induction of hepatic metabolic abnormalities; and (5) immune-mediated following reconstitution of immune activity in patients coinfected with HIV and HCV or HBV.[106] A retrospective study of 132 HCV-HIV coinfected patients who had been observed for a mean of 35 months after interferon therapy identified 49 episodes of hepatotoxicity (9.7% per year).[107] The annual incidence of hepatotoxic events was greater in patients who had not achieved an SVR than in those who did (14.4%/year vs 3.1%/year; $P<.001$). Failure to achieve SVR (OR 6.13, 95% CI 1.83–37.45; $P = .003$) or HAART regimens containing didanosine or stavudine (OR 3.59, 95% CI 1.23–10.42; $P = .02$) were significant independent predictors of hepatotoxicity.[107] Although recognition of hepatotoxicity remains important, it should not dissuade physicians or patients from prescribing HAART.[108]

ORTHOTOPIC LIVER TRANSPLANTATION IN HCV-HIV COINFECTED PATIENTS

Prior to the development of HAART becoming capable of controlling HIV infection and preventing AIDS-related complications, HIV infection was considered an absolute contraindication to OLT as well as transplantation of other solid organs.[109] As discussed earlier, the improved survival of patients receiving HAART for HIV infection resulted in recognition of an increased morbidity and mortality due to hepatitis C cirrhosis and its complications in HCV-HIV coinfected patients. To date, OLT has been performed in several hundred selected patients with HCV-HIV coinfection, with mixed results.[110]

Although long-term data remain limited, HCV-HIV coinfected patients may have a worse outcome following OLT than cirrhotic patients with HCV infection alone. A study of 79 consecutive patients transplanted between 1999 and 2005 (35 with HCV-HIV coinfection and 44 with HCV infection alone) reported 2- and 5-year survival rates of 73% and 51% in HCV-HIV coinfected patients compared with 91% and 81% in HCV monoinfected patients ($P = .004$).[111] Two other studies, each containing only small numbers of patients, also showed a trend toward worse survivals after OLT for cirrhotic patients with HCV-HIV coinfection; however, survival differences were not statistically significant. Testillano and colleagues[112] reported that the 1-, 2-, and 3-year survival rates of 12 patients with HCV-HIV coinfection after OLT were 83%, 75%, and 62%, respectively, whereas the survival rates of 59 patients with HCV infection alone were 98%, 89%, and 84%, respectively ($P = .09$). In a retrospective case-control study of 27 HCV-HIV coinfected patients matched with 27 HCV monoinfected patients, de Vera and colleagues observed 1-, 3-, and 5-year survival rates in the HCV-HIV coinfected patients of 67%, 56%, and 33%, respectively, compared with survival rates of 76%, 72%, and 72%, respectively, in HCV monoinfected patients ($P = .07$). de Vera and colleagues also noted that HCV-HIV coinfected patients had a statistically significantly higher risk of developing cirrhosis and dying from complications of recurrent HCV infection after OLT than did HCV monoinfected patients (RR 2.6, 95% CI 1.06–6.35; $P = .03$).[113] Risk factors for inferior survival included African American race ($P = .02$), post-OLT intolerance of HAART OLT ($P = .01$), pre-OLT MELD score greater than 20 ($P = .05$), and a viral load greater than 30 million IU/mL ($P = .000$). In contrast, a prospective study of 11 HIV-infected patients undergoing OLT (6 with HCV-HIV coinfection and 5 with HBV-HIV coinfection) showed 1- and 3-year survival rates of 91% and 64%, respectively, which were similar to those in the UNOS 1999–2004 database.[114] Four of the 6 HCV-HIV coinfected patients had recurrent HCV infection, while no recurrent HBV infections occurred.

Additional studies are required to determine the applicability of OLT in HIV-infected patients, the majority of whom have HCV-HIV coinfection. Data from the NIH-sponsored multicenter group assessing OLT in HIV-infected patients are eagerly awaited.[115]

SUMMARY

The issue of HIV and the liver is dominated by the high frequency of HCV-HIV coinfections, due to the fact that both viruses are parenterally transmitted. Prior to the introduction of HAART, premature deaths due to AIDS-related complications obscured the impact of HCV infection. As HAART led to control of HIV infections and prevention of AIDS-related complications, it became clear that HCV infection was associated with an accelerated progression to cirrhosis and an increase in liver-related morbidity and mortality in patients with HCV-HIV coinfection. In addition, HAART has been implicated in drug-induced liver injury. Unfortunately, antiviral therapy with pegylated interferon and ribavirin for HCV in HCV-HIV coinfected patients has been less successful than in patients with HCV monoinfections. Multiple barriers, including decompensated liver disease, substance abuse, socioeconomic condition, and compliance, also limit the number of HCV-HIV coinfected patients who receive antiviral therapy for HCV. The incidences of decompensated cirrhosis and HCC are increased in HCV-HIV coinfected patients. In cirrhosis caused by HCV or other etiological factors in HIV-infected patients, the role of OLT remains controversial. Clinical trials of HCV-specific protease or polymerase inhibitors combined with pegylated interferon and ribavirin are needed urgently in coinfected patients both before and after OLT.

REFERENCES

1. Thomas DL. Hepatitis C and human immunodeficiency virus infection. Hepatology 2002;36(5 Suppl 1):S201–9.
2. Sherman KE, Rouster SD, Chung RT, et al. Hepatitis C virus prevalence among patients infected with human immunodeficiency virus: a cross-sectional analysis of the US adult AIDS Clinical Trials Group. Clin Infect Dis 2002;34(6):831–7.
3. Sulkowski MS, Thomas DL. Hepatitis C in the HIV-infected patient. Clin Liver Dis 2003;7(1):179–94.
4. Merchante N, Giron-Gonzalez JA, Gonzalez-Serrano M, et al. Survival and prognostic factors of HIV-infected patients with HCV-related end-stage liver disease. AIDS 2006;20(1):49–57.

5. Pineda JA, Romero-Gomez M, az-Garcia F, et al. HIV coinfection shortens the survival of patients with hepatitis C virus-related decompensated cirrhosis. Hepatology 2005;41(4):779–89.

6. Fleming CA, Craven DE, Thornton D, et al. Hepatitis C virus and human immunodeficiency virus coinfection in an urban population: low eligibility for interferon treatment. Clin Infect Dis 2003;36(1):97–100.

7. Thomas DL. The challenge of hepatitis C in the HIV-infected person. Annu Rev Med 2008;59:473–85.

8. Lau DT, Kleiner DE, Ghany MG, et al. 10-Year follow-up after interferon-alpha therapy for chronic hepatitis C. Hepatology 1998;28(4):1121–7.

9. Poynard T, McHutchison J, Manns M, et al. Impact of pegylated interferon alfa-2b and ribavirin on liver fibrosis in patients with chronic hepatitis C. Gastroenterology 2002;122(5):1303–13.

10. Singal AK, Anand BS. Management of hepatitis C virus infection in HIV/HCV co-infected patients: clinical review. World J Gastroenterol 2009;15(30):3713–24.

11. Rockstroh JK, Mocroft A, Soriano V, et al. Influence of hepatitis C virus infection on HIV-1 disease progression and response to highly active antiretroviral therapy. J Infect Dis 2005;192(6):992–1002.

12. Mohsen AH, Murad S, Easterbrook PJ. Prevalence of hepatitis C in an ethnically diverse HIV-1-infected cohort in south London. HIV Med 2005;6(3):206–15.

13. Larsen C, Pialoux G, Salmon D, et al. Prevalence of hepatitis C and hepatitis B infection in the HIV-infected population of France, 2004. Euro Surveill 2008; 13(22):18888.

14. Polis CB, Shah SN, Johnson KE, et al. Impact of maternal HIV coinfection on the vertical transmission of hepatitis C virus: a meta-analysis. Clin Infect Dis 2007; 44(8):1123–31.

15. Thomas DL, Villano SA, Riester KA, et al. Perinatal transmission of hepatitis C virus from human immunodeficiency virus type 1-infected mothers. Women and Infants Transmission Study. J Infect Dis 1998;177(6):1480–8.

16. Dionne-Odom J, Osborn MK, Radziewicz H, et al. Acute hepatitis C and HIV co-infection. Lancet Infect Dis 2009;9(12):775–83.

17. Thomas DL, Astemborski J, Rai RM, et al. The natural history of hepatitis C virus infection: host, viral, and environmental factors. JAMA 2000;284(4):450–6.

18. Shores NJ, Maida I, Soriano V, et al. Sexual transmission is associated with spontaneous HCV clearance in HIV-infected patients. J Hepatol 2008;49(3): 323–8.

19. Alter MJ, Margolis HS, Krawczynski K, et al. The natural history of community-acquired hepatitis C in the United States. The Sentinel Counties Chronic non-A, non-B Hepatitis Study Team. N Engl J Med 1992;327(27):1899–905.

20. Villano SA, Vlahov D, Nelson KE, et al. Persistence of viremia and the importance of long-term follow-up after acute hepatitis C infection. Hepatology 1999;29(3):908–14.

21. Garcia-Samaniego J, Soriano V, Castilla J, et al. Influence of hepatitis C virus genotypes and HIV infection on histological severity of chronic hepatitis C. The Hepatitis/HIV Spanish Study Group. Am J Gastroenterol 1997;92(7):1130–4.

22. Romeo R, Rumi MG, Donato MF, et al. Hepatitis C is more severe in drug users with human immunodeficiency virus infection. J Viral Hepat 2000;7(4):297–301.

23. Greub G, Ledergerber B, Battegay M, et al. Clinical progression, survival, and immune recovery during antiretroviral therapy in patients with HIV-1 and hepatitis C virus coinfection: the Swiss HIV Cohort Study. Lancet 2000;356(9244): 1800–5.

24. Sullivan PS, Hanson DL, Teshale EH, et al. Effect of hepatitis C infection on progression of HIV disease and early response to initial antiretroviral therapy. AIDS 2006;20(8):1171–9.
25. Miller MF, Haley C, Koziel MJ, et al. Impact of hepatitis C virus on immune restoration in HIV-infected patients who start highly active antiretroviral therapy: a meta-analysis. Clin Infect Dis 2005;41(5):713–20.
26. Peters L, Mocroft A, Soriano V, et al. Hepatitis C virus coinfection does not influence the CD4 cell recovery in HIV-1-infected patients with maximum virologic suppression. J Acquir Immune Defic Syndr 2009;50(5):457–63.
27. Rotman Y, Liang TJ. Coinfection with hepatitis C virus and human immunodeficiency virus: virological, immunological, and clinical outcomes. J Virol 2009; 83(15):7366–74.
28. Smit C, van den BC, Geskus R, et al. Risk of hepatitis-related mortality increased among hepatitis C virus/HIV-coinfected drug users compared with drug users infected only with hepatitis C virus: a 20-year prospective study. J Acquir Immune Defic Syndr 2008;47(2):221–5.
29. Pineda JA, Garcia-Garcia JA, Guilar-Guisado M, et al. Clinical progression of hepatitis C virus-related chronic liver disease in human immunodeficiency virus-infected patients undergoing highly active antiretroviral therapy. Hepatology 2007;46(3):622–30.
30. Weber R, Sabin CA, Friis-Moller N, et al. Liver-related deaths in persons infected with the human immunodeficiency virus: the D:A:D study. Arch Intern Med 2006; 166(15):1632–41.
31. Cacoub P, Geffray L, Rosenthal E, et al. Mortality among human immunodeficiency virus-infected patients with cirrhosis or hepatocellular carcinoma due to hepatitis C virus in French Departments of Internal Medicine/Infectious Diseases, in 1995 and 1997. Clin Infect Dis 2001;32(8):1207–14.
32. Rosenthal E, Salmon-Ceron D, Lewden C, et al. Liver-related deaths in HIV-infected patients between 1995 and 2005 in the French GERMIVIC Joint Study Group Network (Mortavic 2005 study in collaboration with the Mortalite 2005 survey, ANRS EN19). HIV Med 2009;10(5):282–9.
33. Puoti M, Bonacini M, Spinetti A, et al. Liver fibrosis progression is related to CD4 cell depletion in patients coinfected with hepatitis C virus and human immunodeficiency virus. J Infect Dis 2001;183(1):134–7.
34. Benhamou Y, Bochet M, Di M, et al. Liver fibrosis progression in human immunodeficiency virus and hepatitis C virus coinfected patients. The Multivirc Group. Hepatology 1999;30(4):1054–8.
35. Mohsen AH, Easterbrook PJ, Taylor C, et al. Impact of human immunodeficiency virus (HIV) infection on the progression of liver fibrosis in hepatitis C virus infected patients. Gut 2003;52(7):1035–40.
36. Bonnard P, Lescure FX, Amiel C, et al. Documented rapid course of hepatic fibrosis between two biopsies in patients coinfected by HIV and HCV despite high CD4 cell count. J Viral Hepat 2007;14(11):806–11.
37. Sulkowski MS, Mehta SH, Torbenson MS, et al. Rapid fibrosis progression among HIV/hepatitis C virus-co-infected adults. AIDS 2007;21(16):2209–16.
38. Thomson EC, Nastouli E, Main J, et al. Delayed anti-HCV antibody response in HIV-positive men acutely infected with HCV. AIDS 2009;23(1): 89–93.
39. Rodger AJ, Roberts S, Lanigan A, et al. Assessment of long-term outcomes of community-acquired hepatitis C infection in a cohort with sera stored from 1971 to 1975. Hepatology 2000;32(3):582–7.

40. Pol S, Lamorthe B, Thi NT, et al. Retrospective analysis of the impact of HIV infection and alcohol use on chronic hepatitis C in a large cohort of drug users. J Hepatol 1998;28(6):945–50.
41. Graham CS, Baden LR, Yu E, et al. Influence of human immunodeficiency virus infection on the course of hepatitis C virus infection: a meta-analysis. Clin Infect Dis 2001;33(4):562–9.
42. Thein HH, Yi Q, Dore GJ, et al. Natural history of hepatitis C virus infection in HIV-infected individuals and the impact of HIV in the era of highly active antiretroviral therapy: a meta-analysis. AIDS 2008;22(15):1979–91.
43. Poynard T, Mathurin P, Lai CL, et al. A comparison of fibrosis progression in chronic liver diseases. J Hepatol 2003;38(3):257–65.
44. Ragni MV, Eghtesad B, Schlesinger KW, et al. Pretransplant survival is shorter in HIV-positive than HIV-negative subjects with end-stage liver disease. Liver Transpl 2005;11(11):1425–30.
45. Shaw E, Castellote J, Santin M, et al. Clinical features and outcome of spontaneous bacterial peritonitis in HIV-infected cirrhotic patients: a case-control study. Eur J Clin Microbiol Infect Dis 2006;25(5):291–8.
46. Sherman M. Surveillance for hepatocellular carcinoma and early diagnosis. Clin Liver Dis 2007;11(4):817–37, viii.
47. McGinnis KA, Fultz SL, Skanderson M, et al. Hepatocellular carcinoma and non-Hodgkin's lymphoma: the roles of HIV, hepatitis C infection, and alcohol abuse. J Clin Oncol 2006;24(31):5005–9.
48. Giordano TP, Kramer JR, Souchek J, et al. Cirrhosis and hepatocellular carcinoma in HIV-infected veterans with and without the hepatitis C virus: a cohort study, 1992–2001. Arch Intern Med 2004;164(21):2349–54.
49. Garcia-Garcia JA, Romero-Gomez M, Giron-Gonzalez JA, et al. Incidence of and factors associated with hepatocellular carcinoma among hepatitis C virus and human immunodeficiency virus co-infected patients with decompensated cirrhosis. AIDS Res Hum Retroviruses 2006;22(12):1236–41.
50. Ghany MG, Strader DB, Thomas DL, et al. Diagnosis, management, and treatment of hepatitis C: an update. Hepatology 2009;49(4):1335–74.
51. Chung RT, Andersen J, Volberding P, et al. Peginterferon Alfa-2a plus ribavirin versus interferon alfa-2a plus ribavirin for chronic hepatitis C in HIV-coinfected persons. N Engl J Med 2004;351(5):451–9.
52. Torriani FJ, Rodriguez-Torres M, Rockstroh JK, et al. Peginterferon Alfa-2a plus ribavirin for chronic hepatitis C virus infection in HIV-infected patients. N Engl J Med 2004;351(5):438–50.
53. Carrat F, Bani-Sadr F, Pol S, et al. Pegylated interferon alfa-2b vs standard interferon alfa-2b, plus ribavirin, for chronic hepatitis C in HIV-infected patients: a randomized controlled trial. JAMA 2004;292(23):2839–48.
54. Laguno M, Murillas J, Blanco JL, et al. Peginterferon alfa-2b plus ribavirin compared with interferon alfa-2b plus ribavirin for treatment of HIV/HCV co-infected patients. AIDS 2004;18(13):F27–36.
55. Cargnel A, Angeli E, Mainini A, et al. Open, randomized, multicentre Italian trial on PEG-IFN plus ribavirin versus PEG-IFN monotherapy for chronic hepatitis C in HIV-coinfected patients on HAART. Antivir Ther 2005;10(2):309–17.
56. Crespo M, Esteban JI, Sauleda S, et al. Early prediction of sustained virological response in patients with chronic hepatitis C and HIV infection treated with IFN + RBV. Hepatology 2004;40(S4):350A. Ref Type: Generic.
57. Kim AI, Dorn A, Bouajram R, et al. The treatment of chronic hepatitis C in HIV-infected patients: a meta-analysis. HIV Med 2007;8(5):312–21.

58. Jacobson IM, Brown RS Jr, Freilich B, et al. Peginterferon alfa-2b and weight-based or flat-dose ribavirin in chronic hepatitis C patients: a randomized trial. Hepatology 2007;46(4):971–81.

59. Soriano V, Nunez M, Camino N, et al. Hepatitis C virus-RNA clearance in HIV-co-infected patients with chronic hepatitis C treated with pegylated interferon plus ribavirin. Antivir Ther 2004;9(4):505–9.

60. Nunez M, Miralles C, Berdun MA, et al. Role of weight-based ribavirin dosing and extended duration of therapy in chronic hepatitis C in HIV-infected patients: the PRESCO trial. AIDS Res Hum Retroviruses 2007;23(8): 972–82.

61. Russmann S, Grattagliano I, Portincasa P, et al. Ribavirin-induced anemia: mechanisms, risk factors and related targets for future research. Curr Med Chem 2006;13(27):3351–7.

62. Grattagliano I, Russmann S, Palmieri VO, et al. Low membrane protein sulfhydrils but not G6PD deficiency predict ribavirin-induced hemolysis in hepatitis C. Hepatology 2004;39(5):1248–55.

63. De FL, Fattovich G, Turrini F, et al. Hemolytic anemia induced by ribavirin therapy in patients with chronic hepatitis C virus infection: role of membrane oxidative damage. Hepatology 2000;31(4):997–1004.

64. Everson GT, Trotter J, Forman L, et al. Treatment of advanced hepatitis C with a low accelerating dosage regimen of antiviral therapy. Hepatology 2005; 42(2):255–62.

65. Prati D, Capelli C, Zanella A, et al. Influence of different hepatitis C virus geno-types on the course of asymptomatic hepatitis C virus infection. Gastroenter-ology 1996;110(1):178–83.

66. Puoti C, Castellacci R, Montagnese F. Hepatitis C virus carriers with persistently normal aminotransferase levels: healthy people or true patients? Dig Liver Dis 2000;32(7):634–43.

67. Martinot-Peignoux M, Boyer N, Cazals-Hatem D, et al. Prospective study on anti-hepatitis C virus-positive patients with persistently normal serum alanine trans-aminase with or without detectable serum hepatitis C virus RNA. Hepatology 2001;34(5):1000–5.

68. Mathurin P, Moussalli J, Cadranel JF, et al. Slow progression rate of fibrosis in hepatitis C virus patients with persistently normal alanine transaminase activity. Hepatology 1998;27(3):868–72.

69. Fonquernie L, Serfaty L, Charrois A, et al. Significance of hepatitis C virus coin-fection with persistently normal alanine aminotransferase levels in HIV-1-in-fected patients. HIV Med 2004;5(5):385–90.

70. Maida I, Babudieri S, Selva C, et al. Liver enzyme elevation in hepatitis C virus (HCV)-HIV-coinfected patients prior to and after initiating HAART: role of HCV genotypes. AIDS Res Hum Retroviruses 2006;22(2):139–43.

71. Maida I, Soriano V, Barreiro P, et al. Liver fibrosis stage and HCV genotype distri-bution in HIV-HCV coinfected patients with persistently normal transaminases. AIDS Res Hum Retroviruses 2007;23(6):801–4.

72. Uberti-Foppa C, De BA, Galli L, et al. Liver fibrosis in HIV-positive patients with hepatitis C virus: role of persistently normal alanine aminotransferase levels. J Acquir Immune Defic Syndr 2006;41(1):63–7.

73. Okanoue T, Makiyama A, Nakayama M, et al. A follow-up study to determine the value of liver biopsy and need for antiviral therapy for hepatitis C virus carriers with persistently normal serum aminotransferase. J Hepatol 2005;43(4): 599–605.

74. Soriano V, Puoti M, Sulkowski M, et al. Care of patients coinfected with HIV and hepatitis C virus: 2007 updated recommendations from the HCV-HIV International Panel. AIDS 2007;21(9):1073–89.
75. Kleiner DE. The liver biopsy in chronic hepatitis C: a view from the other side of the microscope. Semin Liver Dis 2005;25(1):52–64.
76. Shaheen AA, Myers RP. Systematic review and meta-analysis of the diagnostic accuracy of fibrosis marker panels in patients with HIV/hepatitis C coinfection. HIV Clin Trials 2008;9(1):43–51.
77. Macias J, Giron-Gonzalez JA, Gonzalez-Serrano M, et al. Prediction of liver fibrosis in human immunodeficiency virus/hepatitis C virus coinfected patients by simple noninvasive indexes. Gut 2006;55(3):409–14.
78. Nunes D, Fleming C, Offner G, et al. HIV infection does not affect the performance of noninvasive markers of fibrosis for the diagnosis of hepatitis C virus-related liver disease. J Acquir Immune Defic Syndr 2005;40(5):538–44.
79. de L V, Douvin C, Kettaneh A, et al. Diagnosis of hepatic fibrosis and cirrhosis by transient elastography in HIV/hepatitis C virus-coinfected patients. J Acquir Immune Defic Syndr 2006;41(2):175–9.
80. Vergara S, Macias J, Rivero A, et al. The use of transient elastometry for assessing liver fibrosis in patients with HIV and hepatitis C virus coinfection. Clin Infect Dis 2007;45(8):969–74.
81. Benhamou Y, Di Martino V, Bochet M, et al. Factors affecting liver fibrosis in human immunodeficiency virus- and hepatitis C virus-coinfected patients: impact of protease inhibitor therapy. Hepatology 2001;34(2):283–7.
82. Mehta SH, Thomas DL, Torbenson M, et al. The effect of antiretroviral therapy on liver disease among adults with HIV and hepatitis C coinfection. Hepatology 2005;41(1):123–31.
83. Verma S, Wang CH, Govindarajan S, et al. Do type and duration of antiretroviral therapy attenuate liver fibrosis in HIV-hepatitis C virus-coinfected patients? Clin Infect Dis 2006;42(2):262–70.
84. Brau N, Salvatore M, Rios-Bedoya CF, et al. Slower fibrosis progression in HIV/HCV-coinfected patients with successful HIV suppression using antiretroviral therapy. J Hepatol 2006;44(1):47–55.
85. Verma S. HAART attenuates liver fibrosis in patients with HIV/HCV co-infection: fact or fiction? J Antimicrob Chemother 2006;58(3):496–501.
86. Giraudon I, Ruf M, Maguire H, et al. Increase in diagnosed newly acquired hepatitis C in HIV-positive men who have sex with men across London and Brighton, 2002–2006: is this an outbreak? Sex Transm Infect 2008;84(2):111–5.
87. Gerlach JT, Diepolder HM, Zachoval R, et al. Acute hepatitis C: high rate of both spontaneous and treatment-induced viral clearance. Gastroenterology 2003;125(1):80–8.
88. Vogel M, Bieniek B, Jessen H, et al. Treatment of acute hepatitis C infection in HIV-infected patients: a retrospective analysis of eleven cases. J Viral Hepat 2005;12(2):207–11.
89. Dominguez S, Ghosn J, Valantin MA, et al. Efficacy of early treatment of acute hepatitis C infection with pegylated interferon and ribavirin in HIV-infected patients. AIDS 2006;20(8):1157–61.
90. Cacoub P, Rosenthal E, Halfon P, et al. Treatment of hepatitis C virus and human immunodeficiency virus coinfection: from large trials to real life. J Viral Hepat 2006;13(10):678–82.
91. Sylvestre DL. Approaching treatment for hepatitis C virus infection in substance users. Clin Infect Dis 2005;41(Suppl):1S79–82.

92. Nunes D, Saitz R, Libman H, et al. Barriers to treatment of hepatitis C in HIV/HCV-coinfected adults with alcohol problems. Alcohol Clin Exp Res 2006; 30(9):1520–6.

93. Mauss S, Valenti W, Depamphilis J, et al. Risk factors for hepatic decompensation in patients with HIV/HCV coinfection and liver cirrhosis during interferon-based therapy. AIDS 2004;18(13):F21–5.

94. Bani-Sadr F, Carrat F, Pol S, et al. Risk factors for symptomatic mitochondrial toxicity in HIV/hepatitis C virus-coinfected patients during interferon plus ribavirin-based therapy. J Acquir Immune Defic Syndr 2005;40(1):47–52.

95. de MC, Martin-Carbonero L, Barreiro P, et al. Mitochondrial DNA depletion in HIV-infected patients with chronic hepatitis C and effect of pegylated interferon plus ribavirin therapy. AIDS 2007;21(5):583–8.

96. Cote HC, Brumme ZL, Craib KJ, et al. Changes in mitochondrial DNA as a marker of nucleoside toxicity in HIV-infected patients. N Engl J Med 2002; 346(11):811–20.

97. Perronne C. Antiviral hepatitis and antiretroviral drug interactions. J Hepatol 2006;44(Suppl 1):S119–25.

98. Brau N, Rodriguez-Torres M, Prokupek D, et al. Treatment of chronic hepatitis C in HIV/HCV-coinfection with interferon alpha-2b+ full-course vs. 16-week delayed ribavirin. Hepatology 2004;39(4):989–98.

99. Bani-Sadr F, Denoeud L, Morand P, et al. Early virologic failure in HIV-coinfected hepatitis C patients treated with the peginterferon-ribavirin combination: does abacavir play a role? J Acquir Immune Defic Syndr 2007;45(1):123–5.

100. Clark SJ, Creighton S, Portmann B, et al. Acute liver failure associated with antiretroviral treatment for HIV: a report of six cases. J Hepatol 2002;36(2):295–301.

101. Selik RM, Byers RH Jr, Dworkin MS. Trends in diseases reported on U.S. death certificates that mentioned HIV infection, 1987–1999. J Acquir Immune Defic Syndr 2002;29(4):378–87.

102. Saves M, Raffi F, Clevenbergh P, et al. Hepatitis B or hepatitis C virus infection is a risk factor for severe hepatic cytolysis after initiation of a protease inhibitor-containing antiretroviral regimen in human immunodeficiency virus-infected patients. The APROCO Study Group. Antimicrob Agents Chemother 2000; 44(12):3451–5.

103. Saves M, Vandentorren S, Daucourt V, et al. Severe hepatic cytolysis: incidence and risk factors in patients treated by antiretroviral combinations. Aquitaine Cohort, France, 1996–1998. Groupe d'Epidemiologie Clinique de Sida en Aquitaine (GECSA). AIDS 1999;13(17):F115–21.

104. Nunez M, Lana R, Mendoza JL, et al. Risk factors for severe hepatic injury after introduction of highly active antiretroviral therapy. J Acquir Immune Defic Syndr 2001;27(5):426–31.

105. Bonfanti P, Landonio S, Ricci E, et al. Risk factors for hepatotoxicity in patients treated with highly active antiretroviral therapy. J Acquir Immune Defic Syndr 2001;27(3):316–8.

106. Nunez M. Hepatotoxicity of antiretrovirals: incidence, mechanisms and management. J Hepatol 2006;44(Suppl 1):S132–9.

107. Labarga P, Soriano V, Vispo ME, et al. Hepatotoxicity of antiretroviral drugs is reduced after successful treatment of chronic hepatitis C in HIV-infected patients. J Infect Dis 2007;196(5):670–6.

108. Lo RV III, Kostman JR, Amorosa VK. Management complexities of HIV/hepatitis C virus coinfection in the twenty-first century. Clin Liver Dis 2008;12(3): 587–609, ix.

109. Rubin RH, Tolkoff-Rubin NE. The problem of human immunodeficiency virus (HIV) infection and transplantation. Transpl Int 1988;1(1):36–42.
110. Aguero F, Laguno M, Moreno A, et al. Management of end-stage liver disease in HIV-infected patients. Curr Opin HIV AIDS 2007;2(6):474–81.
111. Duclos-Vallee JC, Feray C, Sebagh M, et al. Survival and recurrence of hepatitis C after liver transplantation in patients coinfected with human immunodeficiency virus and hepatitis C virus. Hepatology 2008;47(2):407–17.
112. Testillano M, Fernandez JR, Suarez MJ, et al. Survival and hepatitis C virus recurrence after liver transplantation in HIV- and hepatitis C virus-coinfected patients: experience in a single center. Transplant Proc 2009;41(3):1041–3.
113. de Vera ME, Dvorchik I, Tom K, et al. Survival of liver transplant patients coinfected with HIV and HCV is adversely impacted by recurrent hepatitis C. Am J Transplant 2006;6(12):2983–93.
114. Roland ME, Barin B, Carlson L, et al. HIV-infected liver and kidney transplant recipients: 1- and 3-year outcomes. Am J Transplant 2008;8(2):355–65.
115. Available at: www.clinicaltrials.gov/ct2/show/NCT00074386?term=liver+transplant+and+hiv&rank=4. Accessed March 12, 2010.

Rheumatologic Disease and the Liver

Christine Schlenker, MD[a], Timothy Halterman, MD[a],
Kris V. Kowdley, MD[b,c],*

KEYWORDS

- Rheumatologic diseases • Abnormal liver tests
- Hepatotoxicity • Liver damage

Rheumatologic diseases such as rheumatoid arthritis, systemic lupus erythematosus, Sjögren syndrome (SS), and scleroderma are immunologically mediated disorders that typically have multisystem involvement. Although clinically significant liver involvement is rare, liver enzyme abnormalities may be observed in up to 43% of patients.[1]

In most such cases, further evaluation is unrevealing for an identifiable cause of the biochemical abnormality. Liver biopsy is normal or shows only minor nonspecific histologic changes in 27% to 37% of such patients.[1,2] The biochemical abnormalities are typically mild and transient and the histologic abnormalities are nonprogressive and clinically insignificant.[1] Such biochemical and histologic findings are typically ascribed to the primary rheumatologic condition and require no specific management.

In the remainder of patients with rheumatologic conditions and liver test abnormalities, further evaluation identifies a coexisting, primary liver disease (such as fatty liver disease, viral hepatitis, primary biliary cirrhosis [PBC] or autoimmune hepatitis [AIH][1,2]) or medication-related liver toxicity as the cause of the biochemical abnormality. Liver test abnormalities in patients with a coexisting primary liver disease are more likely to be persistent. The liver damage can be progressive, leading to cirrhosis, complications of portal hypertension, or liver-related death, and therefore must be accurately identified.

This article reviews the spectrum of liver-related abnormalities associated with several rheumatologic diseases (**Table 1**). Hepatotoxicity related to medications commonly prescribed in such conditions is also discussed (**Table 2**).

---

[a] Department of Medicine, University of Washington, 1959 NE Pacific Street, UW Box Number 356424, Seattle, WA, 98195, USA
[b] Center for Liver Disease, Digestive Disease Institute, Virginia Mason Medical Center, Seattle, WA, USA
[c] University of Washington, Seattle, WA, USA
* Corresponding author. Center for Liver Disease, Digestive Disease Institute, Virginia Mason Medical Center, Seattle, WA.
E-mail address: kris.kowdley@vmmc.org

Clin Liver Dis 15 (2011) 153–164
doi:10.1016/j.cld.2010.09.006
1089-3261/11/$ – see front matter © 2011 Elsevier Inc. All rights reserved.

Table 1
Rheumatologic conditions and reported liver abnormalities

Rheumatologic Condition	Reported Liver Test Abnormalities	Reported Coexisting Liver Diseases
Systemic lupus (SLE)	↑ Alkaline phosphatase ↑ AST/ALT	Fatty liver Viral hepatitis NRH PBC AIH
Rheumatoid arthritis	↑ Alkaline phosphatase ↑ GGT	Steatosis NRH Idiopathic pHTN
Felty syndrome	↑ Alkaline phosphatase ↑ GGT ↑ AST/ALT ↑ Bilirubin	NRH
Sjogren syndrome	↑ AST/ALT ↑ Alkaline phosphatase	HCV PBC AIH Fatty liver
Scleroderma	↑ Alkaline phosphatase ↑ AST/ALT	PBC
Ankylosing spondylitis	↑ Alkaline phosphatase ↑ GGT	–

Abbreviations: AIH, autoimmune hepatitis; ALT, alanine aminotransferase; AST, aspartate aminotransferase; GGT, γ-glutamyl-transpeptidase; HCV, hepatitis C virus; NRH, nodular regenerative hyperplasia; PBC, primary biliary cirrhosis; pHTN, portal hypertension.

SYSTEMIC LUPUS ERYTHEMATOSUS

Systemic lupus erythematosus (SLE) is a multisystem immune-mediated disease with variable clinical and immunologic manifestations. Although abnormalities of the skin, joints, kidneys, cardiovascular, central nervous, and hematologic systems are part of the criteria for SLE,[3] other organs may also be involved, including the liver.

Liver test abnormalities have been reported in up to 50% of patients with SLE at some point in the course of their disease.[4,5] In 19 of 45 patients (23%) with SLE and

Table 2
Medication hepatotoxicity in patients with rheumatologic conditions

Medication	Liver Test Abnormality	Clinical Significance
NSAIDs	Mild ↑ AST/ALT	Asymptomatic Resolves with withdrawal
Penicillamine Sulfasalazine	↑ AST/ALT ↑ Alkaline phosphatase	Hypersensitivity reaction
Leflunomide	↑ AST/ALT	Typically normalizes with ongoing medication use
Methotrexate	↑ AST/ALT	Potential fibrosis/cirrhosis
Anti-TNF α agents	↑ AST/ALT	Reactivation of hepatitis B Autoimmune hepatitis

Abbreviations: ALT, alanine aminotransferase; AST, aspartate aminotransferase; TNF, tumor necrosis factor.

liver test abnormalities, no cause for the liver test abnormality was identified and was therefore attributed to SLE.[5] Increases were generally mild (≤2× upper limit of normal) and included abnormalities of serum aminotransferases and alkaline phosphatase. For those patients undergoing liver biopsy, portal inflammation was a common histologic finding. The degree of increase in liver tests has been shown to correlate with disease activity[6] and improve with steroid therapy.[4]

In a histologic review of 73 patients with SLE, Matsumoto and colleagues[2] identified the following coexisting primary liver disorders: fatty liver (72.6%), nodular regenerative hyperplasia (NRH) (6.8%), viral hepatitis (4.1%), PBC (2.7%), and autoimmune hepatitis (2.7%). Case reports of additional liver diseases in patients with SLE include primary sclerosing cholangitis,[7] autoimmune cholangiopathy,[7] granulomatous hepatitis,[8] and idiopathic portal hypertension.[9] Vascular disorders of the liver secondary to antiphospholipid syndrome associated with SLE include Budd-Chiari syndrome,[10] hepatic infarction,[11] and hepatic rupture.[12]

Autoimmune hepatitis (AIH) and lupus-associated hepatitis can be difficult to differentiate given their common clinical and serologic manifestations. Histologic findings may be helpful as AIH characteristically shows periportal inflammation and piecemeal necrosis with dense lymphoid infiltrates, whereas lupus-associated hepatitis shows predominantly mild lobular inflammation without piecemeal necrosis on histology.[13] Antiribosomal P antibodies, which are not found in patients with AIH, are present in a significant proportion (69%) of patients with lupus-associated hepatitis and may aid in differentiating the 2 entities.[14] Clarifying the diagnosis has important prognostic and therapeutic implications, as lupus-associated hepatitis has a more benign course and does not require corticosteroid therapy.

RHEUMATOID ARTHRITIS

Rheumatoid arthritis (RA) is a systemic autoimmune disorder characterized by symmetric polyarticular joint involvement. Extraarticular manifestations, mainly involving the pulmonary, cardiovascular, and hematologic systems, frequently occur. Although liver involvement is not common, abnormalities in liver tests have been reported in 5% to 77% of patients with RA.[1,15–18] Increases in alkaline phosphatase and γ-glutamyl-transpeptidase (GGT) levels are the predominant biochemical abnormality. Although RA is a disorder characterized by erosive synovitis and bony deformities, it has been shown that the predominant source of alkaline phosphatase is the liver.[19] The increase in liver isoenzymes has been shown to correlate with RA activity.[20] Lowe and colleagues[17] found that the degree of increase in GGT corresponded to the level of increase in erythrocyte sedimentation rate (ESR), a surrogate marker for disease activity in patients with RA.

Histologic findings in patients with RA are variable. In a retrospective review of autopsies of 188 patients with RA, Ruderman and colleagues[21] found normal liver parenchyma in only 15 cases; 112 specimens showed hepatic congestion, 42 had steatosis, and 30 had evidence of portal tract inflammation. Rau and colleagues[22] reported mild, generally nonspecific changes in liver biopsies from patients with RA.

Primary liver disorders reported in patients with RA include PBC,[23] autoimmune hepatitis,[24] and autoimmune cholangiopathy.[25] Other rare conditions including NRH,[26] idiopathic portal hypertension,[27] and spontaneous hepatic rupture secondary to vasculitis[28] have also been reported.

Arthropathy and the presence of rheumatoid factor (RF) are defining features of RA. However, polyarthritis similar to that in RA and RF positivity are also common extrahepatic manifestation of primary liver disorders, occasionally presenting a diagnostic dilemma to the clinician. Various serologic autoantibodies have been shown to be beneficial in distinguishing between RA and arthritis associated with liver disorders. Koga and colleagues[29] found that the presence of anticyclic citrullinated peptide antibodies (anti-CCP) is a reliable marker of RA compared with arthropathy associated with chronic hepatitis C (HCV), AIH, or PBC.

FELTY SYNDROME

Felty syndrome is a rare condition characterized by the triad of RA, leucopenia, and splenomegaly. Hepatomegaly has been documented to occur in 42% to 67% of patients with Felty syndrome.[30,31] Abnormal liver tests were found to be present in 10 of 18 patients in a prospective study of patients with Felty syndrome.[31] Abnormalities included increases in alkaline phosphatase, aminotransferases, bilirubin, prothrombin time, and GGT. Histologic changes were nonspecific and included sinusoidal dilation, Kupffer cell hyperplasia, and portal inflammation. An increased prevalence of NRH in Felty syndrome compared with a control population has also been reported.[32] Portal hypertension leading to esophageal variceal bleeding has been noted to develop in several patients with Felty syndrome and NRH.[33,34]

ADULT-ONSET STILLS DISEASE

Adult-onset Stills disease is an acute systemic form of RA characterized by daily spiking fevers, evanescent salmon-colored rash, polyarthralgias, and leukocytosis. Liver test abnormalities, predominantly increases in aminotransferases or alkaline phosphatase, and hepatosplenomegaly occur frequently in those with adult-onset Stills disease and have become part of the diagnostic criteria for this condition.[35] Increases in liver enzymes are generally mild (2–5 times the upper limit of normal), transient, and usually associated with activity of the underlying disease.[36] Fulminant hepatitis requiring liver transplantation has been reported in adult-onset Stills disease.[37] Chronic liver disease secondary to adult-onset Stills disease has not been reported.

SS

SS is an autoimmune disorder characterized by lymphocytic infiltration and destruction of the salivary and lachrymal glands, typically presenting as persistent dryness of the mouth (xerostomia) and eyes (keratoconjunctivitis sicca). SS can be a systemic process, involving organs such as the lungs, kidney, and central nervous system.[38,39] Abnormal liver tests are common, reported to occur in 7% to 49% of patients.[38,40–44] Liver function test (LFT) abnormalities include hepatocellular, cholestatic (primarily increased alkaline phosphatase), and mixed patterns may be persistent or intermittent.

Montano-Loza and colleagues[43] identified a specific liver disease in 50% of patients with SS with liver test abnormalities (26% with HCV, 12% with PBC, 5% with AIH, and 5% with fatty liver disease). No explanation for the liver test abnormality was found in the remaining 50% of patients. Similarly, in a study of 73 patients with SS, 49% of whom had abnormal liver tests, no identifiable cause for the abnormality was found in 60% of patients.[38] In a study of 475 patients with SS, of whom 27% had liver test abnormalities, the main causes were again chronic hepatitis C (13%) and autoimmune liver disease (5%) (PBC in 16 and AIH in 8).[44]

Several studies have reported a higher prevalence of PBC and AIH in patients with primary SS compared with that expected in the general population.[40–42,45] Of 410 patients with SS, Hatzis and colleagues[41] identified 27 patients (6.6%) with PBC. Among 45 patients with SS, Lindgren and colleagues[40] established a diagnosis of PBC in 4 patients (8.8%) and autoimmune hepatitis in 2 (4.4%).

Among 300 patients with SS, 6.6% were antimitochondrial antibody (AMA) positive, 92% of whom demonstrated histologic features consistent with PBC.[42] Therefore, the presence of AMA in a patient with SS and abnormal liver tests, suggests underlying PBC. Differentiating AIH from nonspecific liver test abnormalities associated with SS, however, can be more challenging. Patients with rheumatoid diseases typically demonstrate hypergammaglobulinemia and autoantibodies, findings that are among the criteria used to diagnose AIH.[46] A liver biopsy demonstrating features typical of AIH (interface hepatitis, plasma cell infiltrates, rosette formation) can confirm the diagnosis of coexisting AIH.[1,2] However, because the histologic features of AIH are variable, those patients with SS, biochemical and serologic criteria for AIH, and nonspecific histologic findings are much more difficult to classify.

Several studies have shown that the prevalence of chronic HCV infection among patients with SS is higher than the general population, ranging from 12% to 19%.[43,44,47,48] The presence of sicca symptoms (dryness of the eyes and mouth), lymphocytic infiltration of salivary glands, and serum autoantibodies in patients with HCV infection suggests that HCV may even be the cause of SS in some cases.[47–49] Other investigators, however, point out subtle differences in the clinical, immunologic, and histologic characteristics of patients with HCV-related SS compared with primary SS patients without HCV infection (eg, a lower prevalence of sicca symptoms, a lower frequency of anti-Ro/SS-A and anti-La/SS-B antibodies and a higher prevalence of cryoglobulinemia and hypocomplementemia).[47,48,50] The pathogenic role of HCV in SS remains unclear. HCV infection may be involved in the pathogenesis of SS in a subgroup of patients; conversely, HCV infection may produce extrahepatic manifestations that may mimic SS. In clinical practice, it seems reasonable to recommend that abnormal liver parameters in patients with SS should prompt testing for HCV infection.

There are occasional case reports in the literature describing patients with SS who also have primary sclerosing cholangitis[51] and NRH.[2,52] However, the paucity of such reports suggests that the association may be sporadic rather than causative.

PROGRESSIVE SYSTEMIC SCLEROSIS/SCLERODERMA

Systemic sclerosis (SSc) is a connective tissue disease characterized by fibrosis that involves the skin and various internal organs, including the heart, lungs, kidneys, and gastrointestinal tract. Liver involvement is rare.[53]

PBC is the liver disorder most consistently reported in patients with SSc. Scleroderma occurs in 7% to 12% of patients with PBC.[54,55] Most patients with PBC-SSc have the limited cutaneous type of SSc, rather than the diffuse type. Patients with PBC-SSc generally have a positive AMA.[54,56] Patients with PBC-SSc also commonly have anticentromere Ab (ACA),[54,56] an antibody frequently found in the serum of patients with limited cutaneous SSc. Therefore, testing for ACA may be helpful in evaluating for SSc in patients with known PBC. Although the liver disease in patients with PBC-SSc may progress to cirrhosis and result in liver-related morbidity, mortality is more commonly to the result of other systemic complications of SSc than the liver disease.[54]

SSc has also been reported in rare case reports of patients with other liver diseases, including AIH,[57] NRH,[58] idiopathic portal hypertension,[59] and primary sclerosing cholangitis.[60]

ANKYLOSING SPONDYLITIS

Ankylosing spondylitis (AS) is an inflammatory arthropathy of the sacroiliac joints and spine, typically presenting with back pain and progressive spinal stiffness. Peripheral joints may also be involved. AS is not typically considered a systemic disorder, although extraarticular organs can be affected.

Increased levels of alkaline phosphatase are often seen in patients with AS, occurring in 14% to 47.5% of patients.[61–64] Although the increased levels are often assumed to be derived from the bone,[63] some studies suggest that the liver is the source.[61,62,64] The origin of alkaline phosphatase can be determined by measuring 5-nuceotidase (5-NT) and/or GGT, which are usually increased in parallel with the alkaline phosphatase in liver disorders but are not increased in bone disorders. Bone and liver fractions can also be determined by gel electrophoresis. The increase in alkaline phosphatase is typically an isolated abnormality, with normal aminotransferase and bilirubin levels.[61–64]

The clinical significance of an increased level of alkaline phosphatase of liver origin is uncertain. Some investigators have suggested that the degree of increase in alkaline phosphatase may be a biochemical marker of disease activity and a nonspecific reaction to inflammation.[62,64] Robinson and colleagues[62] found increases in liver alkaline phosphatase to correlate directly with increases in ESR in untreated patients. Reduction in serum alkaline phosphatase, GGT, and ESR was observed after treatment with nonsteroidal anti-inflammatory drugs (NSAIDs).

MEDICATION HEPATOTOXICITY

Many of the medications available for the treatment of rheumatologic diseases have been associated with hepatotoxicity. Medication-related liver injury varies from mild biochemical and histologic abnormalities that reverse on withdrawal of the offending medication to progressive fibrosis/cirrhosis, chronic liver failure or fulminant liver failure. In addition, certain medications may result in liver injury through the exacerbation or induction of primary liver disorders such as viral or autoimmune hepatitis, respectively.

NSAIDs

Nearly all NSAIDs have been reported to cause liver test abnormalities, but serious hepatotoxicity is rare. NSAID-related liver injury is typically characterized by a mild, asymptomatic increase in serum aminotransferase levels that returns to normal on cessation of the suspected NSAID. In a systematic review of 64 randomized controlled trials of commonly used NSAIDs in patients with osteoarthritis or RA, rates of significant aminotransferase increases (>3 times the upper limit of normal) were very low for most NSAIDs (range 0.19%–0.43%) and were similar to the rate in patients receiving placebo (0.29%).[65] Only 1 liver-related hospitalization (out of 37,671 patients taking NSAIDs) and 1 liver-related death (out of 51,942 patients taking NSAIDs) were reported. The risk may be increased, however, in patients who are taking additional potentially hepatotoxic medications.[66]

Disease-modifying Antirheumatic Drugs

Penicillamine and sulfasalazine have both been associated with rare cases of hepatotoxicity.[67,68] The presentation is typically that of a hypersensitivity reaction occurring within the first few weeks of treatment. The injury may be hepatocellular, cholestatic, or mixed. Although liver injury typically resolves with discontinuation of the medication, fatalities have been reported.

Increased liver enzymes, primarily aminotransferases, in patients taking leflunomide has been well documented, ranging from 5.4 %to 14.8%.[69–71] The liver test abnormalities typically normalized during ongoing leflunomide treatment. Serious drug-induced hepatotoxicity with leflunomide is rare,[72] but fatalities as a result of liver failure have been documented.[73]

Methotrexate (MTX) causes increases in liver enzymes and has been associated with an increased risk of fibrosis and cirrhosis in patients receiving long-term therapy.[74] However, there is considerable controversy on the frequency and severity with which progressive fibrosis and cirrhosis occur in patients treated with the doses typically used in rheumatologic disorders. Studies on patients with RA treated with MTX suggest that clinically significant hepatic fibrosis during treatment is rare.[75–77]

Society guidelines differ with regard to how patients on MTX should be monitored to prevent MTX-induced liver fibrosis.[78,79] Management strategies may include 1 or more of the following: pretreatment liver biopsy (could be limited to patients with risk factors for liver disease; eg, history of excessive alcohol use, abnormal baseline aspartate aminotransferase levels, or chronic viral hepatitis); surveillance liver biopsies after each 1.5 to 2 g cumulative MTX dose regardless of liver chemistries; and/or frequent monitoring of LFTs during treatment, with surveillance biopsy reserved for patients with persistent LFT abnormalities. Long-term liver safety with the latter has been demonstrated for patients with RA.[80]

Anti–Tumor Necrosis Factor Therapy

Minor abnormalities of liver enzymes are relatively common with the use of anti–tumor necrosis factor (TNF)-α agents such as infliximab, etanercept, and adalimumab.[81] Severe hepatic reactions are much less common and include jaundice, hepatitis, cholestasis, and acute liver failure.[82,83] AIH is a rare, but increasingly recognized complication of treatment with anti-TNF-α agents.[84,85]

Reactivation of hepatitis B in the setting of TNF-α therapy has been widely reported,[86–88] with 2 cases of fulminant liver failure.[89,90] Although some patients have been treated for 4 to 5 years with no laboratory evidence of reactivation,[88,91] even a single infusion can lead to reactivation.[88]

Patients at risk for reactivation of hepatitis B with anti-TNF therapies include those with chronic inactive hepatitis B (positive hepatitis B surface antigen [HBsAg], normal aminotransferase levels, and low or undetectable serum hepatitis B DNA level) and probably those with occult hepatitis B (HBsAg-negative and hepatitis B core antibody-positive).[92] Current guidelines recommend that all HBsAg-positive patients receive antiviral therapy before or together with the initiation of treatment.[93]

In contrast, case reports suggest that anti-TNF-α therapy in the setting of HCV, either as monotherapy or in combination with other disease-modifying antirheumatic drugs, is safe, based on a lack of significant change in aminotransferase levels and/or HCV viral load after initiation of treatment with TNF agents.[91,94,95] Additional data based on large databases are needed to conclusively establish the safety of anti-TNF-α agents in patients with chronic HCV.

SUMMARY

Abnormal liver tests are common in patients with rheumatologic disorders. Liver test abnormalities include a hepatocellular injury pattern (increased aminotransferases), a cholestatic pattern (increased alkaline phosphatase with or without increased bilirubin), or a mixed picture. Evaluation is often unrevealing for an identifiable cause of the biochemical abnormality. Such nonspecific abnormalities are likely of little clinical significance and no specific management is required. Serious progressive liver injury does occur, more often in the context of a coexisting primary liver disease or pharmacotherapy. An underlying primary liver disease for which treatment might be beneficial (eg, immunosuppressants for autoimmune hepatitis, interferon for viral hepatitis, ursodeoxycolic acid for PBC) should be sought. Testing for AMA, antismooth muscle antibodies, and hepatitis C may be particularly helpful. A new increases in liver tests after initiation of antirheumatic treatment should raise the suspicion for drug-induced liver injury, as many of the antirheumatic drugs have documented hepatotoxicity. In addition, such medications can cause reactivation of hepatitis B.

REFERENCES

1. Kojima H, Uemura M, Sakurai S, et al. Clinical features of liver disturbance in rheumatoid diseases: clinicopathological study with special reference to the cause of liver disturbance. J Gastroenterol 2002;37:617–25.
2. Matsumoto T, Kobayashi S, Shimizu H, et al. The liver in collagen diseases: pathologic study of 160 cases with particular reference to hepatic arteritis, primary biliary cirrhosis, autoimmune hepatitis and nodular regenerative hyperplasia of the liver. Liver 2000;20:366–73.
3. Tan E, Cohen A, Fries J, et al. The 1982 revised criteria for the classification of systemic lupus erythematosus. Arthritis Rheum 1982;25:1271–7.
4. Runyon B, LaBrecque D, Anuras S. The spectrum of liver disease in systemic lupus erythematosus. Report of 33 histologically-proved cases and review of the literature. Am J Med 1980;69:187–94.
5. Gibson T, Myers A. Subclinical liver disease in systemic lupus erythematosus. J Rheumatol 2002;8:752–9.
6. Miller M, Urowitz M, Gladman D, et al. The liver in systemic lupus erythematosus. Q J Med 1984;53:401–9.
7. Mok C. Investigations and management of gastrointestinal and hepatic manifestations of systemic lupus erythematosus. Best Pract Res Clin Rheumatol 2005;19:741–66.
8. Feurle G, Bröker H, Tschahargane C. Granulomatous hepatitis in systemic lupus erythematosus. Report of a case. Endoscopy 1982;14:153–4.
9. Inagaki H, Nonami T, Kawagoe T, et al. Idiopathic portal hypertension associated with systemic lupus erythematosus. J Gastroenterol 2000;35:235–9.
10. Pelletier S, Landi B, Piette J, et al. Antiphospholipid syndrome as the second cause of non-tumorous Budd-Chiari syndrome. J Hepatol 1994;21:76–80.
11. Mor F, Beigel Y, Inbal A, et al. Hepatic infarction in a patient with the lupus anti-coagulant. Arthritis Rheum 1989;32:491–5.
12. Haslock I. Spontaneous rupture of the liver in systemic lupus erythematosus. Ann Rheum Dis 1974;33:482–4.
13. Kaw R, Gota C, Bennett A, et al. Lupus-related hepatitis: complication of lupus or autoimmune association? Case report and review of the literature. Dig Dis Sci 2006;51:813–8.
14. Ohira H, Takiguchi J, Rai T, et al. High frequency of anti-ribosomal P antibody in patients with systemic lupus erythematosus-associated hepatitis. Hepatol Res 2004;28:137–9.
15. Beyeler C, Banks R, Thompson D, et al. Bone alkaline phosphatase in rheumatic diseases. Ann Clin Biochem 1995;32(Pt 4):379–84.
16. Fernandes L, Sullivan S, McFarlane I, et al. Studies on the frequency and pathogenesis of liver involvement in rheumatoid arthritis. Ann Rheum Dis 1979;38:501–6.
17. Lowe J, Pickup M, Dixon J, et al. Gamma glutamyl transpeptidase levels in arthritis: a correlation with clinical and laboratory indices of disease activity. Ann Rheum Dis 1978;37:428–31.
18. Webb J, Whaley K, MacSween R, et al. Liver disease in rheumatoid arthritis and Sjøgren's syndrome. Prospective study using biochemical and serological markers of hepatic dysfunction. Ann Rheum Dis 1975;34:70–81.

19. Thompson P, Houghton B, Clifford C, et al. The source and significance of raised serum enzymes in rheumatoid arthritis. Q J Med 1990;76:869–79.
20. Siede W, Seiffert U, Merle S, et al. Alkaline phosphatase isoenzymes in rheumatic diseases. Clin Biochem 1989;22:121–4.
21. Ruderman E, Crawford J, Maier A, et al. Histologic liver abnormalities in an autopsy series of patients with rheumatoid arthritis. Br J Rheumatol 1997;36: 210–3.
22. Rau R, Karger T, Herborn G, et al. Liver biopsy findings in patients with rheumatoid arthritis undergoing longterm treatment with methotrexate. J Rheumatol 1989;16:489–93.
23. Caramella C, Avouac J, Sogni P, et al. Association between rheumatoid arthritis and primary biliary cirrhosis. Joint Bone Spine 2007;74:279–81.
24. Job-Deslandre C, Feldmann J, Djian Y, et al. Chronic hepatitis during rheumatoid arthritis. Clin Exp Rheumatol 1991;9:507–10.
25. Ogata H, Tsuji H, Hashiguchi M, et al. Autoimmune cholangiopathy associated with rheumatoid arthritis. Hepatogastroenterology 2000;47(36):1533–4.
26. Goritsas C, Roussos A, Ferti A, et al. Nodular regenerative hyperplasia in a rheumatoid arthritis patient without Felty's syndrome. J Clin Gastroenterol 2002;35: 363–4.
27. Sasajima T, Suzuki T, Mori K, et al. A case of idiopathic portal hypertension associated with rheumatoid arthritis. Mod Rheumatol 2006;16:92–6.
28. Hocking W, Lasser K, Ungerer R, et al. Spontaneous hepatic rupture in rheumatoid arthritis. Arch Intern Med 1981;141:792–4.
29. Koga T, Migita K, Miyashita T, et al. Determination of anti-cyclic citrullinated peptide antibodies in the sera of patients with liver diseases. Clin Exp Rheumatol 2008;26(1):121–4.
30. Blendis L, Ansell I, Jones K, et al. Liver in Felty's syndrome. Br Med J 1970;1: 131–5.
31. Thorne C, Urowitz M, Wanless I, et al. Liver disease in Felty's syndrome. Am J Med 1982;73:35–40.
32. Wanless I. Micronodular transformation (nodular regenerative hyperplasia) of the liver: a report of 64 cases among 2,500 autopsies and a new classification of benign hepatocellular nodules. Hepatology 1990;11:787–97.
33. Blendis L, Lovell D, Barnes C, et al. Oesophageal variceal bleeding in Felty's syndrome associated with nodular regenerative hyperplasia. Ann Rheum Dis 1978;37:183–6.
34. Stock H, Kadry Z, Smith J. Surgical management of portal hypertension in Felty's syndrome: a case report and literature review. J Hepatol 2009;50:831–5.
35. Yamaguchi M, Ohta A, Tsunematsu T, et al. Preliminary criteria for classification of adult Still's disease. J Rheumatol 1992;19:424–30.
36. Ohta A, Yamaguchi M, Kaneoka H, et al. Adult Still's disease: review of 228 cases from the literature. J Rheumatol 1987;14:1139–46.
37. Taccone F, Lucidi V, Donckier V, et al. Fulminant hepatitis requiring MARS and liver transplantation in a patient with Still's disease. Eur J Intern Med 2008;19:e26–8.
38. Kaplan MJ, Ike RW. The liver is a common non-exocrine target in primary Sjogren's syndrome: a retrospective review. BMC Gastroenterol 2002;2:21.
39. García-Carrasco M, Ramos-Casals M, Rosas J, et al. Primary Sjögren's syndrome: clinical and immunologic disease patterns in a cohort of 400 patients. Medicine (Baltimore) 2002;81(4):270–80.
40. Lindgren S, Manthorpe R, Eriksson S. Autoimmune liver disease in patients with primary Sjogren's syndrome. J Hepatol 1994;20(3):354–8.

41. Hatzis GS, Fragoulis GE, Karatzaferis A, et al. Prevalence and longterm course of primary biliary cirrhosis in primary Sjogren's syndrome. J Rheumatol 2008;35(10): 2012–6.

42. Skopouli FN, Barbatis C, Moutsopoulos HM. Liver involvement in primary Sjogren's syndrome. Br J Rheumatol 1994;33:745–8.

43. Montano-Loza AJ, Crispin-Acuna JC, Remes-Troche JM, et al. Abnormal hepatic biochemistries and clinical liver disease in patients with primary Sjögren's syndrome. Ann Hepatol 2007;6(3):150–5.

44. Ramos-Casals M, Sanchez-Tapias JM, Pares A, et al. Characterization and differentiation of autoimmune versus viral liver involvement in patients with Sjogren's syndrome. J Rheumatol 2006;33(8):1593–9.

45. Matsumoto T, Morizane T, Aoki Y, et al. Autoimmune hepatitis in primary Sjogren's syndrome: pathological study of the livers and labial salivary glands in 17 patients with primary Sjogren's syndrome. Pathol Int 2005;55(2):70–6.

46. Alvarez F, Berg PA, Bianchi FB, et al. International Autoimmune Hepatitis Group Report: review of criteria for diagnosis of autoimmune hepatitis. J Hepatol 1999;31(5):929–38.

47. Jorgensen C, Legouffe MC, Perney P, et al. Sicca syndrome associated with hepatitis C virus infection. Arthritis Rheum 1996;39(7):1166–71.

48. García-Carrasco M, Ramos M, Cervera R, et al. Hepatitis C virus infection in 'primary' Sjögren's syndrome: prevalence and clinical significance in a series of 90 patients. Ann Rheum Dis 1997;56(3):173–5.

49. Ramos-Casals M, García-Carrasco M, Cervera R, et al. Sjögren's syndrome and hepatitis C virus. Clin Rheumatol 1999;18(2):93–100.

50. Ramos-Casals M, García-Carrasco M, Cervera R, et al. Hepatitis C virus infection mimicking primary Sjögren syndrome. A clinical and immunologic description of 35 cases. Medicine (Baltimore) 2001;80(1):1–8.

51. Montefusco PP, Geiss AC, Bronzo RL, et al. Sclerosing cholangitis, chronic pancreatitis, and Sjogren's syndrome: a syndrome complex. Am J Surg 1984; 147(6):822–6.

52. González-Alvaro I, Carmona-Ortell L, Amigo-Etxenagusia A, et al. Nodular regenerative hyperplasia of the liver and primary Sjögren's syndrome. J Rheumatol 1994;21(1):168–9.

53. D'Angelo WA, Fries JF, Masi AT, et al. Pathologic observations in systemic sclerosis (scleroderma). A study of fifty-eight autopsy cases and fifty-eight matched controls. Am J Med 1969;46(3):428–40.

54. Rigamonti C, Shand LM, Feudjo M, et al. Clinical features and prognosis of primary biliary cirrhosis associated with systemic sclerosis. Gut 2006;55(3):388–94.

55. Marasini B, Gagetta M, Rossi V, et al. Rheumatic disorders and primary biliary cirrhosis: an appraisal of 170 Italian patients. Ann Rheum Dis 2001;60(11): 1046–9.

56. Akimoto S, Ishikawa O, Takagi H, et al. Immunological features of patients with primary biliary cirrhosis (PBC) overlapping systemic sclerosis: a comparison with patients with PBC alone. J Gastroenterol Hepatol 1998;13(9):897–901.

57. Ishikawa M, Okada J, Shibuya A, et al. CRST syndrome (calcinosis cutis, Raynaud's phenomenon, sclerodactyly, and telangiectasia) associated with autoimmune hepatitis. Intern Med 1995;34(1):6–9.

58. Kaburaki J, Kuramochi S, Fujii T, et al. Nodular regenerative hyperplasia of the liver in a patient with systemic sclerosis. Clin Rheumatol 1996;15(6):613–6.

59. Moschos J, Leontiadis GI, Kelly C, et al. Idiopathic portal hypertension complicating systemic sclerosis: a case report. BMC Gastroenterol 2005;5:16.

60. Fraile G, Rodríguez-García JL, Moreno A. Primary sclerosing cholangitis associated with systemic sclerosis. Postgrad Med J 1991;67(784):189–92.
61. Smith DH, Spencer DG, Allam BF, et al. Serum alkaline phosphatase in ankylosing spondylitis. J Clin Pathol 1979;32(8):853–4.
62. Robinson AC, Teeling M, Casey EB. Hepatic function in ankylosing spondylitis. Ann Rheum Dis 1983;42(5):550–2.
63. Kendall MJ, Lawrence DS, Shuttleworth GR, et al. Haematology and biochemistry of ankylosing spondylitis. Br Med J 1973;2(5860):235–7.
64. Sheehan NJ, Slavin BM, Kind PR, et al. Increased serum alkaline phosphatase activity in ankylosing spondylitis. Ann Rheum Dis 1983;42(5):563–5.
65. Rostom A, Goldkind L, Laine L. Nonsteroidal anti-inflammatory drugs and hepatic toxicity: a systematic review of randomized controlled trials in arthritis patients. Clin Gastroenterol Hepatol 2005;3(5):489–98.
66. García Rodríguez LA, Williams R, Derby LE, et al. Acute liver injury associated with nonsteroidal anti-inflammatory drugs and the role of risk factors. Arch Intern Med 1994;154(3):311–6.
67. Jobanputra P, Amarasena R, Maggs F, et al. Hepatotoxicity associated with sulfasalazine in inflammatory arthritis: A case series from a local surveillance of serious adverse events. BMC Musculoskelet Disord 2008;9:48.
68. Rosenbaum J, Katz WA, Schumacher HR. Hepatotoxicity associated with use of D-penicillamine in rheumatoid arthritis. Ann Rheum Dis 1980;39(2):152–4.
69. Emery P, Breedveld FC, Lemmel EM, et al. A comparison of the efficacy and safety of leflunomide and methotrexate for the treatment of rheumatoid arthritis. Rheumatology (Oxford) 2000;39(6):655–65.
70. Strand V, Cohen S, Schiff M, et al. Treatment of active rheumatoid arthritis with leflunomide compared with placebo and methotrexate. Arch Intern Med 1999;159: 2542–50.
71. van Roon EN, Jansen TL, Houtman NM, et al. Leflunomide for the treatment of rheumatoid arthritis in clinical practice: incidence and severity of hepatotoxicity. Drug Saf 2004;27(5):345–52.
72. Suissa S, Ernst P, Hudson M, et al. Newer disease-modifying antirheumatic drugs and the risk of serious hepatic adverse events in patients with rheumatoid arthritis. Am J Med 2004;117(2):87–92.
73. Alcorn N, Saunders S, Madhok R. Benefit-risk assessment of leflunomide: an appraisal of leflunomide in rheumatoid arthritis 10 years after licensing. Drug Saf 2009;32(12):1123–34.
74. West SG. Methotrexate hepatotoxicity. Rheum Dis Clin North Am 1997;23(4): 883–915.
75. Phillips CA, Cera PJ, Mangan TF, et al. Clinical liver disease in patients with rheumatoid arthritis taking methotrexate. J Rheumatol 1992;19(2):229–33.
76. Erickson AR, Reddy V, Vogelgesang SA, et al. Usefulness of the American College of Rheumatology recommendations for liver biopsy in methotrexate-treated rheumatoid arthritis patients. Arthritis Rheum 1995;38(8):1115–9.
77. Kremer JM, Lee RG, Tolman KG. Liver histology in rheumatoid arthritis patients receiving long-term methotrexate therapy. A prospective study with baseline and sequential biopsy samples. Arthritis Rheum 1989;32(2):121–7.
78. Visser K, Katchamart W, Loza E, et al. Multinational evidence-based recommendations for the use of methotrexate in rheumatic disorders with a focus on rheumatoid arthritis: integrating systematic literature research and expert opinion of a broad international panel of rheumatologists in the 3E Initiative. Ann Rheum Dis 2009;68(7):1086–93.

79. Menter A, Korman NJ, Elmets CA, et al. Guidelines of care for the management of psoriasis and psoriatic arthritis: section 4. Guidelines of care for the management and treatment of psoriasis with traditional systemic agents. J Am Acad Dermatol 2009;61(3):451–85.

80. Kremer JM, Kaye GI, Kaye NW, et al. Light and electron microscopic analysis of sequential liver biopsy samples from rheumatoid arthritis patients receiving long-term methotrexate therapy. Followup over long treatment intervals and correlation with clinical and laboratory variables. Arthritis Rheum 1995;38(9):1194–203.

81. Leonardi CL, Powers JL, Matheson RT, et al. Etanercept as monotherapy in patients with psoriasis. N Engl J Med 2003;349:2014–22.

82. Tobon G, Cañas C, Jaller JJ, et al. Serious liver disease induced by infliximab. Clin Rheumatol 2007;26:578–81.

83. Thiéfin G, Morelet A, Heurgué A, et al. Infliximab-induced hepatitis: absence of cross-toxicity with etanercept. Joint Bone Spine 2008;75(6):737–9.

84. Ozorio G, McGarity B, Bak H, et al. Autoimmune hepatitis following infliximab therapy for ankylosing spondylitis. Med J Aust 2007;187(9):524–6.

85. Ramos-Casals M, Roberto-Perez-Alvarez, Diaz-Lagares C, et al. Autoimmune diseases induced by biological agents: a double-edged sword? Autoimmun Rev 2010;9(3):188–93.

86. Wendling D, Di Martino V, Prati C, et al. Spondyloarthropathy and chronic B hepatitis. Effect of anti-TNF therapy. Joint Bone Spine 2009;76(3):308–11.

87. Chung SJ, Kim JK, Park MC, et al. Reactivation of hepatitis B viral infection in inactive HBsAg carriers following anti-tumor necrosis factor-alpha therapy. J Rheumatol 2009;36(11):2416–20.

88. Sakellariou GT, Chatzigiannis I. Long-term anti-TNFalpha therapy for ankylosing spondylitis in two patients with chronic HBV infection. Clin Rheumatol 2007; 26(6):950–2.

89. Esteve M, Saro C, González-Huix F, et al. Chronic hepatitis B reactivation following infliximab therapy in Crohn's disease patients: need for primary prophylaxis. Gut 2004;53(9):1363–5.

90. Michel M, Duvoux C, Hezode C, et al. Fulminant hepatitis after infliximab in a patient with hepatitis B virus treated for an adult onset still's disease. J Rheumatol 2003;30(7):1624–5.

91. Li S, Kaur PP, Chan V, et al. Use of tumor necrosis factor-alpha (TNF-alpha) antagonists infliximab, etanercept, and adalimumab in patients with concurrent rheumatoid arthritis and hepatitis B or hepatitis C: a retrospective record review of 11 patients. Clin Rheumatol 2009;28(7):787–91.

92. Kim YJ, Bae SC, Sung YK, et al. Possible reactivation of potential hepatitis B virus occult infection by tumor necrosis factor-alpha blocker in the treatment of rheumatic diseases. J Rheumatol 2010;37(2):346–50.

93. Lok AS, McMahon BJ. Chronic hepatitis B: update 2009. Hepatology 2009;50(3): 661–2.

94. Ferri C, Ferraccioli G, Ferrari D, et al. Safety of anti-tumor necrosis factor-alpha therapy in patients with rheumatoid arthritis and chronic hepatitis C virus infection. J Rheumatol 2008;35(10):1944–9.

95. Peterson JR, Hsu FC, Simkin PA, et al. Effect of tumour necrosis factor alpha antagonists on serum transaminases and viraemia in patients with rheumatoid arthritis and chronic hepatitis C infection. Ann Rheum Dis 2003;62(11):1078–82.

Dermatologic Disorders and the Liver

Sanjaya K. Satapathy, MD, DM[a], David Bernstein, MD, AGAF[b,c],*

KEYWORDS

- Cirrhosis • Chronic liver disease • Hepatitis
- Dermatologic disorder

Dermatologic manifestations are one of the most common extrahepatic manifestations and often provide the first clues of the underlying liver disease. An understanding of these various manifestations and their underlying disorder will better prepare nonder-matologists for these diagnostic challenges and appropriate care can be instituted in a timely manner. This review focuses on the dermatologic manifestations of liver diseases in general and of various infectious, autoimmune, metabolic, hereditary, developmental, and neoplastic liver disorders. In addition, hepatotoxicity of the dermatologic drugs is reviewed.

LIVER DISEASE AND THE SKIN

Manifestations of the liver and skin disorders are inter-related in various ways. For a better understanding of the pathophysiologic process involved in this inter-relation, they are divided into the following five categories:

1. Dermatologic manifestations of liver cirrhosis.
2. Systemic diseases affecting both liver and the skin
3. Primary skin disorders affecting the liver
4. Dermatologic manifestations of specific liver diseases
5. Drugs used by dermatologists causing hepatotoxicity.

[a] Long Island Jewish Medical Center at Albert Einstein College of Medicine, North Shore-Long Island Jewish Health system, 270-05 76th Avenue, New Hyde Park, NY 11040, USA
[b] Digestive Disease Institute, Department of Medicine, North Shore University Hospital and Long Island Jewish Medical Center, North Shore University Hospital, 300 Community Drive, Manhasset, NY 11030, USA
[c] Department of Medicine, Albert Einstein College of Medicine, 1300 Morris Park Avenue, Bronx, NY 10461, USA
* Corresponding author. Digestive Disease Institute, Department of Medicine, North Shore University Hospital and Long Island Jewish Medical Center, North Shore University Hospital, 300 Community Drive, Manhasset, NY 11030.
E-mail address: dbernste@nshs.edu

Clin Liver Dis 15 (2011) 165–182
doi:10.1016/j.cld.2010.09.001
1089-3261/11/$ – see front matter © 2011 Elsevier Inc. All rights reserved.

liver.theclinics.com

Dermatologic Manifestations of Liver Cirrhosis

Jaundice

Jaundice (icterus) is the clinical manifestation of hyperbilirubinemia and presents as yellow discoloration of the skin and mucous membranes. It is the most obvious sign of liver disease and is best seen in the conjunctivae. It is usually detectable when the serum level of bilirubin exceeds 2 mg/dL (34 μmol/L). Elevation of both unconjugated and conjugated bilirubin occurs in patients with hepatocellular disease due to impaired canalicular excretion or biliary obstruction.

Palmar erythema

Palmar erythema, or liver palms, is a nonspecific red discoloration of the palms and fingertips of the hands. Twenty-three percent of patients with cirrhosis, from varying causes, manifest palmar erythema.[1] Abnormal serum estradiol levels[1] and regional differences in the peripheral circulation of patients with cirrhosis have been attributed as causes.[2] Palmar erythema can occur in conditions unrelated to liver disease, such as pregnancy, rheumatoid arthritis, thyrotoxicosis, diabetes mellitus, gestational syphilis, and human T-lymphotropic virus 1–associated myelopathy.[1] Drugs, such as amiodarone, gemfibrozil, cholestyramine, topiramate, and albuterol (salbutamol), have been reported to cause palmar erythema.[1]

Spider nevi

Spider nevi, or spider angiomas, are telangiectases consisting of a central arteriole with superficially radiating small vessels (**Fig. 1**), resembling spider's legs, and are mainly observed in the superior vena cava distribution area (ie, in the face, V of the neck, and upper part of the trunk above the nipple line and arms). Spider nevi occur in healthy people, especially at puberty, in pregnant women, or in women using hormonal contraception. Approximately 33% of patients with cirrhosis have spider angiomas.[3] Many factors have been associated with the pathogenesis of spider nevi in patients with cirrhosis. Young age, elevated plasma vascular endothelial growth factor, and basic fibroblast growth factor have been attributed as significant independent predictors of spider nevi in cirrhotic patients.[4] The presence of spider nevi is accompanied by an increased serum estradiol/free testosterone ratio in male

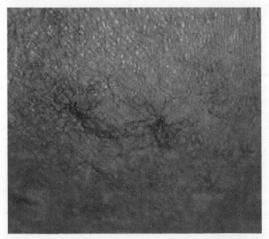

Fig. 1. Spider nevi. They are characterized by a vascular, central body with symmetrically radiating thin branches, the central vessel being an arteriole.

cirrhotic patients.[5] People who have significant hepatic impairment cannot detoxify estrogen from the blood, resulting in high levels of estrogen. An increase in number or size of spider nevi may suggest progressive liver damage. The spider angiomas associated with liver disease may resolve when liver function improves or when a liver transplant is performed. Spider nevi can be successfully treated with laser therapy for cosmetic reasons.[6]

White nails (Terry nails)

Terry nails is a physical finding in which fingernails and/or toenails appear white with a characteristic ground glass appearance with a dark band at the tip and the absence of a lunula. Terry nails are associated with several diseases and advancing age.[7–10] Type 2 diabetes mellitus, congestive heart failure, chronic renal failure, and cirrhosis are all systemic diseases that are associated with Terry nails.[7–10] The pathogenesis of these nail changes is unclear but is thought to be due to a decrease in vascularity and an increase in connective tissue within the nail bed. In a study conducted by Holzberg and Walker,[8] biopsies of nail beds that were performed on several patients showed dilated vasculature in the dermis of the distal band. Holzberg postulated that these vascular changes were related to the premature aging of the nail bed, which resulted in the abnormal appearance of the nail.[7] Although aging is a common cause of Terry nails, it is important for physicians to consider other disease entities that can lead to this abnormal nail appearance, especially in younger patients.

Systemic Disorders Affecting Both Liver and the Skin

Many of the systemic diseases, including autoimmune and rheumatoid-related disorders, affect both the skin and the liver, such as systemic lupus erythematosus (SLE), psoriasis, sarcoidosis, and lichen planus (LP) (**Table 1**).

Systemic lupus erythematosus

SLE is a chronic, immunologically mediated disease classically involves the skin, kidneys, cardiovascular system, and central nervous system. Abnormalities of liver function are not included in the diagnostic criteria of SLE. Patients with SLE, however, have a 25% to 50% chance of developing abnormal liver tests.[11,12] Harvey and colleagues[11] reported hepatomegaly in 35% of patients but without any evidence of impairment of liver function. Histologically, the most common findings were fatty infiltration and "atrophy and necrosis of the central hepatic cells." Previous studies have shown that[12,13] advanced liver disease is not usually seen in SLE patients. A large pathologic series[14] of 73 patients with SLE showed hepatic arteritis in 15.1%, primary biliary cirrhosis (PBC) in 2.7%, nodular regenerative hyperplasia in 6.8%, and autoimmune hepatitis in 2.7%. Other causes of liver disease included fatty liver (73%), viral chronic hepatitis or cirrhosis (4.1%), and drug-induced hepatitis or cholangitis (2.7%). A higher prevalence of autoimmune liver disease (9.8%) in patients with juvenile SLE compared with adult patients (1.3%) has been reported.[15]

Sjögren syndrome

Sjögren syndrome is a chronic autoimmune disorder that can be classified as primary or secondary. Primary Sjögren syndrome consists of the association of keratoconjunctivitis sicca, xerostomia, and swelling of the salivary glands, whereas secondary Sjögren syndrome describes the former in association with rheumatoid arthritis. Other clinical features include Raynaud phenomenon, achlorhydria (from atrophic gastritis), alopecia, splenomegaly, and leukopenia. The dermatologic manifestations range from dryness (sicca) and its complications to vasculitis. Seven percent of patients with Sjögren syndrome have evidence of liver disease—either subclinical (2%) or

Table 1
Associated hepatic manifestations of systemic and primary skin diseases

Systemic/Primary Skin Disease	Hepatic Manifestations
SLE	Hepatic arteritis PBC Nodular regenerative hyperplacia Autoimmune hepatitis Fatty liver Cirrhosis
Sjögren syndrome	PBC Hepatitis C
Scleroderma	PBC (with systemic sclerosis)
Sarcoidosis	Chronic intrahepatic cholestatis Micronodular billiary cirrhosis Budd-Chiari syndrome
Psoriasis	NAFLD Risk for methotrexate-induced cirrhosis
DHS and toxic epidermal necrolysis	Mild liver chemistry abnormality to fulminant hepatic failure
Dermatitis herpetiformis	Nonspecific liver chemistry abnormality PBC PSC Drug-induced hepatitis (with Dapson)
Mastocytosis	Cholestasis Venooclusive disease Cirrhosis
Malignant dermatologic disorders	Hepatic metastasis from melanoma and basal cell carcinoma (rare) Hepatic lymphoma with cutaneous T-cell lymphoma

asymptomatic (5%)—manifested by elevated liver enzyme levels and positive test results for anti-mitochondrial antibody (AMA).[16] Positive titers for AMA are usually accompanied by histopathologic abnormalities consistent with PBC.[16] Ninety-two percent of patients with a positive AMA have liver involvement with features similar to stage I PBC, even in the presence of normal liver enzyme levels. An association of hepatitis C and Sjögren syndrome has been suggested as well.[17]

Scleroderma
Scleroderma (systemic sclerosis) is a chronic systemic disease that targets the skin, lungs, heart, gastrointestinal tract, kidneys, and musculoskeletal system. The disorder is characterized by three features: tissue fibrosis, small blood vessel vasculopathy, and an autoimmune response associated with specific autoantibodies. Scleroderma is classified into two major subsets, which are distinguished by the extent of skin thickening: limited and diffuse cutaneous scleroderma The CREST (calcinosis cutis, Raynaud phenomenon, esophageal dysfunction, sclerodactyly, and telangiectasia) syndrome is a form of limited scleroderma that is associated with anticentromere antibodies. Two population-based studies showed association of PBC with systemic sclerosis.[18,19] Such an association of PBC has not been confirmed, however, with limited cutaneous involvement.[18]

Sarcoidosis

Sarcoidosis is a multisystem disease characterized by noncaseating granulomas in the affected organs, including skin, heart, nervous system, and joints. Sarcoidosis of the skin may have an extremely heterogeneous clinical presentation and is capable of imitating a variety of diseases; consequently, in dermatology it is often called The Great Imitator, or a clinical chameleon.[20] The clinical morphology of cutaneous sarcoidosis may vary within a wide range. Many cutaneous lesions can mimic sarcoidosis of the skin either clinically or/and pathologically, a detailed review of which is beyond the scope of this review and is described elsewhere.[20,21]

Approximately 50% to 79% of livers are involved by biopsy and 67% to 70% by autopsy.[21–24] Patients with sarcoidosis are infrequently symptomatic due to liver disease and may present with pruritus, abdominal pain, and fever[25] Hepatomegaly is found in approximately 21% to 50% of the patients.[26–28] Abnormal liver chemistries are found in only 35% of patients.[29,30] Liver involvement may occur without lung involvement in up to 26% of the patients.[30] Jaundice is rare[26] and may be due to intrahepatic cholestasis, hemolysis, hepatocellular dysfunction, or obstruction of the extrahepatic bile ducts by granulomatous hepatic hilar lymph nodes. Alkaline phosphatase is more reliable than γ-glutamyl transpeptidase in predicting liver involvement.[31] Hyperglobulinemia is common.

In sarcoidosis, the histologic abnormalities include noncaseating granulomas, chronic intrahepatic cholestasis, progressive diminution in the number of interlobular bile ducts, periportal fibrosis, and micronodular biliary cirrhosis.[32] Progressive liver disease due sarcoidosis may lead to the development of portal hypertension.[33,34] Development of cirrhosis is not a prerequisite of portal hypertension.[35] Severe liver dysfunction and jaundice are uncommon.[33] Because such patients have little hepatic dysfunction, they do not develop encephalopathy after portasystemic shunts.[27] Other vascular complications include portal vein thrombosis because of stasis from obliteration of small portal veins[33] and Budd-Chiari syndrome because of extrinsic compression of hepatic veins by sarcoid granulomas, causing narrowing of venous vessels, venous stasis, and subsequent thrombosis.[36]

Primary Skin Disorders Affecting the Liver

Many primary skin disorders have a variety of systemic manifestations, and the liver is not spared from its brunt. These various manifestations are summarized in **Table 1**.

Psoriasis

Psoriasis is a chronic inflammatory skin disease that affects 1% to 3% of the general population. It is characterized by epidermal hyperproliferation, abnormal keratinocyte differentiation, angiogenesis with vasodilatation, and activated CD4+ and CD8+ T-cell infiltrates in the dermis and epidermis, respectively.[37] The clinical presentation is highly variable in terms of lesion localization and severity, and in nearly one-third of all cases the skin lesions are associated with an inflammatory joint disease known as psoriatic arthritis (PsA). Hepatotoxicity of the drugs used in the treatment for psoriasis is a major concern for hepatologists. Methotrexate is the most widely used drug in the treatment of psoriasis. Previous studies on hepatotoxicity after long-term methotrexate therapy in patients with PsA found that the risk of developing cirrhosis may be as high as 25%.[38] The risk of serious liver disease among patients with rheumatoid arthritis who receive low-dose methotrexate has been reported to be less than 1 per 1000 cases after 5 years of treatment.[39] Due to the cost and morbidity associated with liver biopsy and the relatively low incidence of serious methotrexate-induced liver toxicity, the British Association of Dermatologists has questioned the appropriateness of routine liver biopsy.[40] Other safety concerns in regard to the hepatoxicity are related to therapy with infliximab,[41,42] etenercept,[43] and vitamin A.[44] Recent studies have linked psoriasis to nonalcoholic fatty liver disease (NAFLD). The authors reported that NAFLD is highly prevalent among psoriasis patients, where it is closely associated with obesity (overall and abdominal), metabolic syndrome, and PsA and more likely to cause severe liver fibrosis (compared with nonpsoriasis NAFLD).[40] Routine work-up for NAFLD may thus be warranted in patients with psoriasis, especially when potentially hepatotoxic drug therapy is considered.

Drug-induced hypersensitivity and toxic epidermal necrolysis

The incidence of drug-induced hypersensitivity (DHS) and toxic epidermal necrolysis is unclear because of their variable presentations, diverse clinical features, and laboratory abnormalities. DHS starts within the first 2 to 8 weeks after initial drug exposure. The reaction usually begins with low- or high-grade fever followed by development of a cutaneous eruption, lymphadenopathy, and in some cases pharyngitis. The skin rash is most commonly an exanthema with or without pruritus. Rarely, generalized follicular pustules or more severe skin reactions, such as exfoliative dermatitis, Stevens-Johnson syndrome, or toxic epidermal necrolysis, may occur. The incidence of these severe skin reactions as part of anticonvulsant-induced hypersensitivity syndrome was found as high as 9% among 53 patients with anticonvulsant-induced hypersensitivity syndrome induced by phenytoin, carbamazepine, or phenobarbital, as reported by Shear and Spielberg.[45] Angioedema (especially facial or periorbital swelling) may be a sign of a systemic and potentially severe life-threatening reaction. The liver is the most frequently involved internal organ in DHS and the rate is reported to be 34% to 94%. The organ involvement can vary from mild elevations in liver enzymes to marked abnormalities in function tests with hepatomegaly and fulminant hepatic necrosis.[46] Laboratory features of the syndrome are leukocytosis with eosinophilia and atypical lymphocytosis. Treatment is primarily symptomatic and hospitalization is required in life-threatening situations. The efficacy of corticosteroids is debatable, but some investigators recommend the use of prednisone at a dosage of 1 to 2 mg/kg per day if symptoms are severe.[47] Silver sulfadiazine is not usually recommended in cases of toxic epidermal necrolysis because it has been reported to cause leukopenia and sulfonamides are associated with severe cutaneous adverse reactions.[48]

Dermatitis herpetiformis

Dermatitis herpetiformis (DH) is an intensely pruritic, chronic blistering disease that often appears suddenly, mainly between the ages of 20 and 55, and is more common in men than women.[49] Overall prevalence is estimated at between 10 and 39 cases per 100,000 annually.[49] Erythematous papulovesicular lesions are characteristically distributed symmetrically on extensor body surfaces and on the buttocks and back. Granular deposits of IgA (normally involved in immunoprotection of the body's mucosal surfaces, especially the respiratory and gastrointestinal tracts) at the dermoepidermal junction are the immunologic marker of this disease, and patients have a gluten-sensitive enteropathy that is histologically apparent but generally asymptomatic.[49] Previous studies have shown abnormalities of bilirubin or elevated liver enzyme levels in 17% of the patients in a series of 60 cases of DHS. Hepatic disease occurs more often in patients with celiac disease than in those with DH (approximately 45% compared with 17%) and is thought to be related to the degree of gut mucosal damage, which is greater in celiac disease than in DH. The incidence of liver chemistry abnormalities was higher (19%) in those on a normal diet than those on a gluten-free diet (9%).[50] Liver tests improve in these patients as does the small bowel when a gluten-free diet is adhered to. Uncommonly, liver impairment in DH may be caused by either of two autoimmune disorders, PBC[51,52] and primary sclerosing cholangitis (PSC).[53,54] Both DH and PSC are strongly associated with certain HLA types. Reports of autoantibody abnormalities in PSC and the known association of α-gliadin and antiendomysial antibodies in DH suggest a possible underlying immune mechanism. Dapsone used in treating DH may increase bilirubin (indirect) because of drug-induced hemolytic anemia but can also directly cause liver function test abnormalities in isolation or as part of the dapsone syndrome.[55,56] Dapsone hypersensitivity syndrome typically presents with a triad of fever, skin eruption, and internal organ (lung, liver, neurologic, and other systems) involvement, occurring several weeks to as late as 6 months after the initial administration of the drug.[57] If not promptly identified and treated, DHS could be fatal.

Mastocytosis

Mastocytosis is characterized by an excessive number of apparently normal mast cells in the skin and in various tissues.[58] The exact cause has not been elucidated. Clinical manifestations of systemic mastocytosis vary depending on the mast cell burden in different tissues, the host response to mast cell mediators, or the presence of an underlying non–mast cell hematologic process.[59,60] Gastrointestinal and liver involvement is common in systemic mastocytosis.[61–65] The prevalence of gastrointestinal symptoms is estimated to be 51% (range 14%–85%), but the only prospective study reports an 80% prevalence.[62,63] Abdominal pain and diarrhea are the two most common gastrointestinal symptoms, occurring in 51% and 43% of patients, respectively.[63] Manifestations of liver involvement include hepatomegaly (48%), portal hypertension, and ascites (5%–50%).[63] The most common liver test abnormalities is an elevated alkaline phosphatase.[63] Studies have shown that the degree of hepatomegaly varies with the type of systemic mastocytosis and that the degree of alkaline phosphatase elevation correlates with liver size, fibrosis, and mast cell infiltrate.[63,65] Reported liver biopsy findings include the following: (1) bridging fibrosis, (2) cirrhosis, (3) inflammatory cell infiltrates in the portal tracts and lobules, (4) venoocclusive disease, and, rarely, (5) cholestasis.[61,64] Four published case report series describe the cholestatic liver manifestations of systemic mastocytosis.[66–69] From these series, three distinct histologic patterns of cholestatic livers manifesting systemic mastocytosis have emerged—intrahepatic cholestasis, autoimmune cholangitis, and sclerosing cholangitis. Clinicians and pathologists need to have a high index of clinical suspicion for systemic mastocytosis in proper clinical context with multisystemic symptoms and signs to avoid its attendant morbidity and mortality.

Malignant dermatologic disorders and the liver

Malignant melanoma occurs most frequently in skin but also in many organs and tissues of the body, including the retina, anorectal canal, genital tract, gastrointestinal tract, accessory nasal cavity, and parotid gland. Primary hepatic malignant melanoma is exceedingly rare.[70] Basal cell carcinoma is a malignant but slow-growing tumor and is locally invasive, rarely extending beyond basal layer; hepatic metastases have been described.[71,72] Another uncommon yet important entity is the cutaneous T-cell lymphomas (mycosis fungoides and Sézary syndrome). In Huberman and colleagues'[73] series of 43 patients with cutaneous T-cell lymphomas (mycosis fungoides and Sézary syndrome), seven patients (16%) had biopsy-documented hepatic lymphoma. Liver transplant recipients are at increased risk of developing cancer, mainly as a consequence of immunosuppressant treatment, although a variety of other factors are involved. Skin cancers have been reported to be high as 40% in liver transplant recipients and are the most frequently encountered cancer.[74–76] The most common skin cancer type was nonmelanoma skin cancer, with a higher frequency of basal cell cancer than melanoma. Skin cancer education should be integrated into the care of transplant patients as part of their numerous visits to the transplant clinic to reduce their risk of skin cancer.[77]

Cutaneous Manifestations of Specific Liver Diseases

Direct extension from infective hepatic lesions
The skin is mostly involved indirectly in infectious liver diseases, although rarely involvement could be direct through transcutaneous extension/fistulization of hepatic infections, such as actinomycosis,[78] amoebiasis,[79] and hydatid cysts.[80]

Dermatologic manifestations of hepatitis B virus infection
Hepatitis B virus (HBV) infection can produce or induce various dermatologic manifestations (**Table 2**). Most of the dermatologic manifestations described in HBV infections are

Table 2
Dermatologic manifestations associated with specific liver diseases

Liver Disease	Associated Dermatologic Conditions
Autoimmune liver disease (mostly with PBC)	Xanthomatous lesions Melanosis LP Scleroderma CREST
Hereditary and developmental disorder	Xanthomas
Hepatitis C infection	LP MC PCT Sicca syndrome Anecdotal observations Psoriasis PAN Behçet syndrome Leukocytoclastic reactions Myositis/dermatomyositis Chronic urticaria Chronic pruritus Kaposi's pseudosarcoma Vitiligo Mooren corneal ulcer Acral necrolytic erythema
Hepatitis B infection	Papular eruption Gianotti-Crosti syndrome Erythema nodosum LP Lecocytoclastic vasculitis PAN MC Dermatomyositis-like syndrome Pyoderma gangreonosum PCT Skin neoplacia
Hepatic neoplasm	Dermatomyositis Cutaneous metastasis

immune complex–related illnesses.[81] These disorders include serum sickness–like prodrome,[82] some recurrent papular eruptions,[83] Gianotti-Crosti syndrome, erythema nodosum,[84] LP,[85,86] leukocytoclastic vasculitis,[87] polyarteritis nodosa (PAN),[88] mixed cryoglobulinemia (MC),[89] dermatomyositis-like syndrome,[90] pyoderma gangrenosum,[91] porphyria cutanea tarda (PCT),[92] and increased susceptibility to skin neoplasia.[93] Manifestations, such as erythema nodosum, LP, PAN, MC, are common in HBV and hepatitis C virus (HCV) infections.[94]

Approximately 7% to 8% of acute HBV infection patients develop PAN.[95] Although HBV-associated PAN shares the characteristics of classic PAN, it is not an antineutrophil cytoplasmic antibody–mediated vasculitis. The majority of the HBV/PAN cases are associated with wild-type HBV infection, characterized by hepatitis B e (HBe) antigenemia and high HBV replication, supporting the concept that lesions could result from the deposit of viral antigen-antibody (Ag/Ab) complexes soluble in Ag excess, possibly involving HBeAg.[96] These observations have been challenged, however, because cases of PAN have been reported in patients with precore mutations. This may suggest that other, still undefined, circulating HBV-related Ags distinct from HBeAg could be involved. The first-line treatment for HBV-associated PAN is short-term steroid therapy, antiviral agents, and plasma exchanges. This therapy surpasses the conventional treatment of PAN (which consists of corticosteroids and cyclophosphamide), facilitates seroconversion, and prevents the development of long-term hepatic complications of chronic HBV infection.[97]

Dermatologic manifestations of hepatitis C virus infection

Among the many cutaneous manifestations associated with chronic hepatitis C (CHC), the most important are summarized in **Table 2**. It is now well established that approximately 80% of MC is secondary to HCV infection.[98,99] Patients with essential mixed cryoglobulinemia (EMC) display palpable purpura in the legs (which is worse distally and inferiorly), livido reticularis, ulcerations, urticaria, symmetric polyarthritis, myalgias, cutis marmorata, and fatigue.[100] Evidence of HCV RNA has been found with high frequency in organs affected in cryoglobulinemia, particularly in the skin and kidney.[99] Antiviral treatment of CHC is the therapy of first choice for all patients with MC complicating hepatitis C infection.[99]

LP is an idiopathic inflammatory disease with characteristic clinical and pathologic features affecting the skin, mucous membranes, nails, and hair (**Fig. 2**). An increased prevalence of chronic liver diseases has been reported in patients with LP, including PBC and chronic active hepatitis or cirrhosis of unknown origin.[101,102] Many studies have confirmed a significant association of LP with HCV[101–105]; other investigations have failed to document this finding.[106–108] In a recent metanalysis including 33 studies comparing the seroprevalence of HCV in LP patients and six reporting the prevalence of LP in patients with HCV infection, the investigators concluded that LP patients have significantly higher risk than controls of being HCV seropositive.[109] A similar relationship of having LP was found among HCV patients in the same study.[109] In view of that possible association, screening patients with oral LP for antibodies to HCV needs consideration.

Acral necrolytic erythema is a papulosquamous and sometimes vesiculobullous eruption bearing clinical and histologic similarity to other necrolytic erythemas, such as necrolytic migratory erythema, pseudoglucagonoma, and nutritional deficiency syndromes.[110–113] Chronic lesions are hyperkeratotic plaques with erosions and peripheral erythema preferring the acral parts of the legs. Response to interferon-based regimen has been documented.[113]

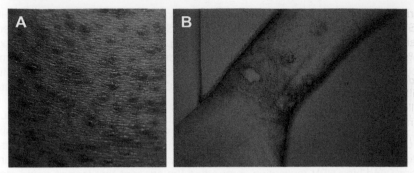

Fig. 2. (A) LP. Papulosquamous skin lesions. They are often characterized by the six Ps: pruritus, polygonal shape, planar, purple color, papules, and plaques. Images depict some of the cardinal features. (B) LP. Hypertrophic lesions are often chronic; residual pigmentation and scarring can occur when the lesions eventually clear.

CHC is also a risk factor for PCT (**Fig. 3**).[114] The frequent association of both CHC infection and HLA-linked, hereditary hemochromatosis with PCT has two implications: all patients with PCT should be screened for HCV infection with measurement of antibodies against HCV, and all should undergo HFE gene mutational analysis to look for either of the two mutations (C282Y or the H63D) that have been linked with iron overload. The initial management of PCT should continue to be vigorous iron removal, to the point of mild iron deficiency.[115] After this has been accomplished, patients who are HCV positive should be considered for treatment of HCV infection with interferon-based therapies.

Considering the proved association between EMC, PCT, LP, and CHC (see **Table 1**), all patients with these disorders should be tested for HCV, and all cases of CHC should be investigated for the presence of these disorders.[116]

Autoimmune liver diseases

Autoimmune liver diseases, especially the cholestatic autoimmune liver diseases like PBC, are associated with many skin manifestations. In 38.7% of the patients with PBC, dermatologic lesions are the presenting signs and symptoms.[117] Dermatologic manifestations commonly associated with PBC are xanthomatous lesions and melanosis.[117] At the late stages, nonspecific skin lesions typically seen in patients with advanced liver disease can also be found. Various case reports exist in the literature

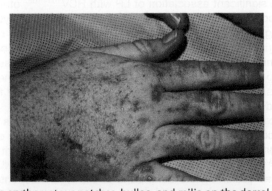

Fig. 3. PCT. Erosive erythematous patches, bullae, and milia on the dorsal side of right hand.

describing a more frequent association of PBC with LP,[118,119] scleroderma,[120,121] and CREST syndrome.[122] In a series 49 cases, Koulentaki and colleagues[117] reported fungal skin infections (31.5%), neoplastic lesions (18.4%), dermatitis-urticaria (15.7%), and disturbances of pigmentation (12.4%).

Hereditary and developmental liver disease
Alagille syndrome
Alagille syndrome (arteriohepatic dysplasia)[123] is a genetic disorder with autosomal dominant transmission (chromosome 20p). A nonsyndromic type associated with α1-antitrypsin deficiency and viral infections, such us congenital rubella, cytomegalovirus, or HBV, occurs less frequently and has a worse prognosis than the syndromic type. The syndromic type is characterized by five main features: (1) chronic cholestasis, (2) peculiar facies, (3) cardiovascular abnormalities, (4) vertebral arch defects, and (5) posterior embryotoxon. Less frequently, some of the following can be observed: growth retardation, renal disturbances, mental retardation, bone abnormalities, and high-pitched voice.[123] Cutaneous manifestations include jaundice, pruritus, and widespread xanthomata. Xanthomas (29%) are caused by chronic cholestasis and severe hypercholesterolemia and are seen on the extensor surfaces of the fingers, acral creases (striate palmar and plantar xanthomas), nape, popliteal fossae, inguinal areas, helixes, gluteal areas, and elbows and knees, where they are usually confluent. Xanthelasma and tuberous xanthomas are also present. Many aspects of the syndrome, including cholestasis, pruritus, and hypercholesterolemia, improve after liver transplantation.[124]

Hepatic neoplasm
Hepatocellular carcinoma (HCC) rarely involves the skin, and the occurrence of cutaneous metastasis as the disease may be seen in 1% to 5% of cases.[125–127] Cutaneous metastasis may occur through local invasion, the lymphatics, a hematologic route, or as a result of seeding after percutaneous invasive procedures, such as percutaneous ethanol injection, fine-needle aspiration, and percutaneous microwave coagulation therapy. Cutaneous HCC lesions may be solitary or multiple and are usually firm, painless, reddish-blue, and nodular lesions of 1 to 5 cm without ulceration.[125,128] They may be necrotic or purulent and may exhibit massive bleeding when ulcerated or traumatized.[128] Previous investigators[128] have observed that lesions may clinically resemble a pyogenic granuloma (also known as granuloma telangiectaticum), mostly because of the tumor's hypervascularity. Cutaneous HCC should be considered in the context of a fast-growing nodule on the head, shoulders, or chest, especially in patients with chronic or recently diagnosed liver disease.[127] A case of dermatomyosistis after HCC in a patient with hepatitis B has been described.[129] Cutaneous metastases of hepatic tumors, such as epithelioid hemangioendothelioma,[130] leiomyosarcoma,[131] and sarcomatoid carcinoma,[132] or as a complication of hepatic intraarterial chemotherapy[133] or cutaneous seeding after fine-needle biopsy of liver metastases[134] have been reported. Primary hepatic cancers may rarely be associated with a PCT-like picture.[135]

Hepatotoxicity of Dermatologic Drugs

Hepatic toxicity may occasionally occur as a result of systemic drugs prescribed by dermatologists. The drugs commonly used in dermatology that present a significant risk of direct hepatic toxicity include azathioprine, dapsone, methotrexate, and acitretin.[136] Other uncommon causes include chlorambucil, cyclophosphamide, mycophenolate mofetil, cyclosporine, isotretinoin, hydroxychloroquine, chloroquine, itraconazole, and fluconazole. Hepatotoxicity secondary to methotrexate and dapsone is discussed previously. A close monitoring of the liver function tests during the initial phase of therapy is of paramount importance in to order to detect hepatotoxicities in a timely fashion.[136] In addition to dapsone, azathioprine and minocycline are associated with DHS. A characteristic morbilliform or erythrodermic cutaneous eruption is present concomitantly with symptoms resembling infectious mononucleosis (fever, fatigue, pharyngitis, and adenopathy) in patients who have DHS.[136] Patients receiving dapsone, azathioprine, and minocycline should be encouraged to report these signs and symptoms promptly. Concomitant CBC values are pivotal to the diagnosis of this subset of hepatic toxicity. It is common for the absolute eosinophil count to exceed 1000/mm^3 and rarely reaches levels higher than 10,000/mm^3 in the presence of fulminant DHS.

SUMMARY

In conclusion, patients with liver disorders have a wide array of cutaneous manifestations. These manifestations may be liver specific and sometimes reflect the severity of the liver diseases. Also, many of the systemic diseases, especially autoimmune and related disorders, have common involvement of skin and the liver. Thus, recognition of these associations is of utmost importance in diagnosing these conditions early so as to initiate timely interventions with a curative intention.

REFERENCES

1. Serrao R, Zirwas M, English JC. Palmar erythema. Am J Clin Dermatol 2007;8: 347–56.
2. Okumura H, Aramaki T, Katsuta Y, et al. Regional differences in peripheral circulation between upper and lower extremity in patients with cirrhosis. Scand J Gastroenterol 1990;25:883–9.
3. Khasnis A, Gokula RM. Spider nevus. J Postgrad Med 2002;48:307–9.
4. Li CP, Lee FY, Hwang SJ, et al. Spider angiomas in patients with liver cirrhosis: role of vascular endothelial growth factor and basic fibroblast growth factor. World J Gastroenterol 2003;9:2832–5.
5. Li CP, Lee FY, Hwang SJ, et al. Spider angiomas in patients with liver cirrhosis: role of alcoholism and impaired liver function. Scand J Gastroenterol 1999;34:520–3.
6. Scheepers JH, Quaba AA. Treatment of nevi aranei with the pulsed tunable dye laser at 585 nm. J Pediatr Surg 1995;30:101–4.
7. Terry R. White nails in hepatic cirrhosis. Lancet 1954;266:757–9.
8. Holzberg M, Walker HK. Terry's nails: revised definition and new correlations. Lancet 1984;1:896–9.
9. Nabai H. Nail changes before and after heart transplantation: personal observation by a physician. Cutis 1998;61:31–2.
10. Jemec GB, Kollerup G, Jensen LB, et al. Nail abnormalities in nondermatologic patients: prevalence and possible role as diagnostic aids. J Am Acad Dermatol 1995;32:977–81.
11. Harvey AM, Shulman LE, Tumulty PA, et al. Systemic lupus erythematosus: review of the literature and clinical analysis of 138 cases. Medicine 1954;33: 291–437.
12. Kofman S, Johnson GC, Zimmerman HJ. Apparent hepatic dysfunction in lupus erythematosus. Arch Intern Med 1955;95:669–76.
13. Chowdhary VR, Crowson CS, Poterucha JJ, et al. Liver involvement in systemic lupus erythematosus: case review of 40 patients. J Rheumatol 2008;35: 2159–64.
14. Matsumoto T, Kobayashi S, Shimizu H, et al. The liver in collagen diseases: pathologic study of 160 cases with particular reference to hepatic arteritis,

primary biliary cirrhosis, autoimmune hepatitis and nodular regenerative hyperplasia of the liver. Liver 2000;20:366–73.

15. Irving KS, Sen D, Tahir H, et al. A comparison of autoimmune liver disease in juvenile and adult populations with systemic lupus erythematosus—a retrospective review of cases. Rheumatology (Oxford) 2007;46:1171–3.

16. Skopouli FN, Barbatis C, Moutsopoulos HM. Liver involvement in primary sjogren's syndrome. Br J Rheumatol 1994;338:745–8.

17. Garcia-Carrasco M, Ramos M, Cervera R, et al. Hepatitis C virus infection in primary sjogren's syndrome: prevalence and significance in a series of 90 patients. Ann Rheum Dis 1997;56:173–7.

18. Assassi S, Fritzler MJ, Arnett FC, et al. Primary biliary cirrhosis (PBC), PBC autoantibodies, and hepatic parameter abnormalities in a large population of systemic sclerosis patients. J Rheumatol 2009;36:2250–6.

19. Jacobsen S, Halberg P, Ullman S, et al. Clinical features and serum antinuclear antibodies in 230 danish patients with systemic sclerosis. Br J Rheumatol 1998; 37:39–45.

20. Tchernev G. Cutaneous sarcoidosis: the great imitator: etiopathogenesis, morphology, differential diagnosis, and clinical management. Am J Clin Dermatol 2006;7:375–82.

21. Ricker W, Clark M. Sarcoidosis: a clinicopathologic review of three hundred cases, including twenty-two autopsies. J Clin Pathol 1949;19:725–49.

22. Hercules H, Bethlem NM. Value of liver biopsy in sarcoidosis. Arch Pathol Lab Med 1984;108:831–4.

23. Irani SK, Dobbins WO 3rd. Hepatic granulomas: review of 73 patients from one hospital and survey of the literature. J Clin Gastroenterol 1979;1:131–43.

24. Iwai K, Oka H. Sarcoidosis: report of ten autopsy cases in Japan. Am Rev Respir Dis 1964;90:612–22.

25. Nolan JP, Klatskin G. The fever of sarcoidosis. Ann Intern Med 1964;61:455–61.

26. Branson JH, Park JH. Sarcoidosis—hepatic involvement: presentation of a case with fatal liver involvement, including autopsy findings and review of the evidence for sarcoid involvement of the liver as found in the literature. Ann Intern Med 1954;40:111–45.

27. Rosenberg JC. Portal hypertension complicating hepatic sarcoidosis. Surgery 1971;69:294–9.

28. Warshauer DM, Molina PL, Hamman SM, et al. Nodular sarcoidosis of the liver and spleen: analysis of 32 cases. Radiology 1995;195:757–62.

29. Vatti R, Sharma OP. Course of asymptomatic liver involvement in sarcoidosis: role of therapy in selected cases. Sarcoidosis Vasc Diffuse Lung Dis 1997;14: 73–6.

30. Kennedy PT, Zakaria N, Modawi SB, et al. Natural history of hepatic sarcoidosis and its response to treatment. Eur J Gastroenterol Hepatol 2006;18:721–6.

31. Lebacq EG, Heller F. LP-X test in sarcoidosis patients with liver involvement: comparison with other liver function tests. Ann N Y Acad Sci 1976;278:439–44.

32. Rudzki C, Ishak KG, Zimmerman HJ. Chronic intrahepatic cholestasis of sarcoidosis. Am J Med 1975;59:373–87.

33. Moreno-Merlo F, Wanless IR, Shimamatsu K, et al. The role of granulomatous phlebitis and thrombosis in the pathogenesis of cirrhosis and portal hypertension in sarcoidosis. Hepatology 1997;26:554–60.

34. Maddrey WC, Johns CJ, Boitnott JK, et al. Sarcoidosis and chronic hepatic disease: a clinical and pathologic study of 20 patients. Medicine 1970;49: 375–95.

35. Valla D, Pessegueiro-Miranda H, Degott C, et al. Hepatic sarcoidosis with portal hypertension. A report of seven cases with a review of the literature. QJM 1987; 63:531–44.
36. Russi EW, Bansky G, Pfaltz M, et al. Budd-chiari syndrome in sarcoidosis. Am J Gastroenterol 1986;81:71–5.
37. Griffiths CE, Barker JN. Pathogenesis and clinical features of psoriasis. Lancet 2007;370:263–71.
38. Roenigk HH Jr, Auerbach R, Maibach H, et al. Methotrexate in psoriasis: consensus conference. J Am Acad Dermatol 1998;38:478–85.
39. Walker AM, Funch D, Dreyer NA, et al. Determinants of serious liver disease among patients receiving low-dose methotrexate for rheumatoid arthritis. Arthritis Rheum 1993;36:329–35.
40. Gawkrodger DJ. on behalf of the therapy guidelines and audit subcommittee of the British association of dermatologists. Current management of psoriasis. J Dermatolog Treat 1997;8:27–55.
41. Fairhurst DA, Sheehan-Dare R. Autoimmune hepatitis associated with infliximab in a patient with palmoplantar pustular psoriaisis. Clin Exp Dermatol 2009;34: 421–2.
42. Germano V, Picchianti Diamanti A, Baccano G, et al. Autoimmune hepatitis associated with infliximab in a patient with psoriatic arthritis. Ann Rheum Dis 2005;64:1519–20.
43. Leak AM, Rincon-Aznar B. Hepatotoxicity associated with etanercept in psoriatic arthritis. J Rheumatol 2008;35:2286–7.
44. Nollevaux MC, Guiot Y, Horsmans Y, et al. Hypervitaminosis A-induced liver fibrosis: stellate cell activation and daily dose consumption. Liver Int 2006;26:182–6.
45. Shear NH, Spielberg SP. Anticonvulsant hypersensitivity syndrome: in vitro assessment of risk. J Clin Invest 1988;82:1826–32.
46. Syn WK, Naibitt DJ, Holt AP, et al. Carbamazepine-induced acute liver failure as part of the DRESS syndrome. Int J Clin Pract 2005;59:988–91.
47. Chopra S, Levell NJ, Cowley G, et al. Systemic corticosteroids in the phenytoin hypersensitivity syndrome. Br J Dermatol 1996;134:1109–12.
48. Fremia ML. Use of silver sulfadiazine in Stevens-Johnson syndrome. Ann Pharmacother 1994;28:736.
49. Hall RP 3rd. Dermatitis herpetiformis. J Invest Dermatol 1992;99:873–81.
50. Wojnarowska F, Fry L. Hepatic injury in dermatitis herpetiformis. Acta Derm Venereol 1981;61:165–8.
51. Walton C, Walton S. Primary biliary cirrhosis in a diabetic male with dermatitis herpetiformis. Clin Exp Dermatol 1987;12:46–7.
52. Gabrielsen TO, Hoel PS. Primary biliary cirrhosis associated with celiac disease and dermatitis herpetiformis. Dermatologica 1985;170:31–4.
53. Lewis HM, Goldin R, Leonard JN. Dermatitis herpetiformis and primary sclerosing cholangitis. Clin Exp Dermatol 1993;18:363–5.
54. Kirby B, Keaveney A, Brophy D, et al. Abnormal liver function tests induced by dapsone in a patient with dermatitis herpetiformis and primary sclerosing cholangitis. Br J Dermatol 1999;14:172–3.
55. Coleman MD. Dapsone: modes of action, toxicity and possible strategies for increasing patient tolerance. Br J Dermatol 1993;129:507.
56. Stone SP, Goodwin RM. Dapsone-induced jaundice. Arch Dermatol 1978;114:947.
57. Kosseifi SG, Guha B, Nassour DN, et al. The Dapsone hypersensitivity syndrome revisited: a potentially fatal multisystem disorder with prominent hepatopulmonary manifestations. J Occup Med Toxicol 2006;1:9.

58. Valent P, Akin C, Sperr WR, et al. Mastocytosis: pathology, genetics, and current options for therapy. Leuk Lymphoma 2005;46:35–48.
59. Golkar L, Bernhard JD. Mastocytosis. Lancet 1997;349:1379–85.
60. Akin C, Metcalfe DD. Systemic mastocytosis. Annu Rev Med 2004;55:19–32.
61. Yam LT, Chan CH, Li CY. Hepatic involvement in systemic mast cell disease. Am J Med 1986;80:819–26.
62. Horny HP, Kaiserling E, Campbell M, et al. Liver findings in generalized mastocytosis. A clinicopathologic study. Cancer 1989;63:532–8.
63. Cherner JA, Jensen RT, Dubois A, et al. Gastrointestinal dysfunction in systemic mastocytosis. A prospective study. Gastroenterology 1988;95:657–67.
64. Jensen RT. Gastrointestinal abnormalities and involvement in systemic mastocytosis. Hematol Oncol Clin North Am 2000;14:579–623.
65. Mican JM, di Bisceglie AM, Fong TL, et al. Hepatic involvement in mastocytosis: clinicopathologic correlations in 41 cases. Hepatology 1995;22:1163–70.
66. Baron TH, Koehler RE, Rodgers WH, et al. Mast cell cholangiopathy: another cause of sclerosing cholangitis. Gastroenterology 1995;109:1677–81.
67. Marbello L, Anghilieri M, Nosari A, et al. Aggressive systemic mastocytosis mimicking sclerosing cholangitis. Haematologica 2004;89:ECR35.
68. Kyriakou D, Kouroumalis E, Konsolas J, et al. Systemic mastocytosis: a rare cause of noncirrhotic portal hypertension simulating autoimmune cholangitis—report of four cases. Am J Gastroenterol 1998;93:106–8.
69. Safyan EL, Veerabagu MP, Swerdlow SH, et al. Intrahepatic cholestasis due to systemic mastocytosis: a case report and review of literature. Am J Gastroenterol 1997;92:1197–200.
70. Furuta M, Suto H, Nakamoto S, et al. MRI of malignant melanoma of liver. Radiat Med 1995;13:143–5.
71. Gold JF, Boudreaux DJ, Rupard EJ. Basal cell carcinoma with hepatic metastases. Am J Clin Oncol 2007;30:661–3.
72. Affleck AG, Gore A, Millard LG, et al. Giant primary basal cell carcinoma with fatal hepatic metastases. J Eur Acad Dermatol Venereol 2007;21:262–3.
73. Huberman MS, Bunn PA Jr, Matthews MJ, et al. Hepatic involvement in the cutaneous T-cell lymphomas: results of percutaneous biopsy and peritoneoscopy. Cancer 1980;45:1683–8.
74. Aberg F, Pukkala E, Höckerstedt K, et al. Risk of malignant neoplasms after liver transplantation: a population-based study. Liver Transpl 2008;14:1428–36.
75. Tallón Aguilar L, Barrera Pulido L, Bernal Bellido C, et al. Causes and predisposing factors of de novo tumors in our series of liver transplant recipients. Transplant Proc 2009;41:2453–4.
76. Marqués Medina E, Jiménez Romero C, Gómez de la Cámara A, et al. Malignancy after liver transplantation: cumulative risk for development. Transplant Proc 2009;41:2447–9.
77. Feuerstein I, Geller AC. Skin cancer education in transplant recipients. Prog Transplant 2008;18:232–41.
78. Buyukavci M, Caner I, Eren S, et al. A childhood case of primary hepatic actinomycosis presenting with cutaneous fistula. Scand J Infect Dis 2004;36:62–3.
79. Thomas JE. Cutaneous amoebiasis due to liver abscess. Cent Afr J Med 1972;18:190–1.
80. Bastid C, Pirro N, Sahel J. Cutaneous fistulation of a liver hydatid cyst. Gastroenterol Clin Biol 2005;29:748–9.
81. Pyrsopoulos NT, Reddy KR. Extrahepatic manifestations of chronic viral hepatitis. Curr Gastroenterol Rep 2001;3:71–8.

82. Weiss TD, Tsai CC, Baldassare AR, et al. Skin lesions in viral hepatitis: histologic and immunofluorescent findings. Am J Med 1978;64:269–73.
83. Martinez MI, Sanchez JL, Lopez-Malpica F. Peculiar papular skin lesions occurring in hepatitis B carriers. J Am Acad Dermatol 1987;16:31–4.
84. Maggiore G, Grifeo S, Marzani M. Erythema nodosum and hepatitis B infection. J Am Acad Dermatol 1983;9:602–3.
85. Lichen planus and liver diseases. A multicentre case-control study. Gruppo italiano studi epidemiologici in dermatologia (GISED). BMJ 1990;300:227–30.
86. Rebora A, Rongioletti F. Lichen planus and chronic active hepatitis. A retrospective survey. Acta Derm Venereol 1984;64:52–6.
87. Gower RG, Sausker WF, Kohler PF, et al. Small vessel vasculitis caused by hepatitis B virus immune complexes. Small vessel vasculitis and HBsAg. J Allergy Clin Immunol 1978;62:222–8.
88. Lowosky MS. The clinical course of viral hepatitis. Clin Gastroenterol 1980;9:1–21.
89. Levo Y, Gorevic PD, Kassab HJ, et al. Association between hepatitis B virus and essential mixed cryoglobulinemia. N Engl J Med 1977;296:1501–4.
90. Pittsley RA, Shearn MA, Kaufman L. Acute hepatitis B simulating dermatomyositis. JAMA 1978;239:959.
91. Chevrant-Breton J, Logeais B, Pibouin M. Pyoderma gangrenosum (phagedenic pyoderma). Ann Dermatol Venereol 1989;116:577–89.
92. Malina L, Stránský J, Havlícková M, et al. Chronic hepatic porphyria and hepatitis B and C virus infections. Cas Lek Cesk 1998;137:561–4.
93. Hsueh YM, Cheng GS, Wu MM, et al. Multiple risk factors associated with arsenic-induced skin cancer: effects of chronic liver disease and malnutritional status. Br J Cancer 1995;71:109–14.
94. Parsons ME, Russo GG, Millikan LE. Dermatologic disorders associated with viral hepatitis infections. Int J Dermatol 1996;35(2):77–81.
95. Guillevin L, Lhote F, Cohen P, et al. Polyarteritis nodosa related to hepatitis B virus. A prospective study with long-term observation of 41 patients. Medicine 1995;74:238–53.
96. Trepo C, Guillevin L. Polyarteritis nodosa and extrahepatic manifestations of HBV infection: the case against autoimmune intervention in pathogenesis. J Autoimmun 2001;16:269–74.
97. Guillevin L, Mahr A, Callard P, et al. Hepatitis B virus–associated polyarteritis nodosa: clinical characteristics, outcome, and impact of treatment in 115 patients. Medicine (Baltimore) 2005;84:313–22.
98. Agnello V. The etiology and pathophysiology of mixed cryoglobulinemia secondary to hepatitis C virus infection. Semin Immunopathol 1997;19:111–29.
99. Levey JM, Bjornsson B, Banner B, et al. Mixed cryoglobulinemia in chronic hepatitis C infection. A clinicopathologic analysis of 10 cases and review of recent literature. Medicine 1994;73:53–67.
100. Meltzer M, Franklin EC, Elias K, et al. Cryoglobulinemia—a clinical and laboratory study. II. Cryoglobulins with rheumatoid factor activity. Am J Med 1966;40:837–56.
101. Sanchez-Perez J, De Castro M, Buezo GF, et al. Lichen planus and hepatitis C virus: prevalence and clinical presentation of patients with lichen planus and hepatitis C virus infection. Br J Dermatol 1996;134:715–9.
102. Jubert C, Pawlotsky J-M, Pouget F, et al. Lichen planus and hepatitis C virus-related chronic active hepatitis. Arch Dermatol 1994;130:73–6.
103. Arrieta JJ, Rodriguez-Inigo E, Casqueiro M, et al. Detection of hepatitis C virus replication by in situ hybridization in epithelial cells of anti-hepatitis C virus-positive patients with and without oral lichen planus. Hepatology 2000;32:97–103.

104. Nagao Y, Kawasaki K, Sata M. Insulin resistance and lichen planus in patients with HCV-infectious liver diseases. J Gastroenterol Hepatol 2008;23:580–5.

105. Chuang TY, Stitle L, Brashear R, et al. Hepatitis C virus and lichen planus: a case-control study of 340 patients. J Am Acad Dermatol 1999;41:787–9.

106. Gimenez-García R, Pérez-Castrillón JL. Lichen planus and hepatitis C virus infection. J Eur Acad Dermatol Venereol 2003;17:291–5.

107. Dupin N, Chosidow O, Lunel F, et al. Oral lichen planus and hepatitis C virus infection: a fortuitous association? Arch Dermatol 1997;133:1052–3.

108. Tucker SC, Coulson IH. Lichen planus is not associated with hepatitis C virus infection in patients from North West England. Acta Derm Venereol 1999;79:378–9.

109. Lodi G, Pellicano R, Carrozzo M. Hepatitis C virus infection and lichen planus: a systematic review with meta-analysis. Oral Dis 2010;16:601–12.

110. El Darouti M, Abu El Ela M. Necrolytic acral erythema: a cutaneous marker of viral hepatitis C (report). Int J Dermatol 1996;35:252–6.

111. Chastain MA. The glucagonoma syndrome: a review of its features and discussion of new perspectives. Acad Dermatol 1990;23:850–4.

112. Miller DJ. Nutritional deficiency and the skin. J Am Acad Dermatol 1989;21: 1–30.

113. Khanna VJ, Shieh S, Benjamin J, et al. Necrolytic acral erythema associated with hepatitis C: effective treatment with interferon alfa and zinc. Arch Dermatol 2000;136(6):755–7.

114. Hivnor CM, Yan AC, Junkins-Hopkins JM, et al. Necrolytic acral erythema: response to combination therapy with interferon and ribavirin. J Am Acad Dermatol 2004;50:S121–4.

115. Bonkovsky HL, Poh-Fitzpatrick M, Pimstone N, et al. Porphyria cutanea tarda, hepatitis C, and HFE gene mutations in North America. Hepatology 1998;27: 1661–9.

116. Bonkovsky HL, Mehta S. Hepatitis C: a review and update. J Am Acad Dermatol 2001;44:159–82.

117. Koulentaki M, Ioannidou D, Stefanidou M, et al. Dermatological manifestations in primary biliary cirrhosis patients: a case control study. Am J Gastroenterol 2006; 101:541–6.

118. Graham-Brown RA, Sarkany I, Sherlock S. Lichen planus and primary biliary cirrhosis. Br J Dermatol 1982;106:699–703.

119. Powell FC, Rogers RS, Dickson ER. Lichen planus, primary biliary cirrhosis and penicillamine. Br J Dermatol 1982;107:616.

120. Murray-Lyon IM, Thompson RP, Ansell ID, et al. Scleroderma and primary biliary cirrhosis. BMJ 1970;1:258–9.

121. Marasini B, Gagetta M, Rossi V, et al. Rheumatic disorders and primary biliary cirrhosis: an appraisal of 170 Italian patients. Ann Rheum Dis 2001;60:1046–9.

122. Powell FC, Schroeter AL, Dickson ER. Primary biliary cirrhosis and the CREST syndrome: a report of 22 cases. QJM 1987;62:75–82.

123. Garcia MA, Ramonet M, Ciocca M, et al. Alagille syndrome: cutaneous manifestations in 38 children. Pediatr Dermatol 2005;22:11–4.

124. Kamath BM, Schwarz KB. Hadzić N. Alagille syndrome and liver transplantation. J Pediatr Gastroenterol Nutr 2010;50:11–5.

125. Amador A, Monforte NG, Bejarano N, et al. Cutaneous metastasis from hepatocellular carcinoma as the first clinical sign. J Hepatobiliary Pancreat Surg 2007; 14:328.

126. de Agustin P, Conde E, Alberti N, et al. Cutaneous metastasis of occult hepatocellular carcinoma: a case report. Acta Cytol 2007;51:214.

127. Okusaka T, Okada S, Ishii H, et al. Prognosis of hepatocellular carcinoma patients with extrahepatic metastases. Hepatogastroenterology 1997;44:251.
128. Kubota Y, Koga T, Nakayama J. Cutaneous metastasis from hepatocellular carcinoma resembling pyogenic granuloma. Clin Exp Dermatol 1999;24:78.
129. Kee SJ, Kim TJ, Lee SJ, et al. Dermatomyositis associated with hepatitis B virus-related hepatocellular carcinoma. Rheumatol Int 2009;29:595–9.
130. Vignon-Pennamen MD, Varroud-Vial C, Janssen F, et al. Cutaneous metastases of hepatic epithelioid hemangioendothelioma. Ann Dermatol Venereol 1989;116:864–6.
131. Pequignot R, Thevenot T, Permal S, et al. Hepatic leiomyosarcoma revealed by cutaneous metastasis. Gastroenterol Clin Biol 1999;23:991–2.
132. Nishie W, Iitoyo M, Koshiyama T, et al. Sarcomatoid carcinoma of the liver with skin and pleural metastases. Br J Dermatol 2003;148:1069–71.
133. O'Hagan S, Diamond T. Cutaneous metastasis as a complication of hepatic intra-arterial chemotherapy. Ulster Med J 1997;66:136–7.
134. McGrath FP, Gibney RG, Rowley VA, et al. Cutaneous seeding following fine needle biopsy of colonic liver metastases. Clin Radiol 1991;43:130–1.
135. Siersema PD, ten Kate FJ, Mulder PG, et al. Hepatocellular carcinoma in porphyria cutanea tarda: frequency and factors related to its occurrence. Liver 1992;12:56–61.
136. Wolverton SE, Remlinger K. Suggested guidelines for patient monitoring: hepatic and hematologic toxicity attributable to systemic dermatologic drugs. Dermatol Clin 2007;25:195–205, vi–ii.

Hepatobiliary Manifestations of Critically Ill and Postoperative Patients

Andrew Aronsohn, MD, Donald Jensen, MD*

KEYWORDS

- Critical illness • Hypoxic liver injury • Sepsis
- Post operative liver dysfunction

Liver dysfunction is common in the intensive care unit (ICU) and in the postoperative patient. A recent prospective study of 38,036 patients admitted to 32 ICUs over a 4-year period showed that 10.9% of patients exhibited hepatic dysfunction defined as hyperbilirubinemia in the absence of preexisting liver disease.[1] In addition, early liver dysfunction was found to be an independent risk factor for increased mortality.[1] Severe metabolic derangements found in the critically ill cause hepatic injury by means of reduced perfusion, insufficient oxygenation, vulnerability to infection, insufficient support of increased metabolic demands, and as a side effect of therapies employed to treat critical illness. Patients with hypoxic liver injury, sepsis-induced cholestasis, and those with complicated postoperative courses often suffer from one or more of these derangements causing deterioration of hepatic function. Limited hepatic function, in turn, often exacerbates the severity of the underlying disease process, creating a vicious cycle that leads to high rates of morbidity and mortality. The aim of this review is to describe the pathogenesis and clinical manifestations of liver dysfunction in patients without preexisting liver disease who are critically ill or are in the immediate postoperative period (**Box 1**).

HYPOXIC LIVER INJURY

The term "ischemic hepatitis" was first used by Bynum and colleagues[2] in 1979 to describe centrilobular necrosis seen in conjunction with markedly elevated serum aminotransferase levels in the setting of cardiac failure. Two years after the publication of this study, Arcidi and colleagues[3] elaborated on the pathogenesis of hypoxic liver

The authors have nothing to disclose.
Center for Liver Disease, Section of Gastroenterology, Hepatology and Nutrition, University of Chicago Medical Center, 5841 South Maryland Avenue, MC 7120, Chicago, IL 60637, USA
* Corresponding author.
E-mail address: djensen@medicine.bsd.uchicago.edu

Clin Liver Dis 15 (2011) 183–197
doi:10.1016/j.cld.2010.09.004
1089-3261/11/$ – see front matter © 2011 Elsevier Inc. All rights reserved.
liver.theclinics.com

Box 1
Etiology of liver dysfunction in postoperative and critically ill patients

Hypoxic Liver Injury

    Congestive heart failure

    Acute cardiac failure

    Acute respiratory failure

Liver Dysfunction in Sepsis

    Primary hepatic dysfunction due to hypoperfusion of the liver

    Secondary hepatic dysfunction due to hepatic response to infection

    Cholestasis in sepsis

        Hemolysis

        Hepatocyte dysfunction

        Bile duct dysfunction

Postoperative Liver Dysfunction

    Ischemic injury

    Bilirubin overproduction

    Benign postoperative jaundice

    Acalculous cholecystitis

    Anesthetic agents

Total Parenteral Nutrition

---

injury by suggesting that circulatory shock was necessary to induce this clinical and histologic pattern. Subsequent to this landmark article this disease process was known as "shock liver"; however, more recent evidence suggests that circulatory shock and severe hypotension are common, but not absolute prerequisites for this type of liver injury, and the term hypoxic hepatitis or hypoxic liver injury is now favored.[4] The pathophysiologic mechanism of inadequate oxygen uptake by the liver is defined as occurring (1) commonly, but not always, in the clinical setting of cardiac or circulatory shock, (2) with marked increase in serum aminotransferase levels that are reversible with restoration of adequate hepatic oxygenation, and (3) in the absence of other forms of acute liver damage.[5,6] Hypoxic liver injury is not uncommon in the ICU setting and carries a high mortality risk. A large, multicenter, retrospective analysis of more than 32,000 ICU patients found that approximately 1% of all admissions met criteria for hypoxic liver injury, which was defined as sudden 10-fold or greater increase in lactate dehydrogenase (LDH), alanine aminotransferase, or aspartate aminotransferase. Of these patients, 45% died during the hospitalization.[7]

Under normal physiologic conditions the liver receives approximately 20% of total cardiac output, which is delivered by the portal vein and the hepatic artery.[8] In addition, the liver has a high affinity for oxygen and is able to extract up to 95% of the oxygen from blood.[8] Although these factors are generally protective from hypoxic injury, severe physiologic derangements causing congestion of the liver, severe hypoxemia, inadequate oxygen extraction, or increased hepatic metabolic demand can overcome these protective mechanisms and precipitate hypoxic liver injury.

Hypoxic Liver Injury in the Setting of Congestive Heart Failure

Hypoxic liver injury related to cardiac dysfunction is relatively common. When defined as serum aminotransferase levels greater than 20 times the upper limit of normal in the absence of any underlying cause of hepatic necrosis, this type of injury was seen in 2.6% of 766 patients admitted to a coronary care unit over a 1-year period.[9] In a large series of 142 patients with hypoxic liver injury, 80 (56%) were classified as having liver injury related to congestive heart failure.[4] Although systemic hypoperfusion was seen in most of these patients (92.5%), shock was observed in only 41%.[4] Hemodynamic parameters of these patients included low systemic arterial pressure, low cardiac index, low oxygen delivery, and high central venous pressure.[4] The correlation of congestive heart failure with hypoxic liver injury has been demonstrated by the presence of clinical features of right-sided heart failure (ankle edema, hepatojugular reflex, liver tenderness) in patients with hypoxic liver injury in addition to a significant association between higher central venous pressure and confirmed hypoxic liver injury (90% vs 38%, $P<.001$).[9] Seeto and colleagues[10] have supported this relationship by showing that underlying cardiac disease in conjunction with systemic hypotension is often necessary to cause liver injury. In a case-controlled study of patients who had systolic blood pressures of less than 75 mm Hg for at least 15 minutes, 94% of the patients who exhibited hypoxic liver injury had evidence of preexisting right-sided heart failure whereas none of the patients who had systemic hypotension alone exhibited hypoxic liver injury.[10]

Hypoxic Liver Injury Related to Acute Cardiac Failure

Although less common, hypoxic liver injury secondary to acute cardiac failure in patients without known underlying cardiac disease has been reported after myocardial infarction, pulmonary embolism, pericardial tamponade, and sudden arrhythmia.[4] These patients tend to have similar hemodynamic features to patients with hypoxic liver injury who have preexisting congestive heart failure, except that shock was more common (70% vs 41%), indicating that the mechanism for liver injury in many of these patients is attributed to sudden decreased cardiac output and poor hepatic perfusion.[4] Biochemical features of patients with acute cardiac disease causing hypoxic liver injury include elevation of bilirubin, prothrombin time, and significantly increased aminotransferase levels.[11,12] Similar to patients with preexisting cardiac disease who have hypoxic liver injury, patients with acute cardiac failure also have a high in-hospital mortality rate.[13]

Hypoxic Liver Injury Related to Respiratory Failure

Hypoxic liver injury has also been described in patients with respiratory failure. Henrion and colleagues[14] described 17 patients with hypoxic liver injury after an acute or chronic exacerbation of respiratory failure in the absence of cardiac failure. Patients with hypoxic hepatitis secondary to respiratory failure had similarly elevated aminotransferase levels; however, hemodynamic parameters of patients with respiratory causes of hypoxic injury differed from those with cardiac failure induced hypoxic injury. Patients with cardiac disease were found to have relatively low cardiac index and high systemic vascular resistance, whereas those with respiratory failure–induced hypoxic injury conversely had high cardiac index and low systemic vascular resistance, leading to low values of hepatic oxygen delivery and causing hypoxic rather than ischemic damage.[14]

In summary, hypoxic liver injury is common in the ICU among patients with derangement of circulatory and respiratory function due to cardiac or pulmonary failure.

Management should be focused on treating the underlying cardiac and/or pulmonary disease while simultaneously supporting hepatic perfusion with careful volume management and, if needed, use of vasopressors and mechanical ventilation (**Table 1**).

LIVER DYSFUNCTION IN SEPSIS

Sepsis is a systemic inflammatory response to infection characterized by disequilibrium of pro- and anti-inflammatory cytokines, which can lead to multiorgan failure and death.[15,16] Rates of sepsis have been estimated as 3 cases per 1000 people, and this diagnosis carries a mortality rate ranging from 38% to 59%.[17–19] The liver plays important role in the pathophysiology of sepsis in that it clears endotoxin and removes bacteria from the circulation, in addition to acting as both a target and source of inflammatory mediators.

The Liver as a Protective Organ in Sepsis

Kupffer cells in the liver make up the largest mass of macrophages in the body and play a key role in detoxification of bacterial endotoxin or lipopolysaccharide, a key mediator of the septic response. A classic study that described the relationship between the liver and endotoxin clearance was performed in an experimental rabbit model where approximately half of radiolabeled lipopolysaccharide was found to accumulate in the liver within 5 minutes of intravenous injection, graphically depicting the role of Kupffer cells in sepsis.[20] The mechanism of hepatic detoxification of lipopolysaccharide occurs via lipoprotein micelle binding, which allows lipopolysaccharide to be transported from Kupffer cells to the hepatic parenchyma where it ultimately can be excreted into the bile.[21–23]

In addition to hepatic removal of endotoxin, the liver is involved in removal of bacteria from the circulation.[22] The mechanism of hepatic bacterial clearance is thought to be predominantly through the reticuloendothelial system of the liver, where Kupffer cells clear bacteria from the bloodstream.[24] The role of the liver in bacterial clearance has been demonstrated in experimental rat models, by showing a high hepatic affinity for radiolabeled *Escherichia coli* within 10 minutes of injection.[25] In addition, similar studies have reported decreased ability to take up bacteria in experimental models that have undergone partial hepatectomy or portocaval shunts whereby bacteria was shunted to the lung and spleen.[22,26]

The importance of the liver's role in defense against systemic infections may help explain the increased incidence and severity of sepsis in patients with limited hepatic function.[27,28] In an analysis of data from the National Hospital Discharge Survey consisting of 175 million discharges from 1995 to 1999, 1% or 1.7 million patients carried

Table 1	
Approach to patients with hypoxic liver injury	
Clinical setting	• Acute on chronic exacerbations of congestive heart failure, acute cardiac failure, and/or acute respiratory failure • Circulatory shock often seen
Diagnosis	• Elevated aminotransferase levels (usually >10 × upper limit of normal) • Histologic pattern of centrilobular necrosis
Therapy	• Correct underlying cause of ischemic injury • Support circulation and oxygenation to maintain adequate hepatic oxygenation and perfusion

a diagnosis of cirrhosis. When compared with patients without end-stage liver disease after adjustment for age, race, and gender, patients with cirrhosis were more likely to have hospitalizations associated with sepsis (adjusted risk ratio 2.7, 95% confidence interval [CI] 2.3–3.1) and had a increased likelihood of death from sepsis (adjusted relative risk ratio 2.0, 95% CI 1.3–2.6).[29] Independent risk factors for mortality in the setting of patients with sepsis and cirrhosis have been evaluated in several smaller studies and include pulmonary infiltrates, renal dysfunction, decreased cholesterol, increased lactate, APACHE III score, mechanical ventilation, and vasopressor support.[30–32]

The Liver as a Target of Sepsis

Hepatic dysfunction as a result of sepsis can be divided into 2 phases. The primary phase of dysfunction occurs in the initial stages of septic shock and is a result of hepatic hypoperfusion whereby low cardiac output and mesenteric arterial vasoconstriction diminish both portal and systemic circulation.[33,34] This type of injury leads to synthetic dysfunction of the liver, causing a decrease in protein synthesis, lactate clearance, gluconeogenesis, glycogenolysis, and serum glucose levels. Elevated aminotransferase levels are common in primary hepatic dysfunction because of enzyme leakage from acute cellular and mitochondrial injury. Clinically, disseminated intravascular coagulation and bleeding may also be seen.[35] Because this injury is primarily a hemodynamic phenomenon, many of these insults can be reversed with proper resuscitation.[34]

Secondary hepatic dysfunction describes the liver injury that occurs with the interaction between Kupffer cells, hepatocytes, neutrophils, and endothelial cells as a response to systemic infection. Kupffer cells make up approximately 70% of the liver's macrophages, and play a crucial role in bacterial clearance and endotoxin detoxification. This process causes local inflammation, and as a result these cells become activated and produce proinflammatory cytokines, eicosanoid mediators, reactive oxygen products, and nitric oxide, all of which act as mediators of sepsis.[22] Kupffer cells have been shown to respond to endotoxin stimulation by recruiting neutrophils to the liver and activating them through a release of leukotriene B4 and tumor necrosis factor (TNF)-α. Neutrophils then bind to sinusoidal cells, migrate to hepatic parenchyma, and injure hepatocytes via oxygen-derived radical and protease production.[34,36] Finally, endothelial cells interact with Kupffer cells, neutrophils, and sepsis mediators, causing increases in inflammation and coagulation activities.[22,37]

Cholestasis in Sepsis

Sepsis is the most common cause of jaundice in ICU patients.[38,39] In addition, the severity of jaundice has been associated with more extensive organ failure and increased mortality.[40] Intra-abdominal sources of infection are the most common cause of cholestasis but this phenomenon has also been reported in patients with pneumonia, endocarditis, urinary tract infection, and meningitis.[38,41,42] Jaundice in sepsis is primarily caused by increased bilirubin load from hemolysis, hepatocyte dysfunction, and decreased bile flow (**Fig. 1**).[38]

Hemolysis is the primary mechanism of the increased bilirubin load observed in sepsis. Hemolysis of normal red blood cells has been demonstrated by direct bacterial injury and by immune-mediated hemolysis, which includes IgM- or IgG-mediated antibody destruction of red blood cells, polyagglutination, and formation of antigen/antibody complexes.[38,43–45] Other causes of hemolysis commonly seen in sepsis include increased oxidative stress injury and subsequent injury in patients with underlying

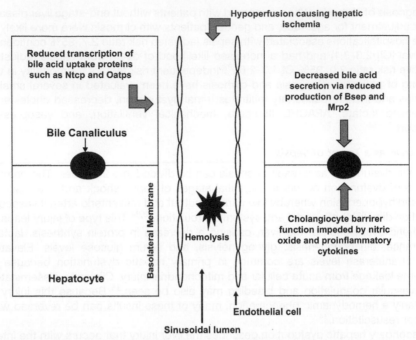

Fig. 1. Mechanisms of hepatic dysfunction and cholestasis in sepsis.

G-6-PD deficiency, microangiopathic hemolytic anemia secondary to infection, disseminated intravascular coagulation, antibiotics used in treatment of sepsis, blood transfusions, and resorption of large hemotomas.[38,46–49]

Hepatocyte dysfunction resulting in reduced bilirubin uptake, intrahepatic processing, and canalicular excretion also contributes to cholestasis in sepsis; this has been shown grossly by Roelofsen and colleagues[50] in an animal model, where rats were injected with an intravenous bolus of lipopolysaccharide followed by hepatectomy and measurement of single-pass perfusion of bilirubin. Decreased uptake and canalicular excretion of bilirubin was observed in rats exposed to endotoxin when compared with controls. Similar excretion kinetics were described when the investigators compared conjugated bilirubin with unconjugated bilirubin, suggesting that intrahepatic conjugation of bilirubin is not a rate-limiting step in bilirubin metabolism during sepsis. More specifically, exposure to lipopolysaccharide induces Kupffer cell release of inflammatory mediators such as TNF-α and interleukin-6, which likely act to decrease both basolateral and canalicular transport mechanisms by decreasing basolateral membrane fluidity and reducing expression of several key bile acid transporters.[38,51,52] On the basolateral side, there is reduced transcription of bile acid uptake proteins such as Ntcp and Oatps, and on the canalicular side decreased production of Bsep and Mrp2 impairs bile acid excretion.[38,53] These changes impede normal flow of bile salts through the liver to form bile in the biliary canaliculus, contributing to cholestasis seen in sepsis.

The bile ducts are also involved in cholestasis of sepsis, as nitric oxide (NO) and proinflammatory cytokines released in sepsis interfere with cholangiocyte barrier functions and tight junctions.[54,55] Cholangiocytes themselves can also produce cytokines such as interferon-γ and TNF as well as growth factors that can lead to cholangitis and inflammatory cholestasis.[54,56] Bile duct injury from sepsis and trauma may also lead to progressive sclerosing cholangitis, which is characterized by bile duct strictures seen on endoscopic retrograde cholangiopancreatography as well as histologic findings of bile duct proliferation and portal and periductal fibrosis.[54,57,58] Although there is some variability, many patients with progressive sclerosing cholangitis rapidly progress to cirrhosis after the critical illness resolves, and carry a poor prognosis.[58]

Serologic findings in sepsis-induced cholestasis include elevated bilirubin from 5 mg/dL to 50 mg/dL, with minimally elevated or normal alkaline phosphatase and aminotransferase levels.[59] With appropriate management of sepsis through antibiotic therapy, hyperbilirubinemia usually resolves.[54] Persistently elevated bilirubin levels with elevated alkaline phosphatase and γ-glutamyltranspeptidase levels should raise concern for progressive sclerosing cholangitis.[58] Although patients with sepsis induced cholestasis rarely undergo liver biopsy, histology findings include intrahepatic cholestasis with Kupffer cell hyperplasia, focal hepatocyte dropout, and portal mononuclear cell infiltrates.[59]

The liver plays an important role in clearance of bacteria and endotoxin from the bloodstream, acting as a protective organ in sepsis; however, a cascade of endotoxin-induced inflammatory cytokine-mediated events causes hepatic dysfunction, primarily manifesting as cholestasis. Patients with sepsis-induced hepatic injury often have concomitant multiorgan system failure and should be managed aggressively in an ICU, where they will benefit from antimicrobial therapy and cardiopulmonary support (**Table 2**).

POSTOPERATIVE LIVER DYSFUNCTION

Abnormal liver chemistries are a common finding in the postoperative setting, and can be seen in patients without preexisting liver disease.[60,61] Careful evaluation of a patient with postoperative liver dysfunction is necessary, because self-limited, hepatic decompensation may arise, especially in patients with preexisting liver disease. Ischemic injury, bilirubin overproduction, cholestasis, acalculous cholecystitis, and anesthesia-related liver dysfunction are all potential causes of postoperative liver dysfunction, and are discussed in detail here.

Postoperative Ischemic Injury

Postoperative ischemic liver injury occurs as a result of decreased hepatic blood flow followed by reperfusion, causing ischemia-reperfusion injury characterized by centrilobular sinusoidal congestion and necrosis.[3] Similar to ischemic liver injury in the nonsurgical patient, this type of injury is typically caused by cardiogenic or respiratory

Table 2	
Approach to patients with liver dysfunction in sepsis	
Clinical setting	• Systemic infection on the continuum from systemic inflammatory response syndrome to sepsis • Septic shock physiology often noted
Diagnosis	• Bacteremia (usually gram-negative) is common • Primary hepatic dysfunction due to initial hypoperfusion manifested by elevated aminotransferases • Secondary hepatic dysfunction from endotoxin-mediated damage resulting in cholestasis
Therapy	• Aggressive antimicrobial therapy • Support sepsis associated hypotension and hypoxia

failure and is clinically characterized by markedly elevated aminotransferase and LDH levels for up to 10 days after the initial insult followed by late-onset development of hyperbilirubinemia.[60] Patients undergoing cardiovascular bypass surgery and those with preexisting right and/or left heart failure are at increased risk for this type of injury. Treatment involves vigilant optimization of hemodynamic status; however, mortality can be high, especially in the presence of multiple concomitant surgical and medical comorbidities.[60]

Bilirubin Overproduction

Bilirubin overproduction is a relatively benign factor of postoperative jaundice, characterized by unconjugated hyperbilirubinemia with normal or near normal aminotransferase and alkaline phosphatase levels.[62] A normally functioning liver conjugates and excretes approximately 250 mg of bilirubin daily; however, hematoma formation and transfusions, which are common during surgery, can create a state of bilirubin overproduction that may overwhelm hepatic capacity to conjugate and excrete bilirubin, causing clinical jaundice.[62] Hematomas formed during surgery are eventually degraded into bilirubin. A liter of blood resorption into tissue produces approximately 5 g of bilirubin, which may be insufficiently conjugated and excreted.[63] Hemolysis from fasting or from underlying genetic conditions such as G6PD deficiency or sickle cell anemia may also be exacerbated due to the physiologic stress of surgery, creating an increased bilirubin load.[62,64] Finally, multiple blood transfusions often required during extensive surgeries also may overload hepatic capacity for bilirubin excretion.[62]

Benign Postoperative Cholestasis

Benign postoperative cholestasis is a term associated with progressive conjugated hyperbilirubinemia up to 40 mg/dL that occurs within 2 to 10 days after surgery.[60,65,66] The etiology of benign postoperative cholestasis is multifactorial and includes increased pigment load, decreased operative hepatic perfusion due to hypotension, anesthetic agent effect, passive liver congestion, hypoxemia, and infection.[60] Liver biopsy findings are often nonspecific and treatment is supportive; however, the contributing factors to this condition are sometimes indicative of high operative and postoperative morbidity, and mortality may be high.[60]

Acalculous Cholecystitis

Acute acalculous cholecystitis accounts for approximately half of all cases of cholecystitis following major surgery, and carries a mortality rate of up to 50%.[62,67,68] Surgical patients may encounter volume depletion, hypotension, a hypercoagulable state, and bowel rest, in addition to being exposed to narcotics and parenteral nutrition as part of the management of their critical illness. These factors cause bile stasis, gallbladder ischemia, and infection, leading to acalculous cholecystitis.[67] Clinical presentation of acalculous cholecystitis is nonspecific and includes fever, leukocytosis, and jaundice. Right upper quadrant pain and Murphy's sign are sometime present; however, postoperative patients in the ICU are frequently unable to report these symptoms. Because serologic studies are often nonspecific, diagnosis of acalculous cholecystitis usually relies on imaging studies. Ultrasonography is the most common radiographic study used to diagnose acalculous cholecystitis because it is noninvasive and can be done at the bedside. Using specific major and minor criteria, ultrasound sensitivity has been reported to be as high as 94% to 98%.[69] Computed tomography may also be used to diagnose acalculous cholecystitis with similar sensitivity and specificity; however, transportation of patients with this degree of critical illness is often logistically difficult.[70] Treatment ideally includes broad-spectrum anti-biotics and cholecystectomy; however, because many patients are poor surgical candidates due to severe critical illness, cholecystostomy is a less invasive approach to gallbladder decompression.[71] Even with optimal management in the ICU, the mortality rate in acalculous cholecystitis remains high.[60]

Anesthetic Agents and Liver Dysfunction

Volatile anesthetic agents such as halothane have been widely reported as a cause of liver injury.[60] A large epidemiologic study conducted in 1969 found fatal hepatic necrosis attributed to halothane in 1 in 35,000 cases.[72] Although safety concerns have curtailed halothane use in adults in the United States, it continues to be a commonly used induction agent worldwide.[73] Halothane continues to be used in the United States pediatric population, due to fewer reports of hepatic toxicity.[74] Female gender, age greater than 30 years, obesity, and multiple exposures to halothane have been reported as risk factors in developing liver dysfunction.[60,75,76] Halothane hepatotoxicity can be divided into 2 categories based on degree of toxicity and mechanism of injury. Mild/moderate injury or type 1 hepatotoxicity appears 1 to 3 days after exposure, and results in mild increases in aminotransferase levels along with leth-argy, nausea, and fever. Liver injury is thought to be caused by direct injury, and histology reveals centrilobular necrosis and mononuclear infiltrate.[60] This pattern of injury is usually self limited, as symptoms and aminotransferase levels usually resolve within 2 weeks. Severe acute hepatitis and acute liver failure, also known as type 2 injury, occur more commonly after multiple halothane exposures.[77] Type 2 injury pres-ents within 2 weeks of exposure and is characterized by eosinophilia, marked eleva-tions in aminotransferase levels, and jaundice in patients presenting with fever, rash, arthralgias, and tender hepatomegaly.[78] In contrast to type 1 hepatotoxicity, type 2 injury is thought to be immune mediated and involving a metabolite of halothane, tri-fluoroacetyl, which binds to the endoplasmic reticulum of the hepatocyte to form a protein complex that invites an immune response, causing hepatocyte injury.[60,79] Liver biopsy in severe cases shows massive necrosis. Treatment for type 2 halothane hepatotoxicity is supportive; however, liver transplantation has been reported in patients who suffer from acute liver failure.[80] Safer alternatives to halothane have been introduced, including enflurane, isoflurane, desflurane, and sevoflurane. Although the risk of liver injury is smaller, these agents have been reported to have

Table 3 Approach to patients with postoperative liver dysfunction	
Clinical setting	• May occur within days of surgery and may last several weeks
Diagnosis	• Ischemic injury characterized by elevated aminotransferase levels due to ischemia-reperfusion injury • Cholestasis from bilirubin overproduction, benign postoperative cholestasis, acalculous cholecystitis • Anesthetic agents causing damage ranging from mild aminotrans-ferase elevation to severe hepatitis and acute liver failure
Therapy	• Cardiopulmonary support in ischemia • Antimicrobial therapy and/or cholecystectomy/cholecystostomy in cholecystitis • Avoidance of repeated exposure to halothane and halothane-based anesthetic agents if evidence of liver dysfunction

Table 4	
Approach to patients with TPN related liver dysfunction	
Clinical setting	• Short-term or long-term TPN
Diagnosis	• Mild hepatomegaly, abdominal pain
	• Elevated aminotransferase levels due to steatosis, rarely cholestasis
Therapy	• Avoidance of excessive calories
	• Avoidance of dextrose as the sole form of carbohydrate
	• Appropriate dosing and formulation of lipids

similar cross-reactivity properties to halothane, and hepatotoxicity has been reported in patients who have had multiple exposures to these agents.[81–83]

Postoperative liver dysfunction can be a result of operative ischemia, bilirubin overproduction, and volatile anesthetic agents. Identification of the mechanism of injury is crucial in the management of the postoperative patient because therapy should be specifically tailored to treat the underlying cause of liver dysfunction (**Table 3**).

TOTAL PARENTERAL NUTRITION

Total parenteral nutrition (TPN) is a commonly employed method used to deliver nutrition to postoperative and critically ill patients who are unable to tolerate enteral feeding. Grau and colleagues[84] studied nutritional parameters of a cohort of 3409 patients in 40 ICUs. Of the 303 patients who received TPN, 30% had evidence of liver dysfunction, which included cholestasis, hepatic necrosis, a mixed pattern of cholestasis and necrosis, and acalculous cholecystitis.[84] A univariate analysis showed a significant association between TPN administration and liver dysfunction.[84] The most common form of TPN-induced liver injury involves hepatic steatosis, which can manifest as mild hepatomegaly, vague right upper quadrant pain, elevated aminotransferase levels, and occasional cholestasis.[85] Liver histology shows periportal fat, which may progress to panlobular steatosis in more severe cases.[86] Although this process is multifactorial, evidence suggests that TPN, especially with dextrose as the sole form of carbohydrate, may increase the insulin/glucagon ratio, which increases lipogenesis and retards hepatocyte excretion of triglycerides.[85,87] In addition, patients on TPN also undergo prolonged bowel rest with subsequent bacterial overgrowth, which may also contribute to hepatic steatosis and cholestasis.[85,88] Liver dysfunction may be self limited, especially after the discontinuation of TPN; however, patients exposed to long-term TPN (>6 months) may progress to steatohepatitis and micronodular cirrhosis.[60,89] Avoidance of excessive calories, cycling of TPN (if possible), and appropriate dosing and formulation of lipids may help decrease TPN-associated liver injury (**Table 4**).[85]

SUMMARY

Liver dysfunction is common in both the critically ill and postoperative patient, and can be independently associated with high mortality rates. Through a variety of mechanisms, the complex milieu of metabolic perturbations seen in critical illness result in liver injury, which leads to impairment of hepatic function. Most therapies that are currently employed to treat liver dysfunction in critical illness are aimed at treating the underlying disease state and are not liver specific. Further study is needed to address a targeted approach to therapy for liver dysfunction in these patients.

REFERENCES

1. Kramer L, Jordan B, Druml W, et al. Incidence and prognosis of early hepatic dysfunction in critically ill patients—a prospective multicenter study. Crit Care Med 2007;35(4):1099–104.
2. Bynum TE, Boitnott JK, Maddrey WC. Ischemic hepatitis. Dig Dis Sci 1979;24(2): 129–35.
3. Arcidi JM Jr, Moore GW, Hutchins GM. Hepatic morphology in cardiac dysfunction: a clinicopathologic study of 1000 subjects at autopsy. Am J Pathol 1981; 104(2):159–66.
4. Henrion J, Schapira M, Luwaert R, et al. Hypoxic hepatitis: clinical and hemodynamic study in 142 consecutive cases. Medicine (Baltimore) 2003;82(6):392–406.
5. Henrion J, Schapira M, Heller FR. Ischemic hepatitis: the need for precise criteria. J Clin Gastroenterol 1996;23(4):305.
6. Kamiyama T, Miyakawa H, Tajiri K, et al. Ischemic hepatitis in cirrhosis. clinical features and prognostic implications. J Clin Gastroenterol 1996;22(2):126–30.
7. Birrer R, Takuda Y, Takara T. Hypoxic hepatopathy: pathophysiology and prognosis. Intern Med 2007;46(14):1063–70.
8. Ebert EC. Hypoxic liver injury. Mayo Clin Proc 2006;81(9):1232–6.
9. Henrion J, Descamps O, Luwaert R, et al. Hypoxic hepatitis in patients with cardiac failure: incidence in a coronary care unit and measurement of hepatic blood flow. J Hepatol 1994;21(5):696–703.
10. Seeto RK, Fenn B, Rockey DC. Ischemic hepatitis: clinical presentation and pathogenesis. Am J Med 2000;109(2):109–13.
11. Batin P, Wickens M, McEntegart D, et al. The importance of abnormalities of liver function tests in predicting mortality in chronic heart failure. Eur Heart J 1995; 16(11):1613–8.
12. Myers RP, Cerini R, Sayegh R, et al. Cardiac hepatopathy: clinical, hemodynamic, and histologic characteristics and correlations. Hepatology 2003;37(2):393–400.
13. Fuhrmann V, Kneidinger N, Herkner H, et al. Hypoxic hepatitis: underlying conditions and risk factors for mortality in critically ill patients. Intensive Care Med 2009;35(8):1397–405.
14. Henrion J, Minette P, Colin L, et al. Hypoxic hepatitis caused by acute exacerbation of chronic respiratory failure: a case-controlled, hemodynamic study of 17 consecutive cases. Hepatology 1999;29(2):427–33.
15. Bone RC, Balk RA, Cerra FB, et al. Definitions for sepsis and organ failure and guidelines for the use of innovative therapies in sepsis. The ACCP/SCCM Consensus Conference Committee. American College of Chest Physicians/ Society of Critical Care Medicine. Chest 1992;101(6):1644–55.
16. Plank LD, Hill GL. Sequential metabolic changes following induction of systemic inflammatory response in patients with severe sepsis or major blunt trauma. World J Surg 2000;24(6):630–8.
17. Angus DC, Linde-Zwirble WT, Lidicker J, et al. Epidemiology of severe sepsis in the United States: analysis of incidence, outcome, and associated costs of care. Crit Care Med 2001;29(7):1303–10.
18. Brun-Buisson C, Doyon F, Carlet J, et al. Incidence, risk factors, and outcome of severe sepsis and septic shock in adults. A multicenter prospective study in intensive care units. French ICU Group for Severe Sepsis. JAMA 1995;274(12):968–74.
19. Finfer S, Bellomo R, Lipman J, et al. Adult-population incidence of severe sepsis in Australian and New Zealand intensive care units. Intensive Care Med 2004; 30(4):589–96.

20. Mathison JC, Ulevitch RJ. The clearance, tissue distribution, and cellular localization of intravenously injected lipopolysaccharide in rabbits. J Immunol 1979; 123(5):2133–43.
21. Pastor CM, Billiar TR, Losser MR, et al. Liver injury during sepsis. J Crit Care 1995;10(4):183–97.
22. Szabo G, Romics L Jr, Frendl G. Liver in sepsis and systemic inflammatory response syndrome. Clin Liver Dis 2002;6(4):1045–66, x.
23. Van Oosten M, Rensen PC, Van Amersfoort ES, et al. Apolipoprotein E protects against bacterial lipopolysaccharide-induced lethality. A new therapeutic approach to treat gram-negative sepsis. J Biol Chem 2001;276(12):8820–4.
24. Naito M, Hasegawa G, Ebe Y, et al. Differentiation and function of Kupffer cells. Med Electron Microsc 2004;37(1):16–28.
25. Katz S, Jimenez MA, Lehmkuhler WE, et al. Liver bacterial clearance following hepatic artery ligation and portacaval shunt. J Surg Res 1991;51(3):267–70.
26. Matuschak GM, Rinaldo JE. Organ interactions in the adult respiratory distress syndrome during sepsis. Role of the liver in host defense. Chest 1988;94(2): 400–6.
27. Fernandez J, Navasa M, Gomez J, et al. Bacterial infections in cirrhosis: epidemiological changes with invasive procedures and norfloxacin prophylaxis. Hepatology 2002;35(1):140–8.
28. Gustot T, Durand F, Lebrec D, et al. Severe sepsis in cirrhosis. Hepatology 2009; 50(6):2022–33.
29. Foreman MG, Mannino DM, Moss M. Cirrhosis as a risk factor for sepsis and death: analysis of the National Hospital Discharge Survey. Chest 2003;124(3): 1016–20.
30. Singh N, Gayowski T, Wagener MM, et al. Outcome of patients with cirrhosis requiring intensive care unit support: prospective assessment of predictors of mortality. J Gastroenterol 1998;33(1):73–9.
31. Aggarwal A, Ong JP, Younossi ZM, et al. Predictors of mortality and resource utilization in cirrhotic patients admitted to the medical ICU. Chest 2001;119(5): 1489–97.
32. Zauner C, Schneeweiss B, Schneider B, et al. Short-term prognosis in critically ill patients with liver cirrhosis: an evaluation of a new scoring system. Eur J Gastroenterol Hepatol 2000;12(5):517–22.
33. Dahn MS, Lange P, Lobdell K, et al. Splanchnic and total body oxygen consumption differences in septic and injured patients. Surgery 1987;101(1):69–80.
34. Dhainaut JF, Marin N, Mignon A, et al. Hepatic response to sepsis: interaction between coagulation and inflammatory processes. Crit Care Med 2001;29(Suppl 7):S42–7.
35. Maynard ND, Bihari DJ, Dalton RN, et al. Liver function and splanchnic ischemia in critically ill patients. Chest 1997;111(1):180–7.
36. Doi F, Goya T, Torisu M. Potential role of hepatic macrophages in neutrophil-mediated liver injury in rats with sepsis. Hepatology 1993;17(6):1086–94.
37. Marshall JC. Inflammation, coagulopathy, and the pathogenesis of multiple organ dysfunction syndrome. Crit Care Med 2001;29(Suppl 7):S99–106.
38. Chand N, Sanyal AJ. Sepsis-induced cholestasis. Hepatology 2007;45(1): 230–41.
39. Whitehead MW, Hainsworth I, Kingham JG. The causes of obvious jaundice in South West Wales: perceptions versus reality. Gut 2001;48(3):409–13.
40. te Boekhorst T, Urlus M, Doesburg W, et al. Etiologic factors of jaundice in severely ill patients. A retrospective study in patients admitted to an intensive

care unit with severe trauma or with septic intra-abdominal complications following surgery and without evidence of bile duct obstruction. J Hepatol 1988;7(1):111–7.

41. Vermillion SE, Gregg JA, Baggenstoss AH, et al. Jaundice associated with bacteremia. Arch Intern Med 1969;124(5):611–8.

42. Hawker F. Liver dysfunction in critical illness. Anaesth Intensive Care 1991;19(2): 165–81.

43. Batge B, Filejski W, Kurowski V, et al. Clostridial sepsis with massive intravascular hemolysis: rapid diagnosis and successful treatment. Intensive Care Med 1992; 18(8):488–90.

44. Berkowitz FE. Hemolysis and infection: categories and mechanisms of their inter-relationship. Rev Infect Dis 1991;13(6):1151–62.

45. Shander A. Anemia in the critically ill. Crit Care Clin 2004;20(2):159–78.

46. Arndt PA, Garratty G. The changing spectrum of drug-induced immune hemolytic anemia. Semin Hematol 2005;42(3):137–44.

47. Karmali MA, Petric M, Lim C, et al. The association between idiopathic hemolytic uremic syndrome and infection by verotoxin-producing Escherichia coli. J Infect Dis 1985;151(5):775–82.

48. Koster F, Levin J, Walker L, et al. Hemolytic-uremic syndrome after shigellosis. Relation to endotoxemia and circulating immune complexes. N Engl J Med 1978;298(17):927–33.

49. Spolarics Z, Condon MR, Siddiqi M, et al. Red blood cell dysfunction in septic glucose-6-phosphate dehydrogenase-deficient mice. Am J Physiol Heart Circ Physiol 2004;286(6):H2118–26.

50. Roelofsen H, van der Veere CN, Ottenhoff R, et al. Decreased bilirubin transport in the perfused liver of endotoxemic rats. Gastroenterology 1994;107(4):1075–84.

51. Nolan JP. Intestinal endotoxins as mediators of hepatic injury—an idea whose time has come again. Hepatology 1989;10(5):887–91.

52. Wang P, Chaudry IH. Mechanism of hepatocellular dysfunction during hyperdy-namic sepsis. Am J Physiol 1996;270(5 Pt 2):R927–38.

53. Elferink MG, Olinga P, Draaisma AL, et al. LPS-induced downregulation of MRP2 and BSEP in human liver is due to a posttranscriptional process. Am J Physiol Gastrointest Liver Physiol 2004;287(5):G1008–16.

54. Geier A, Fickert P, Trauner M. Mechanisms of disease: mechanisms and clinical implications of cholestasis in sepsis. Nat Clin Pract Gastroenterol Hepatol 2006; 3(10):574–85.

55. Strazzabosco M, Fabris L, Spirli C. Pathophysiology of cholangiopathies. J Clin Gastroenterol 2005;39(4 Suppl 2):S90–102.

56. Spirli C, Nathanson MH, Fiorotto R, et al. Proinflammatory cytokines inhibit secre-tion in rat bile duct epithelium. Gastroenterology 2001;121(1):156–69.

57. Benninger J, Grobholz R, Oeztuerk Y, et al. Sclerosing cholangitis following severe trauma: description of a remarkable disease entity with emphasis on possible pathophysiologic mechanisms. World J Gastroenterol 2005;11(27): 4199–205.

58. Engler S, Elsing C, Flechtenmacher C, et al. Progressive sclerosing cholangitis after septic shock: a new variant of vanishing bile duct disorders. Gut 2003; 52(5):688–93.

59. Moseley RH. Sepsis and cholestasis. Clin Liver Dis 2004;8(1):83–94.

60. Faust TW, Reddy KR. Postoperative jaundice. Clin Liver Dis 2004;8(1):151–66.

61. LaMont JT, Isselbacher KJ. Current concepts of postoperative hepatic dysfunc-tion. Conn Med 1975;39(8):461–4.

62. Molina EG, Reddy KR. Postoperative jaundice. Clin Liver Dis 1999;3(3):477–88.
63. Berg C, Crawford J, Gollan J. Bilirubin metabolism and the pathophysiology of jaundice. In: ER S, MF S, WC M, editors. Schiff's diseases of the liver. 8th edition. Philadelphia: Lippincott-Raven; 1998. p. 147–92.
64. Ketterhagen J, Quackenbush S. Hyperbilirubinemia of fasting. A case of postoperative jaundice. Arch Surg 1983;118(6):756–8.
65. Schmid M, Hefti ML, Gattiker R, et al. Benign postoperative intrahepatic cholestasis. N Engl J Med 1965;272:545–50.
66. Kantrowitz PA, Jones WA, Greenberger NJ, et al. Severe postoperative hyperbilirubinemia simulating obstructive jaundice. N Engl J Med 1967;276(11):590–8.
67. Barie PS, Fischer E. Acute acalculous cholecystitis. J Am Coll Surg 1995;180(2): 232–44.
68. Orlando R 3rd, Gleason E, Drezner AD. Acute acalculous cholecystitis in the critically ill patient. Am J Surg 1983;145(4):472–6.
69. Mirvis SE, Vainright JR, Nelson AW, et al. The diagnosis of acute acalculous cholecystitis: a comparison of sonography, scintigraphy, and CT. AJR Am J Roentgenol 1986;147(6):1171–5.
70. Blankenberg F, Wirth R, Jeffrey RB Jr, et al. Computed tomography as an adjunct to ultrasound in the diagnosis of acute acalculous cholecystitis. Gastrointest Radiol 1991;16(2):149–53.
71. Fox MS, Wilk PJ, Weissmann HS, et al. Acute acalculous cholecystitis. Surg Gynecol Obstet 1984;159(1):13–6.
72. Bunker J, Forrest W, Mosteller F. National Halothane Study. A study of the possible association between halothane anesthesia and postoperative hepatic necrosis. Washington, DC: Government Printing Office; 1969.
73. Wiklund RA, Rosenbaum SH. Anesthesiology. First of two parts. N Engl J Med 1997;337(16):1132–41.
74. Warner LO, Beach TP, Garvin JP, et al. Halothane and children: the first quarter century. Anesth Analg 1984;63(9):838–40.
75. Walton B, Simpson BR, Strunin L, et al. Unexplained hepatitis following halothane. Br Med J 1976;1(6019):1171–6.
76. Benjamin SB, Goodman ZD, Ishak KG, et al. The morphologic spectrum of halothane-induced hepatic injury: analysis of 77 cases. Hepatology 1985;5(6): 1163–71.
77. Wright R, Eade OE, Chisholm M, et al. Controlled prospective study of the effect on liver function of multiple exposures to halothane. Lancet 1975;1(7911):817–20.
78. Holt C, Csete M, Martin P. Hepatotoxicity of anesthetics and other central nervous system drugs. Gastroenterol Clin North Am 1995;24(4):853–74.
79. Brown BR Jr, Gandolfi AJ. Adverse effects of volatile anaesthetics. Br J Anaesth 1987;59(1):14–23.
80. Lo SK, Wendon J, Mieli-Vergani G, et al. Halothane-induced acute liver failure: continuing occurrence and use of liver transplantation. Eur J Gastroenterol Hepatol 1998;10(8):635–9.
81. Nishiyama T, Yokoyama T, Hanaoka K. Liver and renal function after repeated sevoflurane or isoflurane anaesthesia. Can J Anaesth 1998;45(8):789–93.
82. Brunt EM, White H, Marsh JW, et al. Fulminant hepatic failure after repeated exposure to isoflurane anesthesia: a case report. Hepatology 1991;13(6):1017–21.
83. Lewis JH, Zimmerman HJ, Ishak KG, et al. Enflurane hepatotoxicity. A clinicopathologic study of 24 cases. Ann Intern Med 1983;98(6):984–92.
84. Grau T, Bonet A, Rubio M, et al. Liver dysfunction associated with artificial nutrition in critically ill patients. Crit Care 2007;11(1):R10.

85. Chung C, Buchman AL. Postoperative jaundice and total parenteral nutrition-associated hepatic dysfunction. Clin Liver Dis 2002;6(4):1067–84.

86. MacFadyen BV Jr, Dudrick SJ, Baquero G, et al. Clinical and biological changes in liver function during intravenous hyperalimentation. JPEN J Parenter Enteral Nutr 1979;3(6):438–43.

87. Leaseburge LA, Winn NJ, Schloerb PR. Liver test alterations with total parenteral nutrition and nutritional status. JPEN J Parenter Enteral Nutr 1992;16(4):348–52.

88. Pappo I, Bercovier H, Berry EM, et al. Polymyxin B reduces total parenteral nutrition-associated hepatic steatosis by its antibacterial activity and by blocking deleterious effects of lipopolysaccharide. JPEN J Parenter Enteral Nutr 1992; 16(6):529–32.

89. Baker AL, Rosenberg IH. Hepatic complications of total parenteral nutrition. Am J Med 1987;82(3):489–97.

Pregnancy-Related Liver Diseases

Calvin Pan, MD[a],*, Ponni V. Perumalswami, MD[b]

KEYWORDS

- Liver disease • Pregnancy complications
- Nausea and vomiting • Cholestasis
- Abnormal liver function test result • Maternal outcome

Abnormal liver test results are obtained in 3% to 5% of pregnancies because of many potential causes, and the clinical outcomes range from self-limiting to rapidly fatal. There are 4 main conditions that cause abnormal liver tests in pregnant patients: physiologic changes in pregnancy, newly acquired liver disease, preexisting liver disease, and pregnancy-related liver disease. Abnormal liver function test results because of physiologic changes in a pregnant patient without liver dysfunction have a unique pattern and can be recognized when compared with the normal range of liver test results (**Table 1**).

Newly acquired liver disease in pregnant patients, include acute viral hepatitis, drug-induced liver injury, or gallstones, may cause abnormal liver test results. A third cause of abnormal liver test results includes preexisting chronic liver diseases such as cholestatic liver disease, autoimmune hepatitis, Wilson disease, and chronic viral hepatitis. Finally, pregnancy-related causes for liver disease are the most common reasons for abnormalities in liver test results in pregnancy. There are 5 distinct liver diseases unique to pregnancy including hyperemesis gravidarum (HG); intrahepatic cholestasis of pregnancy (ICP); preeclampsia; hemolysis, elevated liver enzymes, and low platelets with or without preeclampsia (HELLP syndrome); and acute fatty liver of pregnancy (AFLP). Unlike newly acquired or preexisting liver diseases, which may

Financial disclosures: Dr C.P. has the following financial relationship with pharmaceutical companies for the past 5 years: he has received research grants from Gilead, Bristol Myers Squibb, Novartis, Idenix, Roche, and Schering Plough. He also serves as a consultant and advisor and serves the speakers bureau for Gilead, Bristol-Myers Squibb, Novartis, Idenix, Roche, Axcan USA, Schering-Plough, Onyx, Three Rivers, and Pharmasset.
Dr P.P. has no financial relationship to be disclosed.

[a] Division of Liver Diseases, Department of Medicine, Mount Sinai Medical Center, Mount Sinai School of Medicine, One Gustave L. Levy Place, PO Box 1123, New York, NY 11355, USA
[b] Division of Liver Diseases, Department of Medicine, Mount Sinai Medical Center, Mount Sinai School of Medicine, 1468 Madison Avenue, Annenberg Building, Room 21-42, PO Box 1123, New York, NY 10029, USA
* Corresponding author. 132-21 Forty First Avenue, Flushing, NY.
E-mail address: cpan100@gmail.com

Clin Liver Dis 15 (2011) 199–208
doi:10.1016/j.cld.2010.09.007
1089-3261/11/$ – see front matter © 2011 Elsevier Inc. All rights reserved.

liver.theclinics.com

Table 1 Physiologic changes in liver test results compared with ranges during normal pregnancy	
Liver Test Results	**Physiologic Changes Compared With Normal Range**
Increased	Alkaline phosphatase (2- to 4-fold), fibrinogen, fetoprotein, white blood cell, ceruloplasmin, cholesterol (2-fold), alpha or/and beta globulins, triglycerides
Unchanged	Aminotransferases, prothrombin time
Decreased	Bilirubin (or unchanged), γ-globulin, hemoglobin (third trimester)

present at any time during pregnancy, pregnancy-related liver diseases have a unique timing of onset (**Table 2**).

This article focuses on the aforementioned causes of pregnancy-induced liver diseases.

LIVER DISEASES RELATED TO PREGNANCY
HG

Nausea with vomiting is common in pregnancy. HG is defined as intractable nausea and vomiting during the first trimester of pregnancy and is the most severe illness within the spectrum of nausea and vomiting in pregnancy.[1] HG often leads to dehydration and electrolyte imbalance and occurs in about 0.3% of pregnancies but usually resolves by weeks 16 to 18 of gestation. In up to 10% of patients with HG, symptoms continue through pregnancy and resolve only with delivery of the fetus.[2,3]

The mechanism for developing HG remains unclear. Proposed mechanisms include hormonal imbalance with increased levels of human chorionic gonadotropin (HCG) and estrogen and decreased levels of prolactin, coupled with overactivity of the hypothalamic-pituitary-adrenal axis.[4,5] It is also proposed that the high level of HCG may stimulate the thyroid gland and upregulate the secretary processes of the upper gastrointestinal tract.[4] Other studies speculate that cytokine, T cell–mediated immune reactivation, immunoglobulin, and complement play an important role in HG because high levels of tumor necrosis factor α, IgG, IgM, C3, C4, natural killer cells, and extrathymic T cells have been observed in patients with HG.[6,7]

Risk factors for the development of HG include molar pregnancy, multiple pregnancies, preexisting diabetes or hyperthyroidism, and psychiatric disorders.[8] An abnormal liver panel is seen in up to 50% of cases. Transaminases are usually elevated to between 2 and 10 times the upper limit of normal but rarely can be up to 20 times the normal with mild jaundice.[2] The diagnosis of HG is clinical and based on exclusion of other underlying or newly acquired liver diseases, especially viral hepatitis.

Table 2 Disease presentation and the timing of onset during pregnancy			
Disease Categories	**First Trimester**	**Second Trimester**	**Third Trimester**
Preexisting Liver Diseases	Chronic hepatitis B or C, autoimmune hepatitis, primary sclerosing cholangitis, Wilson disease, primary biliary cirrhosis, cirrhosis		
Newly Acquired Liver Diseases in Pregnancy	Viral hepatitis, gallstones, drugs, sepsis, Budd-Chiari syndrome (usually post partum)		
Diseases Related to Pregnancy	HG	ICP	ICP, preeclampsia, HELLP syndrome, AFLP

The clinical management of HG is primarily supportive. Patients should be instructed to maintain oral hydration and a high-carbohydrate, low-fat diet. In addition, patients who can tolerate oral intake of food are counseled to take small portioned meals. In patients who cannot maintain their body weight because of intractable vomiting, enteral nutrition and intravenous rehydration may be required. In most patients, HG resolves with the replacement of electrolytes and glucose, rehydration, and nutritional support. Parenteral hydrocortisone may lead to rapid resolution in severe cases, with slow improvement. Rarely, serious complications may occur, which include malnutrition, spontaneous esophageal rupture,[9,10] hyperthyroidism,[3] or even Wernicke encephalopathy caused by vitamin B_{12} deficiency.[11]

ICP

ICP is defined as pruritus and elevated bile acid (BA) levels during the late second or third trimester of pregnancy, with resolution after delivery. ICP is the most common pregnancy-related liver disorder, with a prevalence of about 1 in 1000 to 1 in 10000. ICP is common in South Asia, South America, and Scandinavian countries and has the highest incidence in Chile and Bolivia (5%–15%). However, in North America, the incidence is less than 1%, with a trend of increase in recent reports.[12–14] Risk factors for the development of ICP include multiparity, advancing maternal age, twin pregnancies, and a history of cholestasis due to oral contraceptive use.

While the cause of ICP is not clearly known, it is likely multifactorial, involving genetic, hormonal, and exogenous factors. Studies have demonstrated that sex hormones have known cholestatic effects through inhibition of the hepatocellular bile salt export pump (Bsep).[15] In addition, increased levels of sex hormones in pregnancy have been associated with an abnormal metabolic response with impaired sulfation, which has been a proposed cause for ICP. The hepatic transport systems for biliary excretion can also be affected and saturated by the large amount of sulfated progesterone metabolites.[16,17] Genetic studies to date suggest that at least 10 different multidrug resistance–associated protein (MDR) 3 mutations have been identified in progressive familial intrahepatic cholestasis.[18] MDR3 is the transporter of phospholipids across the canalicular membrane, and mutations (ABCB4/abcb4) may result in loss of function and raised BA levels as a secondary effect.[18] A recent study in Italy identified 5 genes that are expressed differentially in patients with ICP compared with controls. These genes are involved in hepatobiliary transport and cholesterol metabolism (ABCC4 [MRP4 protein] and NR1H3 [LXR-a protein]), protein trafficking and cytoskeleton construction (HAX1 and TTLL5), as well as pathophysiology of pruritus (GABRR1 [GABA receptor type A rho1]).[19] Other studies have suggested the Bsep ABCB11 and the MRP2 ABCC2 as the other candidate proteins that may be involved in ICP.[20] Finally, Reyes and colleagues[21] have reported that exogenous factors associated with ICP include increased intestinal permeability suggesting that there may be enhanced absorption of bacterial endotoxin. Still other studies from Chile have proposed a role for dietary factors (selenium deficiency), seasonal variability, and geographic variations in ICP.[12,22]

Patients with ICP typically present with generalized pruritus, predominately on the palms and the soles of the feet, and the condition is worse at night. Pruritus usually starts during weeks 25 to 32 of pregnancy and resolves after delivery. While skin lesions specific to the disorder are absent, excoriations caused by scratching are often noted on physical examination. In general, serum abnormalities present 4 weeks after the onset of pruritus.[12,23] The most early and specific abnormality in laboratory findings in ICP is the elevation of serum total bilirubin acid level, and it is usually less than 5 mg/dL. Jaundice occurs in approximately 10% to 25% of patients, and some may have diarrhea or steatorrhea as a complication of cholestasis. Aminotransferase levels vary from 2 to 15 times the upper limit of normal. Elevation of alkaline phosphatase levels is not diagnostically helpful because of it is produced by both placenta and bone in pregnancy. The serum γ-glutamyl transferase level is usually normal or modestly elevated. A prolonged prothrombin time (PT) may be noted, which is most often caused by vitamin K deficiency because of the subclinical steatorrhea from cholestasis.

Several atypical presentations of ICP can occur, most notably with variations in the disease course. Some patients can have an early onset of pruritus in the first trimester. In addition, pruritus can resolve spontaneously before delivery with or without an improvement in serum liver test results. Patients can develop pruritus without the usual serum abnormalities. In patients with serum test abnormalities, these laboratory findings may last up to 1 to 2 months after delivery. Finally, rarely, patients may develop abdominal pain or have pruritus and serum abnormality that is exacerbated postpartum with no signs of liver failure. The diagnosis of ICP is based on the clinical feature of pruritus, which is unique to ICP compared with HELLP and AFLP. The differential diagnosis of any pregnant patient with pruritus includes newly acquired viral hepatitis, preexisting liver diseases including primary biliary cirrhosis, choledocholithiasis, or chronic viral hepatitis. Choledocholithiasis can be ruled out with an abdominal sonogram.

A variety of treatment options have been previously studied for ICP. Antihistamines, benzodiazepines, phenobarbital, and epomediol have not shown any significant benefit. Other studies have demonstrated some clinical improvement in ICP with the administration of cholestyramine,[24] dexamethasone,[25] and S-adenosyl-L-methionine.[26] However, these treatments have been proven to be less effective than ursodeoxycholic acid (UDCA) in relieving pruritus and improving liver test result abnormalities, especially aminotransferases and BA levels.[23–28] Therefore, UDCA is the treatment of choice for ICP. It is unclear how UDCA works, but several studies suggest that UDCA can reduce BA levels by increasing the expression of placental BA transporters and facilitating the placental transport of BAs from the fetal to the maternal compartment.[29] Another hypothesis suggests that UDCA promotes BA clearance by facilitating the insertion of transporter proteins such as Bsep (ABCB11) or MRP2 (ABCC2) into the canalicular membranes.[30] UDCA, 10 to 15 mg/kg bodyweight, (up to 2.0 g/d) is usually well tolerated and safe to the fetus without teratogenicity.[27]

Although maternal effects are mild, ICP is associated with a high frequency of fetal distress (20%–40%), with occasional antenatal sudden fetal death and premature labor (60%). Fetal complications are probably caused by elevated fetal levels of BA because of the increased flux of BAs from the mother to the fetus or the impairment of fetal BA transported across the placental membrane to the maternal circulation on top of the immaturity of fetal BA transport systems[31]; high maternal levels of BA correlate with fetal morbidity and mortality.[24,32] Glantz and colleagues[24] have suggested using maternal BA levels of 40 μmol/L as a threshold for early delivery. Close monitoring and early delivery after confirming fetal lung maturity may be the best way to prevent sudden antenatal death. When delivery is not advisable, treatment with UDCA improves maternal pruritus and aminotransferase levels, which may benefit the fetus, because fetal morbidity and mortality are correlated with maternal BA levels. Counseling should be provided to women with a history of ICP because recurrence of cholestasis is common (40%–60%) with future pregnancies or hormonotherapy.

Liver Dysfunction Related to Preeclampsia

Affecting 5% to 10% of pregnancies, preeclampsia is a syndrome of hypertension (blood pressure [BP]≥140/90), edema, and new onset of proteinuria during the late second (>20 weeks of gestation) or third trimester. Proteinuria is defined as more than 300 mg protein per 24-h urine collection or 1+ or greater protein on urine dipstick testing of 2 random urine samples collected at least 4 to 6 hours apart.[33] While the cause is unknown, several factors play a role in the pathogenesis, including abnormal vascular response to placentation, increased systematic vascular resistance, enhanced platelet aggregation, activation of the coagulation system, trophoblast invasion of the spiral arteries, abnormal trophoblast differentiation, and endothelial dysfunction.[34,35]

Clinically, patients can present with symptoms including severe headache, fatigue, epigastric/right upper quadrant abdominal pain, vomiting, changes in vision, and swelling of the face and extremities. Physical exam findings include hypertension, seizures, focal neurologic signs, hyperreflexia, oliguria, oligohydramnios, and intrauterine growth retardation. In addition to proteinuria, patients may have increased serum uric acid levels, liver transaminase level elevation up to 20 times the upper limit of normal, and hyperbilirubinemia. Although there is no specific treatment of hepatic involvement in preeclampsia, these changes may indicate the development of severe preeclampsia, which requires immediate delivery of the fetus. The main complication of preeclampsia is development of eclampsia, which is characterized by intractable seizures. Hepatic complications of preeclampsia include subcapsular hemorrhage and capsular rupture with life-threatening intra-abdominal bleeding. Obstetric complications include placental abruption, fetal demise, and fetal syndrome characterized by fetal growth retardation, reduced amniotic fluid, and abnormal oxygenation.

Definitive therapy for preeclampsia is delivery of the fetus. Patients with severe preeclampsia should be hospitalized. Patients who are at or before their 32nd week of gestation with uncomplicated or moderate preeclampsia (urinary protein excretion≤1 g/24 h, systolic BP≤160 mm Hg) may be managed as outpatients with close follow-up. The use of antihypertensive agents has not been shown to alter the course of maternal disease or decrease perinatal morbidity or mortality. Post partum, hypertension and proteinuria subside within 12 weeks after delivery. In a minority of patients, long-term antihypertensive therapy is required.

In general, maternal and perinatal outcomes are favorable in women with mild preeclampsia developing beyond 34 weeks' gestation but could be worse if preeclampsia occurs before 33 weeks' gestation, in those with preexisting medical conditions, and in those living in developing countries. Women who develop preeclampsia are also at an increased risk of developing cardiovascular disease later in life.

HELLP Syndrome

HELLP syndrome is a multisystem disorder characterized by hemolysis, elevated levels of liver enzymes, and low platelet counts with or without preeclampsia. HELLP syndrome is a potentially life-threatening complication of pregnancy. The prevalence of HELLP syndrome is estimated to be 0.6% of deliveries.[36] Risk factors for the development of HELLP syndrome includes advanced maternal age, Whites and multiparity. The pathogenesis of HELLP syndrome is not known. However, in two-thirds of the patients, the condition occurs in the third trimester, and microangiopathic hemolytic anemia is the hallmark of the syndrome but is not specific to this entity. It is thought that the microangiopathic hemolytic anemia is associated with vascular endothelial injury, fibrin deposition in blood vessels, and platelet activation with platelet consumption. Histopathologically, HELLP syndrome is characterized by periportal or focal parenchymal necrosis with hyaline deposition of fibrin material in the sinusoids.[36,37]

Clinical symptoms of the syndrome include epigastric or right upper quadrant pain, malaise, headache, nausea, and vomiting. On physical examination, hypertension, generalized edema, and weight gain are common signs. Laboratory findings revolve around presence of 3 laboratory criteria: thrombocytopenia, elevated aminotransferase levels, and hemolysis. Several different classifications have been proposed. Generally, platelet count less than 100,000/mm^3, aspartate aminotransferase levels greater than 70 U/L, and L-lactate dehydrogenase (LDH) levels greater than or equal to 600 U/L are helpful to make the diagnosis. The Mississippi classification is based on the degree of thrombocytopenia and the elevation of transaminase and LDH levels, which has been proposed for assessing the severity of the pathologic process (**Table 3**).

Risk factors for preeclampsia include antiphospholipid antibody syndrome, chronic hypertension, chronic renal disease, elevated body mass index, maternal age greater than 40 years, multiple gestation, nulliparity, preeclampsia in a previous pregnancy (particularly if severe or before 32 weeks of gestation), pregestational diabetes mellitus, connective tissue disorders, protein C and S deficiencies, factor V Leiden mutation, and hyperhomocysteinemia.

Serious maternal complications are common in HELLP syndrome. A high index of suspicion and an early diagnosis are key to the management of patients with HELLP syndrome. The most frequent complications are disseminated intravascular coagulopathy (30%), abruptio placentae (16%), acute kidney injury (7.7%), aspiration pneumonia (7%), pulmonary edema (6%), acute respiratory distress syndrome, cardiopulmonary arrest (4%), cerebral hemorrhage (1.2%), and retinal detachment (0.9%). Rarely, severe ascites, subcapsular hematoma, hepatic failure, and hepatic rupture can occur (0.015%).[38,39] Disseminated intravascular coagulation (DIC) may be a late complication, and patients can have a prolonged PT and increased International Normalized Ratio. Proteinuria is a common finding but not required to make the diagnosis. Computed tomography (CT) may show subcapsular hematomas, intraparenchymal hemorrhage, hepatic rupture, or infarction.

Management of the woman with HELLP syndrome begins with hospitalization for stabilization of hypertension and DIC, seizure prophylaxis, and fetal monitoring followed by prompt delivery of the fetus. Transfer to a tertiary care center is advocated, if possible. CT or magnetic resonance image of the liver should be obtained. If the pregnant woman is at or beyond 34 weeks' gestation or if there is any evidence of multiorgan dysfunction or severe complication, immediate induction of labor is recommended. If the gestational age is between 24 to 34 weeks, corticosteroids are administered to accelerate fetal lung maturity in preparation for delivery 48 hours later. After delivery, close monitoring of the mother should continue because studies have shown worsening thrombocytopenia and increasing LDH levels up to 48 hours postpartum. Most laboratory values normalize in 48 hours after delivery of the fetus.

The most frequent severe maternal complications including mortality have been observed in patients with Mississippi class I HELLP syndrome. The perinatal mortality is estimated to be 7% to 22%, with a maternal mortality of 1%.[40]Causes of perinatal mortality include premature detachment of the placenta, intrauterine asphyxia, and prematurity. Subsequent pregnancies in patients with HELLP syndrome carry a high risk of complications including recurrent HELLP.[38,41]

Table 3
Mississippi classification for HELLP syndrome

Class	Platelets (Cells/μL)	Transaminases (IU/L)	LDH (IU/L)
I	≤50,000	≥70	≥600
II	50,000–100,000	≥70	≥600
III	100,000–150,000	≥40	≥600

AFLP

AFLP is a rare condition that is estimated to affect 1 in 7000 to 16000 pregnancies.[42,43] AFLP is associated with microvesicular fatty infiltration of the liver, hepatic failure, and encephalopathy. Most commonly occurring in the third trimester of pregnancy, AFLP carries significant perinatal and maternal mortality.

Recent data suggest that deficiencies of the enzymes of mitochondrial fatty acid beta oxidation (FAO) may play a role in the development of AFLP. The most commonly reported enzyme deficiency in this disorder is a long-chain 2-hydrox-yacyl-CoA dehydrogenase (LCHAD) deficiency. The defect is in the alpha subunit of the mitochondrial protein is associated with G1528C or E474Q mutations.[44,45] Most recently, studies by Natarajan and colleagues[46] demonstrated that placental mitochondrial function is compromised in AFLP, which may lead to free radical production and accumulation of fatty acids in the placenta, resulting in maternal hepatocyte stress and mitochondrial dysfunction leading to acute liver failure.

AFLP has unique clinical features. About 40% to 50% of patients with AFLP are nulliparous with an increased incidence in twin pregnancies.[47] Patients often present with nonspecific symptoms including anorexia, nausea, emesis, malaise, fatigue, and headache. On physical examination, the patient may have jaundice, hypertension, edema, and hepatic encephalopathy. Laboratory findings include serum aminotransferase levels varying from normal to 1000 U/L, but are usually about 300 to 500 U/L. The total bilirubin concentration is typically less than 5 mg/dL. Other laboratory abnormalities include anemia, leukocytosis, normal or low platelet counts, coagulopathy with or without DIC, hypoalbuminemia, hypogly-cemia, and acute kidney injury.

The diagnosis and management of AFLP is a medical and obstetric emergency, and therefore, early diagnosis is the key to improving survival. Management includes hospitalization for stabilization of hypertension and DIC, seizure prophylaxis, and fetal monitoring followed by immediate delivery of the fetus or termination of the pregnancy along with intensive support. The aminotransferase levels and encephalopathy improve within 72 hours of delivery, but continued intensive support may be required to help manage the complications of liver failure. Most patients recover in 1 to 4 weeks post partum.

Maternal mortality in AFLP is 3% to 12% and fetal mortality is 15% to 66%.[48–50] The strong association of AFLP with LCHAD deficiency in the fetus suggests a necessity of neonatal testing for enzymatic defects of FAO. Women who are carriers of the LCHAD mutation have an increased risk of recurrence of AFLP in 20% to 70% of pregnancies.[44,51]

SUMMARY

Liver dysfunction in pregnancy is frequently encountered in clinical practice. Liver disease related to preeclampsia and ICP are common and can affect fetal mortality. Even less common, HELLP syndrome and AFLP may cause severe liver dysfunction, hemorrhage, liver failure, and maternal death. Whereas mechanisms are poorly defined for all causes of pregnancy-related liver disease, recent advances have elucidated new possible mechanisms of disease; genetic defects are detected only in a minority of patients, but further study is needed. Genes expressed differentially in patients with ICP have been further explored. Challenges remain in differentiating liver disease related to pregnancy from other acute liver diseases. Early delivery and advances in supportive management are the only available options for improving the prognosis in liver diseases associated with preeclampsia, which includes liver dysfunction related to preeclampsia, HELLP, and AFLP.

REFERENCES

1. Goodwin TM. Nausea and vomiting of pregnancy: an obstetric syndrome. Am J Obstet Gynecol 2002;186:184–9.
2. Kuscu NK, Koyuncu F. Hyperemesis gravidarum: current concepts and management. Postgrad Med J 2002;78:76–9.
3. Paauw JD, Bierling S, Cook CR, et al. Hyperemesis gravidarum and fetal outcome. JPEN J Parenter Enteral Nutr 2005;29:93–6.
4. Panesar NS, Li CY, Rogers MS. Are thyroid hormones or hCG responsible for hyperemesis gravidarum? A matched paired study in pregnant Chinese women. Acta Obstet Gynecol Scand 2001;80:519–24.
5. Taskin S, Taskin EA, Seval MM, et al. Serum levels of adenosine deaminase and pregnancy-related hormones in hyperemesis gravidarum. J Perinat Med 2009;37:32–5.
6. Kaplan PB, Gucer F, Sayin NC, et al. Maternal serum cytokine levels in women with hyperemesis gravidarum in the first trimester of pregnancy. Fertil Steril 2003;79:498–502.
7. Leylek OA, Toyaksi M, Erselcan T, et al. Immunologic and biochemical factors in hyperemesis gravidarum with or without hyperthyroxinemia. Gynecol Obstet Invest 1999;47:229–34.
8. Fell DB, Dodds L, Joseph KS, et al. Risk factors for hyperemesis gravidarum requiring hospital admission during pregnancy. Obstet Gynecol 2006;107:277–84.
9. Erolu A, Kurkcuolu C, Karaolanolu N, et al. Spontaneous esophageal rupture following severe vomiting in pregnancy. Dis Esophagus 2002;15:242–3.
10. Liang SG, Ooka F, Santo A, et al. Pneumomediastinum following esophageal rupture associated with hyperemesis gravidarum. J Obstet Gynaecol Res 2002;28:172–5.
11. Rastenytė D, Obelienienė D, Kondrackienė J, et al. U sitęsusio nėščiųjų vėmimo sukelta Wernicke encefalopatija. [Wernicke's encephalopathy induced by hyperemesis gravidarum: (case report)]. Medicina (Kaunas) 2003;39:56–61 [in Lithuanian].
12. Lammert F, Marschall HU, Glantz A, et al. Intrahepatic cholestasis of pregnancy: molecular pathogenesis, diagnosis and management. J Hepatol 2000;33:1012–21.
13. Riely CA, Bacq Y. Intrahepatic cholestasis of pregnancy. Clin Liver Dis 2004;8:167–76.
14. Beuers U. Drug insight: mechanisms and sites of action of ursodeoxycholic acid in cholestasis. Nat Clin Pract Gastroenterol Hepatol 2006;3:318–28.
15. Stieger B, Fattinger K, Madon J, et al. Drug- and estrogen-induced cholestasis through inhibition of the hepatocellular bile salt export pump (Bsep) of rat liver. Gastroenterology 2000;118:422–30.
16. Dann AT, Kenyon AP, Seed PT, et al. Glutathione S-transferase and liver function in intrahepatic cholestasis of pregnancy and pruritus gravidarum. Hepatology 2004;40:1406–14.
17. Reyes H, Sjovall J. Bile acids and progesterone metabolites in intrahepatic cholestasis of pregnancy. Ann Med 2000;32:94–106.
18. Floreani A, Carderi I, Paternoster D, et al. Hepatobiliary phospholipid transporter ABCB4, MDR3 gene variants in a large cohort of Italian women with intrahepatic cholestasis of pregnancy. Dig Liver Dis 2008;40:366–70.
19. Floreani A, Caroli D, Memmo A, et al. Gene expression profile in intrahepatic cholestasis of pregnancy [abstract 1546]. Presented at the Annual Meeting of American Association for the Study of Liver Disease. Boston (MA), November 1–4, 2009.

20. Meier Y, Zodan T, Lang C, et al. Increased susceptibility for intrahepatic chole-stasis of pregnancy and contraceptive-induced cholestasis in carriers of the1331T>C polymorphism in the bile salt export pump. World J Gastroenterol 2008;14:38–45.

21. Reyes H, Zapata R, Hernandez I, et al. Is a leaky gut involved in the pathogenesis of intrahepatic cholestasis of pregnancy? Hepatology 2006;43:715–22.

22. Reyes H, Baez ME, Gonzalez MC, et al. Selenium, zinc and copper plasma levels in intrahepatic cholestasis of pregnancy, in normal pregnancies and in healthy individuals, in Chile. J Hepatol 2000;32:542–9.

23. Mullally BA, Hansen WF. Intrahepatic cholestasis of pregnancy: review of the liter-ature. Obstet Gynecol Surv 2002;57:47–52.

24. Glantz A, Marschall HU, Mattsson LA. Intrahepatic cholestasis of pregnancy: relationships between bile acid levels and fetal complication rates. Hepatology 2004;40:467–74.

25. Glantz A, Marschall HU, Lammert F, et al. Intrahepatic Cholestasis of pregnancy: a randomized controlled trial comparing dexamethasone and ursodeoxycholic acid. Hepatology 2005;42:1399–405.

26. Binder T, Salaj P, Zima T, et al. Randomized prospective comparative study of ur-sodeoxycholic acid and S-adenosyl-L-methionine in the treatment of intrahepatic cholestasis of pregnancy. J Perinat Med 2006;34:383–91.

27. Kondrackiene J, Beuers U, Kupcinskas L. Efficacy and safety of ursodeoxycholic acid versus cholestyramine in intrahepatic cholestasis of pregnancy. Gastroenter-ology 2005;129:894–901.

28. Zapata R, Sandoval L, Palma J, et al. Ursodeoxycholic acid in the treatment of intrahepatic cholestasis of pregnancy. A 12-year experience. Liver Int 2005;25: 548–54.

29. Brites D. Intrahepatic cholestasis of pregnancy: changes in maternal–fetal bile acid balance and improvement by ursodeoxycholic acid. Ann Hepatol 2002;1: 20–8.

30. Beuers U, Pusl T. Intrahepatic cholestasis of pregnancy—a heterogeneous group of pregnancy-related disorders? Hepatology 2006;43:647–9.

31. Rodrigues CM, Marin JJ, Brites D. Bile acid patterns in meconium are influenced by cholestasis of pregnancy and not altered by ursodeoxycholic acid treatment. Gut 1999;45:446–52.

32. Mazzella G, Nicola R, Francesco A, et al. Ursodeoxycholic acid administration in patients with cholestasis of pregnancy: effects on primary bile acids in babies and mothers. Hepatology 2001;33:504–8.

33. Sibai B, Dekker G, Kupferminc M. Pre-eclampsia. Lancet 2005;365:785–99.

34. Hanna J, Goldman-Wohl D, Hamani Y, et al. Decidual NK cells regulate key devel-opmental processes at the human fetal-maternal interface. Nat Med 2006;12: 1065–74.

35. Henry CS, Biedermann SA, Campbell MF, et al. Spectrum of hypertensive mer-vencies in pregnancy. Crit Care Clin 2004;20:697–712.

36. Barton JR, Sibai BM. Diagnosis and management of hemolysis, elevated liver enzymes, and low platelets syndrome. Clin Perinatol 2004;31(4):807–33.

37. Hay JE. Liver disease in pregnancy. Hepatology 2008;47:1067–76.

38. Sibai BM, Ramadan MK, Chari RS, et al. Pregnancies complicated by HELLP syndrome (hemolysis, elevated liver enzymes, and low platelets): subsequent pregnancy outcome and long-term prognosis. Am J Obstet Gynecol 1995;172: 125–9.

39. Sibai BM, Ramadan MK, Usta I, et al. Maternal morbidity and mortality in 442 pregnancies with hemolysis, elevated liver enzymes, and low platelets (HELLP syndrome). Am J Obstet Gynecol 1993;169:1000–6.
40. Hepburn IS, Schade RR. Pregnancy-associated liver disorders. Dig Dis Sci 2008; 53(9):2334–58.
41. Baxter JK, Weinstein L. HELLP syndrome: the state of the art. Obstet Gynecol Surv 2004;59:838–45.
42. Reyes H, Sandoval L, Wainstein A, et al. Acute fatty liver of pregnancy: a clinical study of 12 episodes in 11 patients. Gut 1994;35:101–6.
43. Pokros PJ, Peters RL, Reynolds TB. Idiopathic fatty liver of pregnancy: findings in ten cases. Medicine (Baltimore) 1984;63(1):1–11.
44. Yang Z, Zhao Y, Bennett MJ, et al. Fetal genotypes and pregnancy outcomes in 35 families with mitochondrial trifunctional protein mutations. Am J Obstet Gynecol 2002;187:715–20.
45. Shames BD, Fernandez LA, Sollinger HW, et al. Liver transplantation for HELLP syndrome. Liver Transpl 2005;11:224–8.
46. Natarajan SK, Thangaraj KR, Eapen CE, et al. Liver injury in acute fatty liver of pregnancy: possible link to placental mitochondrial dysfunction and oxidative stress. Hepatology 2010;51(1):191–200.
47. Browning MF, Levy HL, Wilkins-Haug LE, et al. Fetal fatty acid oxidation defects and maternal liver disease in pregnancy. Obstet Gynecol 2006;107(1):115–20.
48. Mjahed K, CHarra B, Hamoudi D, et al. Acute fatty liver of pregnancy. Arch Gynecol Obstet 2006;274:349–53.
49. Fesenmeier MF, Coppage KH, Lambers DS, et al. Acute fatty liver of pregnancy in 3 tertiary care centers. Am J Obstet Gynecol 2005;192(5):1416–9.
50. Pereira SP, O'Donahue J, Wendon J, et al. Maternal and perinatal outcome in severe pregnancy-related liver disease. Hepatology 1997;26(5):1258–62.
51. Yang Z, Yamada J, Zhao Y, et al. Prospective screening for pediatric mitochondrial trifunctional protein defects in pregnancies complicated by liver disease. JAMA 2002;288(17):2163–6.

Index

Note: Page numbers of article titles are in **boldface** type.

Clin Liver Dis 15 (2011) 209–222
doi:10.1016/S1089-3261(10)00165-0
1089-3261/11/$ – see front matter © 2011 Elsevier Inc. All rights reserved.

liver.theclinics.com

Moving?

Make sure your subscription moves with you!

To notify us of your new address, find your **Clinics Account Number** (located on your mailing label above your name), and contact customer service at:

Email: journalscustomerservice-usa@elsevier.com

800-654-2452 (subscribers in the U.S. & Canada)
314-447-8871 (subscribers outside of the U.S. & Canada)

Fax number: 314-447-8029

Elsevier Health Sciences Division
Subscription Customer Service
3251 Riverport Lane
Maryland Heights, MO 63043

*To ensure uninterrupted delivery of your subscription, please notify us at least 4 weeks in advance of move.

Printed and bound by CPI Group (UK) Ltd, Croydon, CR0 4YY

03/10/2024

01040448-0019